HOW TO BE
YOUR OWN DOCTOR —
SOMETIMES

HOW TO BE
YOUR OWN DOCTOR —
SOMETIMES

by
Keith W. Sehnert, M.D.

with
Howard Eisenberg

Grosset & Dunlap
A Filmways Company
Publishers   *New York*

Acknowledgment is made to the following individuals and organizations for their cooperation and permission to reprint:

American Academy of Pediatrics, for the infants' and children's weight charts, which appear in the "Family Health Record," from their publication "Child Health Record from Infancy to Adulthood", © 1968 by American Academy of Pediatrics.

Frank S. Caprio, M.D., and *Harper's Bazaar*, for the twenty-question nervous breakdown quiz by Dr. Caprio, published in the November 1974 issue of *Harper's Bazaar*, © 1974 by The Hearst Corporation.

Health Systems, Inc., for forms adapted for the "Family Health Record." The forms originally appeared in *Common Sense — Common Health*, published by Health Systems, Inc., Suite 201, 3131 West State Street, Boise, Idaho 83703.

Methodist Hospital of Indiana, for the Geller-Gesner tables, abbreviated and adapted for use as the Cause of Death Probability Table.

Patient Care, for postural drainage positions and GI drink recipe, adapted from the February 15, 1974, and April 15, 1974, issues, and health hazard appraisal material adapted from articles in the October 1 and October 15, 1974, issues, © 1974 by Miller and Fink Corp., Darien, Connecticut. All rights reserved.

Glenn O. Turner, M.D., and *Medical Office Staff*, published by Science & Medicine Publishing Company, Inc., for Dr. Turner's chest pain screening quiz adapted for use in *The Self-Help Medical Guide*.

The Washington Post, for quoted material from the "Outlook" article by Dr. E. Fuller Torrey, which appeared in the October 12, 1974, issue, © *The Washington Post*.

To all the Activated Patients
who made this book possible
and to two Activated
(and very understanding) Wives —
Colleen and Arlene

ACKNOWLEDGMENTS

THIS BOOK HAD its beginning many years ago when I first read Benjamin Spock's *Baby and Child Care*. Dr. Spock taught in the Department of Pediatrics at what is now Case Western Reserve University, and in med school I attended some of his lectures. I remember thinking, "Someday I'd like to write a Dr. Spock for adults."

After 20 years as a family doctor, teacher and researcher — during which I'm sure I learned as much from my patients as they learned from me — I felt ready to begin. It's been a long pregnancy, but I'm hoping a veterinarian friend of mine was right when he said encouragingly, "The longer the gestation, the longer the life."

If, indeed, *How To Be Your Own Doctor — Sometimes* does have a long and useful life, I'll have a lot of people — and institutions — to thank for it.

Certainly this book could not have been written had it not been for all the patients and interested persons who have enrolled in my Course for the Activated Patient at Georgetown University and elsewhere since its inception in 1970. Their interest and enthusiasm quickly confirmed my feeling that there was a great unmet medical need in the lives of many Americans. I am indebted to them all.

The teaching of such courses required many allies among my medical, nursing and paramedical colleagues.

I am particularly grateful to these fellow trailblazers who helped me at:

Reston-Herndon Medical Center, Herndon, Va.

The late Thomas E. Christopher, M.D., G. E. Arrington, Jr., M.D., David M. Kessner, M.D., John H. Renner, M.D., Helen Pearcy, A.C.S.W. and James Woods, R.P.

Reston-Georgetown Medical Center, Reston, Va.

James Woods, R.P., Arthur Frank, M.D., Al Wilder, P.A., Cesar Caceres, M.D., Stephen I. Granger, M.D., Helen Pearcy, A.C.S.W., Betsy Baldwin, A.C.S.W., Pablo Falo, M.D., Robert R. Huntley, M.D., Maj. Peter Collis, M.C., Joseph T. Nocerino and Aaron Altschul, Ph.D.

Northeast-Georgetown Medical Center, Washington, D.C.

William Fredericks, M.D., Arthur Frank, M.D., John Clausen, Ph.D., Thelma McDonald, R.N., August Godette, M.D., John Syphax, M.D., Fanny Smith, A.C.S.W., Robert R. Huntley, M.D., Gerta Goldberg, Kenwyn Nicholls, M.D., Donald Vickery, M.D., Robert Karpf, M.D., Mary Kay Tucker, R.N., William Flynn, M.D. and Norvell Turner, P.A.

At Georgetown University's Department of Community Medicine and International Health, valuable support came from Professor Bob Huntley, Chairman of the Department and President of the Georgetown University Community Health Plan, and from Asst. Professor Marian Osterweis, who helped so much in course evaluations.

I am indebted to the innovative clinical researchers who developed and refined the concept of clinical algorithms at Harvard, M.I.T., De-Witt Army Hospital, Ft. Belvoir, Va., Beth Israel Hospital, Boston, Mass. and Georgetown's Department of Community Medicine and International Health, Washington, D.C. Among them: Maj. Peter B. Collis, M.C., Anthony L. Komaroff, M.D. and Donald M. Vickery, M.D.

The able and practical clinicians in the family practice training programs at the University of Massachusetts' Family Health Center and the University of Rochester's Highland Hospital performed the original computer studies that identified the kinds of medical problems showing up most often in doctors' offices. Their work helped make possible my *Self-Help Medical Guide* — the book-within-a-book that makes up most of the last half of this volume.

The fine series of patient instructions and diagrams from *Patient Care* was helpful and I am grateful to Lewis A. Miller, Editorial Director of the magazine and his creative staff in Darien, Conn.

My Reader Panel gave me valuable feedback by testing and reviewing *The Self-Help Medical Guide*. I am indebted to: Sonja and Brian Elmer, Phyllis and Ed Sanders, and Sharon and Tillman Neuner of Arlington, Va.; Pat and Frank Gindhart of Alexandria, Va., Loretta Nowakowski, R.N., of Washington, one of my associates at Georgetown University and David Shires, M.D., Dalhousie University, Halifax, Nova Scotia.

I must recognize "the two Joes." Dr. F. Joseph Pettit, my boss and Dean of the School of Summer and Continuing Education at Georgetown University, played a key role in establishing the Center for Continuing Health Education. Joseph T. Nocerino, originator of the concept of tele-health, has served as a director of operations, auditor, evaluator and encourager. His role has been important.

Editor Jess Gorkin of *Parade* published the 1974 magazine article (written by my co-author Howard Eisenberg and his wife, Arlene) that brought my work in patient education to the attention of Grosset & Dunlap. We promptly appropriated Jess' excellent article title for our book — with his consent, of course. Thanks are due, too, my editor, Claire Bazinet, for her sometimes frenzied but always constructive efforts in pulling this book together.

And finally, without the untiring work, comments and vital encouragement of my wife, Colleen, the book would never have been possible. She put up with my innumerable nights away from home teaching and directing the course. She labored through all those initial rough drafts. She typed until her fingers were numb. I am grateful for her help.

And so with a gestation time of 20 years and a labor period of yet another year, birth is about to take place. This "blessed event" finds a weary but proud father. I hope that you, the reader, will consent to be an honorary "Godparent."

KEITH W. SEHNERT, M.D.

August 20, 1975

CONTENTS

HOW TO BE
YOUR OWN DOCTOR —
SOMETIMES

PORTRAIT OF AN ACTIVATED PATIENT

DOLORES MORISSEAU, A mother of two, has learned her medical lessons well.

● Recently, she took her son, who has had more than his share of medical problems in his short lifetime, to a university medical center for some special tests. When the medical student assigned to the boy's case asked what, if any, surgery had been performed on her son, Dolores confidently ticked off the procedures — all seven of them — using all the correct medical terms. Then, just as decisively, without once resorting to "gizmo," "whatsis," or "those little pink pills," she catalogued his medication history. The medical student looked up with interest.

"Excuse me, Ma'am," he asked respectfully, "are you a doctor?"

● When a neighborhood boy was kicked in the kneecap, Mrs. Morisseau heard the clap a half-block away. She ran up to him, and found the boy writhing in agony. She felt for any obvious bone damage. Finding none, she picked him up, carried him to her home, elevated his foot and packed the knee in ice. By the time the boy's working parents returned home, all they had to worry about was whether their son would be able to play in his Little League game the next day.

● Dolores' mother enjoys working in the garden when she visits her daughter. One weekend, the gnats really got to her, and she came in complaining about her neck hurting. Dolores felt it. She explained that the lymph glands were swollen — probably an allergic reaction to the insect bites. Still feeling some discomfort the next day when she returned home, Dolores' mother went in to see her doctor. That evening, she phoned her daughter to say wryly, "I just paid the doctor $10 to tell me what you told me for nothing."

Dolores Morisseau isn't a physician — not even a med school dropout. She is a graduate of a 34-hour Course for Activated Patients at the Reston-Georgetown Medical Center in Reston, Va. The course began experimentally five years ago but has become, as a result of a dozen articles about it in various magazines and medical journals —

I'm proud and still somewhat stunned to say — a model for patient education all over the country.

Dolores isn't about to hang out a shingle and practice medicine. She sums up her view of her limitations and abilities this way: "My medical knowledge is really just a thimbleful. But the understanding you get of how the body works gives you the self-assurance you need to be able to handle a medical problem calmly. My son has a congenital kidney problem, and it's like living with a loaded gun pointed at your head. I used to panic whenever he threw up. Now I know to check for the spiking fever that means the kidney is involved before fearing the worst."

From all indications, the concept of the Activated Patient could be the wave of the health-care future. If that's so, then your surfboard is at the right place at the right time. Read on. Like Dolores Morisseau — and the many men and women who have taken my course — you're about to become an Activated Patient.

1 WHY YOU OUGHT TO BE YOUR OWN DOCTOR — SOMETIMES

MANY OF MY patients already are their own doctors — sometimes. They've learned to handle minor illnesses and emergencies without help, and major ones without panic. They have "black bags" of their own, with everything from stethoscope to sphygmomanometer in them. They examine their youngsters' ears with otoscopes when they complain of earaches. They check husbands' and wives' heartbeats and neighbors' blood pressures.

Strange business? Yes, they are members of that brand-new breed, the Activated Patient — a kind of hearty hybrid who is three-quarters patient and one-quarter physician. They've learned to speak the doctor's own language, and ask him questions rather than passively sit, honor and obey. They've learned to check vital signs, the first signs of a coronary, and how to tell whether a sinus problem is an allergy or a common cold by the color of the mucous membrane of the nose. They've learned Body Talk — that special language of symptoms that enables them to know what an ache or pain is saying. And they are playing an important and needed role in a health partnership with their doctors.

To some extent, you too are your own doctor sometimes — although not always with the best possible results. When your head aches, you reach into your medicine cabinet and silence it with aspirin. You self-medicate for sinus and sneezes, for indigestion and insomnia. When you feel uptight, you prescribe a martini. When you can't stand the rat race any longer, you prescribe yourself a skiing weekend — which is fine if you're in good shape, because you'll return rested and radiant to household or office. If you're not — well, if you're lucky you'll break a leg before you have a coronary. With this book as a guide, you should be able to avoid having to sue yourself for malpractice!

For an Activated Patient, the "thimbleful of medical knowledge" mentioned earlier can go a long way. John Davis, A.P., has two small boys. "They lead a violent existence," he says, smiling. "They are constantly coming home bleeding and cut up. My oldest boy took a mean whack on the head a while back, playing after school. There was no bleeding, but when I got home from the office at 5:30, my wife told

3

me he'd thrown up a couple of times, which is a pretty good sign of concussion. When his pupils didn't respond normally to my pencil flashlight, I bundled him into the car and took him to the doctor, who confirmed my suspicions and recommended bed rest for a couple of days.

"My younger son came home a few weeks later with a fair amount of blood on his head. It looked pretty scary. I saw that the gash wasn't terribly wide or deep, and knowing that the scalp is not very prone to infection, I was able to keep my cool and just clean up the wound. Since I've learned to recognize the difference between what looks alarming but isn't, and what doesn't look alarming but is, my wife and I no longer go running to the doctor or the Emergency Room for every little thing."

This book will not teach you how to remove your own appendix. Nor will it instruct you to do open heart surgery on your friends for fun and profit. But it will show you how, like my other Activated Patients, you can acquire a black bag of your own. And, peeling a layer or two off the medical mystique, The Self-Help Medical Guide — a unique book-within-this-book — will tell you how to put that black bag to good use to improve your family's health care. It will teach you in easy, illustrated step-by-steps how to use that 160-year-old symbol of medical authority, the stethoscope, tell you where to buy one, and how much — surprisingly little — to pay for it.

It will do the same for the sphygmomanometer — more familiar perhaps as the "blood pressure cuff"; the otoscope — a device for inspecting the ear; the thermometer; and a high intensity penlight. It will teach you how to employ these basic tools of the physician's trade, not as gimmicks, and not so that you can compete with your doctor or challenge his diagnoses, but so that you can anticipate and help prevent medical problems. Then, perhaps you won't have to call on him unnecessarily. But, more importantly, you'll be better informed, and more informative, when you do.

From personal medical experience, 20 years of it, I can tell you that for the busy doctor, there's nothing worse than the patient who calls and says with pinpoint inaccuracy, "I ache all over." Or, equally helpful, "I feel so sick." A phone call from a patient who knows how to take vital signs — pulse, respiration, temperature, blood pressure — and to report relevant observations like inflamed throats or reddened eardrums is far more meaningful. I can make a judgment on whether the patient ought to come into the office, or go straight to a hospital. I can usually prescribe confidently on the phone.

I can understand the chagrin of a patient who, sneezing and wheezing all the way, has taken a long and uncomfortable trip in to see me for what proves to be a common cold, requiring little more than the bed rest, juices and aspirin that he could have prescribed himself. He is embarrassed and often not terribly happy that he's paid for nothing more than my reassurance that the cold is running a normal pattern and course. But unless and until he learns to differentiate between a cold and more serious infections, he'll continue to pay me unnecessary visits.

At considerably greater risk is the patient who impatiently dismisses his wife's concern about what ails him with, "It's only a cold. It'll go away by itself!" He stubbornly keeps on working until that wheeze and choking cough have developed into pneumonia. Then there's the patient whose leg cramp — "just a little charley-horse" — turns out to be potentially critical thrombophlebitis. He's got to learn the warning signs — when a visit to the doctor is an urgent necessity, not a luxury.

Activated Patient Orren Cohill encountered just such a patient when — on class assignment — he checked the blood pressure of a 70-year-old neighbor who'd always been so busy taking care of her family she never took care of herself. Her blood pressure was high — very high — and Mr. Cohill warned her to get in to see the doctor. "Oh," she promised, "I'll do that as soon as I get back from vacation." Visiting relatives in North Carolina, the woman became seriously ill, and was hospitalized. Before her condition stabilized, she had spent $11,000 — some of it not covered by health insurance — and had wiped out her savings and part of her daughter's. She's home now, feeling well, seeing her doctor regularly, and on the hypertension medication that her physician would doubtless have put her on in the first place, if she had just listened to her knowledgeable neighbor's good advice.

All my students don't have dramatic stories to tell. Patricia Kurkowski used her otoscope a few times when her kids had earaches, and she handled her broken leg sensibly when an accident occurred. But the big thing to her is a simple one: She's more comfortable now talking to doctors. "I was always afraid to take up their time with questions and little things that worried me," she says. "The course taught me that doctors are human beings."

It is no small thing to be freed from the "Yes, Herr Professor" role based on the European tradition that the patient is passive, clinical "material" and the physician the unquestioned, unchallengeable authority. You come to me. I give you a prescription. You go gratefully on your way.

I find an interesting link in a poem, now framed and hanging on my

5

den wall, presented to me by my then 11-year-old daughter Sarah one Christmas. The chief point of the poem is "M.D. means My Daddy." For too long, most Americans have looked upon their doctors as a kind of benevolent father figure, whose word is, however, law. As Orren Cohill put it: "People have become helplessly, hopelessly dependent upon doctors. It's a far cry from the pioneer tradition where people could splint a leg, treat snakebite, and sometimes even amputate a limb if they had to."

One reason for that, of course, is that health education has long been a national disaster area. Only a handful of states require certification for health ed teachers. The result is that most Americans know more about their automobiles than their own bodies. In elementary and secondary schools, where it could lay the groundwork for better healthier lifetimes, health education is too often a joke — a Mickey Mouse course reluctantly taught by a gym teacher or the football coach, while the kids pass notes, snicker and do homework for other "more important" classes.

But the storm of consumerism that has swept the United States has already established a consumer presence in everything — from department stores and auto assembly lines to health clinics. The next logical step is the patient's right to know — to be educated. As a purchaser of a pair of pajamas for a young daughter, the consumer wants to know what it's made of. Is it safe, flame-resistant, machine-washable? As a health purchaser, he wants to know what kind of pills he's taking, and what side effects they may have on his body. That doesn't mean he wants to bypass the department store and manufacture his own clothes, nor that he wants to bypass the M.D. and be his own doctor all the time. He just wants to be a partner in the things that affect his life — and nothing does, more than his health.

Occasionally, I hear a colleague complain about hypochondriacs who waste his office time. I usually wonder if his "hypochondriacs" aren't just poorly informed patients. As Pat Hunter, another of my Activated Patients, put it: "If the doctor takes the time to show you what the problem is, you're not half as scared of the remedy. The big fear is not knowing what to expect! Doctors have to stop treating us like dummies. This medical mystery stuff has got to go. People are tired of being kept in the dark about their own health and bodies, and getting condescending answers like, 'You don't need to know that, dear.' "

Patient education could go far toward breaking the ever-soaring cost of U.S. health care, which has passed the $100 billion a year mark. The typical family of five can look forward — though hardly with enthusiasm — to 20 mild-to-moderate illnesses or injuries per year requiring primary care, one illness every two years requiring a specialist's care, and one illness in each family member's lifetime demanding the extensive resources of a university medical center. Knowing something about how to stay healthy and how to prevent minor illnesses from becoming major ones can be important, at a time when health care costs are hundreds of dollars a year for the worried well and can run into tens of thousands for the seriously ill.

The internationally known health economist, Prof. Eli Ginzberg of Columbia University, has said, "Programming the American people to do much more about their own health would be a lot more economical and effective in easing the demands on physicians than producing more of them. Patients themselves are an immense, untapped health manpower resource. . . . Unless laymen can be trained to deal with early symptomology — and many ailments require no more than for a citizen of ordinary intelligence to do some very ordinary things — we'll never have enough physicians."

In spite of the billions spent on medical care, it is sometimes difficult, even in affluent suburban communities, to find good, quick emergency medical care — especially for the newcomer. In years gone by, the young couple generally lived in the same town all their lives, and could count on Mom who lived next door, or Aunt Mary who lived across the street, or on the farm near the next section line, for advice in simple medical emergencies. Today they find no one to ask but their next door neighbors who are, most likely, in the same split-level predicament. Their quest for even the simplest counsel may include such options as these:

(1) The family doctor — "I'm sorry, but Dr. Anderson isn't taking any more new patients."
(2) The internist — "No, Mrs. Jackson, the doctor can't work you into his schedule today. I'll be glad to give you an appointment for next week though."
(3) The Army doctor down the street — "Gee, I'm sorry, Jill, but I'm a pathologist. I haven't seen a live patient for ten years!"
(4) The county medical society — "Yes, Mrs. Jackson, here are three names for you to call. No, I can't recommend which is best."
(5) The Yellow Pages number — "This is the answering service for Doctors Jones and Spence. Their calls are being taken by Dr. Holden, but he is busy at the hospital."
(6) The Emergency Room — "Yes, you may come in now, but you can expect a three-hour wait."

The American health machine is breaking down. We can make the machine bigger, but it may still sputter and miss. My idea is to slow the flow of patients into the machine, and, because our problem is not so much a shortage of doctors as an inappropriate use of them, patient education may be the best way to do it.

I'm a family doctor and on any given day, 70% of the people who come to see me have a self-limiting illness or injury. When I say, "This is what you'd expect at this stage of the illness," I remove the thorn of fear. This book is intended to help you handle those fears, giving your physician more time to concentrate on the 30% of his patients with more serious problems.

In suggesting that you be your own doctor sometimes, will this book be hazardous to your health? Not at all. It's known in medical circles that most common illnesses are the self-limiting kind. Essentially, if properly handled, the illness runs its own course. Your body responds. You recover.

In dealing with common illnesses that progress to complications, or with more serious ailments where your body needs more doctoring than you are qualified to give, the when-to-call-the-doctor guidelines in the *Self-Help Medical Guide* will spell out warnings clearly enough so that you are unlikely to miss them. Blood in the urine, for example. A fever that lingers stubbornly. Shivering spells. A history of chronic diseases like diabetes. Possible pregnancy. Given signs like these, it's time to shelve this book and head for your doctor's office with everything he'll need to know ready at your fingertips. But this book will usually help you safely and soundly answer the question: "Is this trip necessary?"

Doctor books have been part of the American scene for almost as long as there's been an America. When I was growing up on the plains of the Dakotas in the Dirty Thirties — where the weather was hardy and the people even hardier — every family had one. I'm not sure whether we had one for animals and one for people, or whether they were combined. But there was a self-help medical book on every living room shelf, and it was as well thumbed through as the family Bible. Doctors were a last resort — partly out of a shortage of doctors, but even more out of a shortage of money. You called upon them only after all else — home remedies, patent medicines, Aunt Mary and the "doctor-on-the-shelf" failed.

Most doctor books are of the encyclopedic kind — a half-million or so words from Acromegaly to Zygote, with a heavy freckling of rare diseases like Psittacosis and Tularemia, authoritative and comprehensive, but sometimes less than practical. One big reason for that is that up to now there's always been a certain amount of uncertainty about precisely what problems affected most people most often. Tay-

Sachs disease is strenuously publicized and promoted, so it's gone into at great length. Hypoglycemia becomes a bridge table conversational biggie so it's there. A type of leukemia is featured in a TV movie so it rates two pages. Yet, since these and other health problems — so rare that the odds of your getting them are almost zero — are included, something else has to go. Unfortunately, it is often the commonplace, everybody-gets-it ailments that are left out.

Prior to the government decision in the late 1960s to expand medical school programs — particularly those producing family practitioners — there really hadn't been an awful lot of thought given to what a family doctor does. Does he see seven cases of sore back a week — or seventeen? Are sprained ankles more frequent than broken fingers? Should a doctor know more about vaginitis or otitis media?

Determined to get more out of the new Family Practitioner — an up-to-date, more highly skilled and sophisticated version of the old whole-person-care G.P. — the directors of Family Practice residencies said, "If we're going to train F.P.s, we need to know what they most need to know."

With the aid of computers, they performed practice analysis that, for the first time, identified the solid mass at the base of the pyramid of medical practice. They learned some interesting things — that, for example, hypertension is No. 1 among the most common illnesses, bronchitis is No. 3, cystitis (bladder infection) is a surprising No. 5 and conjunctivitis (pink eye) figures No. 12. What they learned has proven of immeasurable value in training Family Practitioners, while avoiding the track of the recent past when doctors emerged great on such things as "electrocardiographic abnormalities of intraventricular septum associated with absent Q syndrome," but didn't know how to remove wax from the ear canal. Knowing miles about inches, and only inches about miles. Practice analysis has also made it possible, at last, to write a book like this one, about the medical problems most people encounter most often.

Practice analysis data was of great interest, too, to another medical school group whittling away at the doctor shortage. Instructors training physicians' assistants, nurse practitioners and other medical aides — all of whom can be trained more quickly and economically than physicians themselves — realized that new teaching methods were needed. Again computer technology provided the answer. Apply computer algorithms to determine the steps to be taken for medical diagnosis and treatment.

The clinical algorithm — sometimes called clinical protocol — is a by-the-numbers, one-foot-after-the-other sequence designed to solve a particular medical problem. Given this, this, and this, plus, let's say, a temperature of 101°, the medical aide *must* send the patient to the supervising physician — just as, if my credit card purchases exceed so many dollars, the computer at Woodward & Lothrop's department store calls it to the attention of the credit manager.

How well do protocols work in practice? At Harvard-affiliated Beth Israel Hospital, high school graduates with less than two weeks of part-time training have been using protocols — computer-derived, but without computer support — under the direction of Dr. Anthony Komaroff. In the first 400 diabetics seen by protocol-users, a symptom was missed only 1% of the time. In most cases, low-back pain patients treated according to protocols recovered faster than those treated directly by physicians. Some 80% of women with vaginal complaints didn't even have to see a physician. Users of the protocol did better in getting diabetes patients' blood sugar levels down. And physicians over-ordered antibiotics from eight to twenty times more than personnel using protocols.

The result at Beth Israel: highly trained doctors can concentrate on the 10,000 or so problems that constitute 30% of medical practice, while minimally-trained, lower-salaried protocol-users handle the relatively uncomplicated 15 or so problems that account for 70% of the patient load physicians have traditionally handled.

I'm sure by now you suspect, as I did, that the jump from clinical algorithms for physicians and paramedics to algorithms for patients is not a big one. As editor of *Computer Medicine* I had for several years been reading early success reports about them. It became apparent to me that if we can train medical aides to follow protocols, then, by converting them into patient language, we could train patients, too. Thus converted, as they have been in the *Self-Help Medical Guide,* clinical algorithms have moved from the computer room into your home, and become as easy to use as slapping on a Band-Aid.

Using the *Guide,* you and I can go a long way together toward accomplishing what the Grand Old Man of efficiency engineering and architecture, R. Buckminster Fuller, calls ephemeralization — a long word that means doing *more* with less. Bucky Fuller created the geodesic dome which makes it possible to build a home with 30 tons of building materials instead of the customary 150 tons. A believer in the conservation of natural and human resources, Fuller calculates that the world is being run at a level of about 3% efficiency, though we already have the engineering ability to do at least seven times that well. It is my contention that many of the shortages and problems of modern health care — and its high cost — are also related to inefficiency. Only when the majority of American patients and health care professionals act upon this inefficiency will we get the improvement that Bucky Fuller insists is possible.

In medicine, patient education is a major key to this. Because it can head off minor health problems before they become emergencies, self-help and preventive medicine can mean more than all the exotic, highly technological equipment in our sophisticated medical centers. I remember one patient who came to that realization late — almost too late.

He was suffering from a severe asthma attack and respiratory failure and had been inches away from death. His face, on the sweat-soaked pillow, had turned from an alarming purple to a reassuring pink. His breathing was becoming normal. With the worst over, the intern who'd helped me bring him back and I relaxed a bit. When the patient felt well enough to speak, he beckoned us to his side. He gulped a few deep breaths, removed the mask for a moment, and murmured, "Thank you for saving my life." He paused for a breath, then added, "Now, please teach me to stay well."

That's what this book is all about. Teaching you how to stay well. How to care for yourself when you're not. How to be your own doctor — sometimes.

2 A BLACK BAG OF YOUR OWN

THERE WAS A look about midway between concern and worry on Pat Hunter's face when she stepped up to me, just prior to the start of the evening's session of my Course for the Activated Patient.

"Dr. Sehnert," she said, "you know the stethoscopes you gave us last week to try out on our families? Well, my 15-year-old daughter, Gwen, had a really rapid heartbeat. At first, I figured I must be doing something wrong. And then I thought, well, maybe she was just excited. But when I tried a half-hour later, it was still fast. And it's stayed that way — give or take a few beats — all week long."

I suggested that Gwen might have been under some special kind of stress the past week, and asked Mrs. Hunter to keep a written record in the week ahead. If her heartbeat remained abnormal, I said it might be a good idea to bring Gwen in for an electrocardiogram.

When the ECG confirmed Mrs. Hunter's continued abnormal findings, I did a history. Earlier that month, Gwen had been out of school with a temperature and a sore throat for the better part of a week. She had been taking some tetracycline she had at home, and when the illness seemed to recede, returned to school. The whole episode had been forgotten — until now. Now it was clear that it had been a strep infection and the bacteria had been at work on Gwen's heart for the last three weeks — fortunately not long enough for serious thickening or malfunctioning of the valves to have begun.

I put Gwen on penicillin (tetracycline does not kill the strep bacteria, but penicillin does) for ten days. Later we did a followup ECG — negative — and have rechecked her periodically. Her mother's alertness may well have saved Gwen from serious rheumatic heart disease, and the possibility of a lifetime of trouble. The significant thing to me, as a long-time patient-watcher, was this: Mrs. Hunter couldn't have done it without a black bag of her own.

The contents of the physician's black bag have long been a mystery to the patients they treat. It's past time, I think, to unzip that mystery.

If patients can be trusted to use the thermometer — which is clearly a medical instrument — why not other easy-to-learn-and-use instruments like the stethoscope as well? As you'll see later, you don't need an R.N. or M.D. after your name to master them. And, like Mrs. Hunter's stethoscope, they can do a world of good in the hands of the intelligent able layperson. Gwen and her mother will testify to that.

Take the sphygmomanometer, for example — another instrument that no home should be without. When I gave them to patients in my mostly black class at Northeast-Georgetown Medical Center in Washington, I knew they'd turn up plenty of hypertension, because it runs rampant in the black community. So that was my homework assignment: "Take these blood pressure cuffs home. Try them out on family members, friends, acquaintances — each of you check a minimum of half a dozen people." Nationally, statistics on high blood pressure are 6% for whites and four times that high for blacks, buffeted as they are by inner city stresses and tensions. My students exceeded national figures. A startling 30% of those they examined had this aptly named "silent disease" hypertension — and most didn't even know it.

The third instrument that belongs in your black bag is the otoscope. The first time I saw a patient use one was some 20 years ago, when I was a family doctor in the small Nebraska farming town of York. The city's pride was York College, and I remember making a house call at the home of its president, Mr. Childress who was, needless to say, one of the community's most distinguished citizens. He had a large family of preschool and school-aged kids, and when I sat down, he told me the reason he'd phoned.

"Johnny's eardrum was a bit red yesterday. It's even more inflamed today."

"How do you know that?"

"I have my otoscope. When we lived in Oklahoma, a doctor friend showed me how to use one. Later, I bought my own at a surgical supply house. With as many children as I have, I can't afford to call a doctor every time somebody coughs or sneezes."

President Childress had learned his lesson well. When you look through your otoscope and see that the middle ear is pearly white, you can be reasonably sure all's well within. It's time to call the doctor, with a 95% chance that penicillin will be needed, when your examination discloses a red eardrum. If it's blush-pink, the protocols in the *Self-Help Medical Guide* tell you how to treat your patient — with nosedrops, hot gargles and other tips. And, there's a reasonably good chance that your treatment will make a visit to the doctor's office unnecessary.

When action is necessary though, don't procrastinate. In Alaska, among Eskimo children with a high incidence of ear infection and a low level of medical care, two out of five children are from 20% to 80% deaf. If you fail to take advantage of modern medicines and skills, you

13

might as well be living in the preantibiotic days of my boyhood, where every winter a couple of kids would return from the hospital displaying big holes behind their ears. The doctor had done the only thing he could do to rid the child of an infection that had invaded the mastoid bone. He performed a mastoidectomy, scraping out infected bone in a procedure nobody has to use anymore. My schoolmates also retained another memento: they remain partially deaf in that ear.

In all candor, I must report that not all physicians agree that patients are fit to be their own doctors — sometimes or anytime. Several months ago, one of my Activated Patients brought her son to the pediatrician. As the doctor picked up his otoscope, the child piped up, "Oh, my mommy has one of those!"

Visibly upset at that news, the physician chided the mother sternly. "A medical student," he declared, "has to look into hundreds of ears before he really knows what he's seeing. How can you believe that an evening's training qualifies you to use an otoscope correctly?"

Undismayed, my A.P. explained coolly, "Doctor, I am not a physician. I do not make a diagnosis. I merely report what I see, and then await my doctor's instructions."

I'm afraid that doctor misunderstands the self-help medicine movement. The training a patient gets from this book — or from my course, for that matter — won't qualify anyone as an ENT specialist or a cardiologist. The instruments in the patient's black bag are for preliminary observations only. For screening out the person who needs to see a doctor from the one who may only need to take some simple preventive measures to prevent a spark from becoming a bonfire.

Mrs. Hunter didn't put Gwen on penicillin, I did. The students who found friends and relatives suffering from hypertension didn't treat them. They simply explained that it was important to waste no time getting in to see a doctor.

At-home readings of vital signs can be a significant supplement to office examinations. For example, when my students fanned out to check blood pressures, several of their patients told them, "Well, yes, the doctor did get a high reading on me a few times, but he said it was probably just because I tensed up in his office."

There's some truth to that. Some people are over-reactors. They walk into a doctor's office and their blood pressure automatically soars. With your own black bag, you can take blood pressure readings at home when the patient is relaxed, and get a true measurement. As he fumbled with the cuff the first time, one student remarked, "The person most likely to be nervous isn't the one having his pressure taken, but the one taking the pressure!"

As with all things in science, three observations — taken at different times of the day and on different days — should be made and averaged. Norms should be established for each member of the family. High blood pressure is considered high when it's consistently greater than 150/90 on three separate readings. If the pressure isn't going through the roof, the patient may be spared a lot of doctor bills, costly medication, and possible unpleasant side effects as well.

It's extremely helpful to the physician if norms have been determined on such things as breathing rate as well. For that, no instrument is needed. Just place your hand on the patient's upper chest, with thumb extending up to the collarbone. You can then feel the rise and fall of the chest. With this knowledge, a parent can then tell the doctor, "I know my child's normal sleeping breathing rate is 22 per minute. Since he has a fever, I checked him while sleeping just now and his breathing rate is up to 40."

A family black bag that will last a lifetime can be put together for $40 to $75 — and that price includes a good thermometer, a high-intensity "throwaway" penlight, tongue depressor blades (an ordinary teaspoon handle will do), and an inexpensive airline or gym bag as well. You will find some sources and prices on pages G120 to G126 of the *Self-Help Medical Guide*. That there is a hunger for these instruments has been clear to one enterprising mail order firm for several years. The company has sold well over 50,000 sets of stethoscopes and sphygmomanometers at about $20 the pair. Theirs is not, of course, the highest quality, professional-level equipment. But then, neither are those I recommend in the Guide. They do have one thing in common — they get the job done, at minimal cost. One caution: No matter what you buy, ask your doctor to check it for accuracy against his own. Some of the imported and mail-ordered gauges have been found to be off by as much as 15 points.

In otoscopes, too, we're talking about a stripped-down model, not the "Rolls Royce" you'll find in an ear-nose-throat (ENT) specialist's office. Even the 2× or 3× magnification of the simple $13 British Gowlands that my students use is sufficient to give you a good look at the eardrum — particularly if combined with a high intensity penlight available at the drugstore for $2. But people with young families would be wise to buy a more expensive American otoscope for about $30, like a good Welch-Allyn, with its built-in light and a 10× magnification of the drum.

A utilitarian stethoscope, able to comfortably handle heart and breathing rate measurements, can be picked up for $3 to $5. As a matter of fact, my classes have gotten them free from local hospital Coronary

Care Units. They use $2 disposable stethoscopes, and have been kind enough to dispose of them in my direction.

There are stethoscopes and stethoscopes, of course, with differences between your utilitarian model and the cardiologist's deluxe instrument about as great as between a Piper Cub and a Boeing 727. But his and yours work on the same principle. They concentrate sound, approximately the way an old-fashioned speaking trumpet did. The old man who was nearly deaf would place it to his ear, and you'd speak into it, focusing the sound into the tube instead of allowing it to disperse throughout the room.

Now, of course, your Model T stethoscope isn't going to pick up the subtle murmurs that an internist's sophisticated $60 headset will register any more than you could expect a Hong Kong transistor radio to pick up police calls. But it's just as well, because it takes years of study to understand what those highly refined sounds mean anyway. Cardiology textbooks discuss such things as the pitch and crescendo of a murmur. You almost have to be a classical musician to comprehend their special language.

A mitral valve scarred by rheumatic fever, for example, produces a different sound than a normal one. When blood flows through a healthy valve, you hear a smooth lub-dub, lub-dub. If it's scarred, the blood squirts through, and the turbulence creates a kind of lub-shh-dub, lub-shh-dub. It's a science-and-a-half, and med students sit around with headsets in the cardiology classes of Georgetown's distinguished Professor Proctor Harvey and listen with the concentration of teenagers at a rock concert to the classic cases that he's recorded.

A super-stethoscope in your black bag would be overkill for the sounds you need to hear. The others? Well, as one of my colleagues remarked recently, "Keith, I've been practicing medicine for 20 years, and I still don't know the meaning of the heart sounds I hear." Happily, all you need to know is how to count the beat.

A Baltimore cabbie who drove me to Johns Hopkins Hospital tells me that he's discovered another use for a stethoscope — one that his physician brother-in-law lends him. His cab-driving hours are irregular, and when friends or relatives are hospitalized, there are times when he can't get in to see them during the posted visiting hours. He borrows the stethoscope, jams it in the side pocket of his jacket, with the earpieces trailing conspicuously outside. After hours or not, the stethoscope is his Open Sesame to his sick relative's room. No one dares to challenge him. The nurses all assume he's a doctor.

You'll find the sphygmomanometer easy to handle, too — far more so than the original crude device developed by the Reverend Stephen

Hales in the early 19th century which, with all my enthusiasm for self-help medicine, I would hesitate to recommend. Hales inserted a glass tube into the carotid artery. Blood then spurted up the column, and the level attained — almost 10 feet — measured the blood pressure of his first patient: a horse.

Your sphygmomanometer will give you a reading accurately and with somewhat less risk. Your uncomplicated stethoscope will transmit all the sounds you need to hear. Together with your otoscope, they'll save you many a trip to the doctor's office.

3 PUT A MOON KIT IN YOUR MEDICINE CABINET

I SOMETIMES ASK new patients to do something that really shakes them up.

"Before your next appointment," I say, "take a good sturdy shopping bag to your medicine cabinet at home. Empty all your medications into the bag, and bring it to me."

I'm not running a second-hand pharmacy on the side. Most medicine cabinets are a Hungarian goulash of pharmaceutical odds and ends — half-empty bottles of discolored chemical sludge, never-used tubes of ointments and unguents with the druggist's typed directions and the name of the patient dimmed by time and humidity, a bottle of prescription cough medicine for Uncle Harry that Aunt Rose brought to Cousin Charlie when he just couldn't seem to get rid of his earthquake cough.

What's in the shopping bag as I review it with my patient tells me a lot I should know. It sometimes tells me I'm in the presence of:

Albert Armageddon

Albert is a senior citizen in reasonably good health. He collects tinfoil, Kennedy half-dollars, and has never been known to throw away a bottle of medicine. He and his family have had the usual number of viral and bacterial infections over the years. He owns little brown bottles, jars and tubes representing every one of those illnesses, with anywhere from one-quarter to two-thirds of the original contents still in residence. When I ask Albert why he has squirreled these away so long, he admits that they're probably not as fresh as once they were. But if there should ever be an atomic war, and all the drugstores were bombed out — well, Albert figures even stale antibiotics are better than nothing at all. I explain that they have long since been oxidized into total impotence — two weeks being about maximum shelf life for liquid antibiotics and a year or two for tablets and capsules — and that if any of his hoarded miracle drugs did anything at this point but give the swallower a bellyache, that would be the biggest miracle of all.

Paula Pillpopper

In her bag are prescriptions for six varieties of tranquilizers, three kinds of sleeping pills, four brands of amphetamines. I learn a lot about Ms. Pillpopper as we discuss the health problems that led to her amassing so exotic a selection of pharmaceuticals in her cabinet. I form the definite impression that she is a doctor-shopper who will stay with me a month or so and then move on. This is often a matter of patient personality, but since it may be a matter of communications breakdown — doctor failure to provide sufficient instructions or followup — I am alerted to the fact that this is a mistake I must make a special effort to avoid. The same is, of course, true for Albert.

Having the right medications in your medicine chest is no small matter, since the home medicine cabinet is where self-help medicine begins. During my years of medical practice, patients have often asked me what medications — both prescription and nonprescription, over-the-counter drugs (hereinafter to be referred to as OTC) — they ought to keep there. This happens most often when someone is about to go on a fishing, hiking or hunting trip that will take him (or her) many miles or even days away from a doctor or hospital. Depending on age, state of health, possibility of danger ahead, and other individual factors, I always make the necessary recommendations.

Later, in developing my self-help course, I went a step further and prepared two lists of medications and supplies — one of OTC products and the other prescription drugs — useful for both the first aid emergency kits of the venturesome and for the medicine cabinets of the families they left behind.

Since the problem has long been a familiar one aboard ships at sea — especially merchant vessels without a ship's doctor — before finalizing my list, I reviewed such sources as the *Ship's Medicine Chest and Medical Aid at Sea* (available from the U.S. Public Health Service) and several similar publications.

Then help came from an unexpected source. I came across an article in *Aerospace Medicine* by Dr. Charles Berry, former medical director for the Apollo moon-flight project for NASA, in which he told of facing the same sort of problem — providing emergency medical supplies for men headed for areas where house calls would be inconvenient.

I was pleased to find that the kit Dr. Berry had put together for the astronauts' flight to the moon greatly resembled my own. There were a few differences, but on the theory that his planning budget and staff were a bit larger than mine, I quickly incorporated a few items.

Thereafter, even though my students were going no further than the

19

Appalachian Trail for a week or the Canadian North Woods for a month, I began to call my list of medical supplies the "Moon Kit." This seemed not entirely unreasonable since, insofar as medical help is concerned, there are places in the wilderness where you might as well be on the moon. I explained to students that the list was authentic in every detail save one. I had omitted the electrocardiographic electrode paste for sensor application for monitoring the astronauts' vital signs to the moon and back. Not too many of my patients would be needing that.

I've given copies of my Moon Kit to many patients since its completion. Members of the Peace Corps have taken similar kits with them to Africa and South America. But perhaps its severest test is still in progress. One of my patients gave his list to a friend about to embark on a "round-the-world voyage." As to how well the Moon Kit has served him, the jury is still out. His three year voyage still has two years to go.

Other physicians will disagree with some of my choices. In many cases, there may be others equally good. These represent my personal "clinical trials." I chose them arbitrarily, based on the fact that they are generally available, generally safe, and have been generally effective for my patients. I suggest that you consult your doctor for his choices. He may be able to personalize the list even further for you, knowing as he does any special health problems — allergies and the like — that may exist in your family.

YOUR MEDICINE CABINET MOON KIT

Name of Drug	Price†	Size stock bottle	Adult dosage	Reason
Achromycin caps (250 mg.)	*	—	250 mg. 4× daily	Bacterial infections
Ampicillin	*	—	250 mg. 4× daily	Bacterial infections
Aspirin	varies	Many forms	1 or 2 tabs as needed	Pain, headache
Bacitracin eye ointment	*	—	Apply 3× daily	Conjunctivitis
Band-Aids	varies	Many forms	—	Injuries
Benadryl (50 mg.)	*	—	1 cap every 4 hr.	Allergies
Bronkaid	1.86	30 tabs	1 tab every 4 hr.	Asthma

Name of Drug	Price†	Size stock bottle	Adult dosage	Reason
Caladryl lotion	1.21	6 oz.	As directed	Itching skin
Cepacol gargle	1.19	20 oz.	As directed	Sore throat
Compress, bandage	varies	Many forms	—	Injuries
Darvon compound	*	—	1 cap every 4 hr.	Pain, headache
Di-Gel liquid	1.25	6 oz.	2 tsp. every 2 hr.	Gas, acid indigestion
Debrox drops	2.57	½ oz.	5 drops daily	Ear wax
Dome-Boro tabs	2.28	12 tabs	1 tab in pint of warm water for wet dressing	Itching skin
Emetrol	1.71	3 oz.	1–2 tsp. every hour	Nausea, vomiting
Fleet enema	.53	4½ oz.	As directed	Severe constipation
Lomotil	*	—	2 tabs 3× daily	Diarrhea
Marezine tabs	.94	24	1 tab as needed	Motion sickness
Merthiolate	.75	¾ oz.	As needed	Skin antisepsis
Neosporin ointment	1.63	½ oz.	2–4× daily	Abrasions, skin infections
Neosynephrine Nose drops ¼%	1.09	1 oz.	2–4 drops 3× daily	Nasal congestion, sinusitis
Parepectolin**	2.65	8 oz.	1–2 tbs. 4× daily	Diarrhea
Robitussin CF Syrup	1.79	4 oz.	As directed	Cough control
Seconal (100 mg.)	*	—	1 at bedtime	Insomnia
Senakot Granules	3.89	4 oz.	1 tsp. at bedtime with water	Constipation
Sudafed tabs	1.79	24 tabs	As directed	Colds, allergies
Syrup of ipecac	.50	2 oz.	½ oz. and repeat 1× if needed	Induce vomiting
Tincture Benzion	.39	1 oz.	As needed	Taping skin
Triaminic syrup	1.79	4 oz.	As directed	Colds, allergies

Name of Drug	Price†	Size stock bottle	Adult dosage	Reason
Tylenol	.67	24 tabs	1 or 2 tabs as needed	Pain, headache
Vaseline	.93	7½ oz.	Use as needed	Minor burns, abrasions

*Apollo Medical Kit item: prescription product, price variations depending on local price factors and number of pills in prescription. See your doctor or pharmacist.

**State law usually requires that you sign registry at local pharmacy.

† $ average Metropolitan, Washington, 1975.

Despite his considerable training and skills, the growth of large pharmaceutical houses and the wide distribution of their assembly line products has sometimes unhappily reduced today's chain store pharmacist to being a label-typer who takes tablets from a large bottle and deposits them in small ones. But though some of the mystique of the elixir-compounding apothecary is gone, the neighborhood druggist is still a mighty good man to go to for advice. He's in the front lines. He frequently knows considerably more about the medicines he dispenses than does the doctor who prescribes them, and if something is notorious for producing more side than desired effects, he's often the first to know.

Not all doctors appreciate pharmacists. Consider the physician who asked a new patient if he'd previously consulted anyone about his high blood pressure. "Only the corner druggist," the patient replied. "And what did that simpleton advise?" the doctor asked disdainfully. "He advised me," replied the patient innocently, "to see you."

I feel somewhat differently about Robert Hildebrand, R.P., owner of the Hildebrand Pharmacy in Ames, Iowa, and my good friend and neighbor when I family doctored in York, Nebraska. Bob, whose knowledge of pharmaceuticals is unexcelled, is chiefly responsible for the Prescription Medications table (begins on page 28 at the end of this chapter) which is a comprehensive listing of everything you need to know about how to correctly use the most common prescription medications — antibiotics, corticosteroids, diuretics, etc. — when you take them home and discover that the instructions on them fail to answer your questions. "Should I take the medicine before or after meals? With juice or water? Should I lay off cocktails while I'm on the medication?" These are the kind of questions that ring in my assistant's ears and mine all day long, so I know they're in a great many heads. That table should save a lot of people a lot of fretting, and a lot of doctors a lot of phone calls. Now, let's deal with some other phone-savers.

What to do about side effects

The auto brought us smog. The jet plane gave us jet lag. Modern medications bless us with A.D.R. — Adverse Drug Reaction. A.D.R. can be caused by exaggeration of the known and desired effects of a drug in a toxic reaction. (Barbiturates are prescribed to calm and depress the central nervous system, but an overdose can depress it excessively — causing unconsciousness, coma or death.) A.D.R. can also be caused by effects of the drug — few drugs have only one action — *other* than the desired one. This is what is known as a side effect. Most side effects are so mild they go unnoticed, but in some drugs, side effects can be so severe that dosage must be reduced or discontinued altogether. (Antihistamines given to suppress allergy may also cause dangerous drowsiness.) A.D.R. can result, too, from an unexpected individual response to a drug. (Many people are allergic to penicillin or aspirin.) Some 30% to 40% of adverse drug reactions come, alas, from "causes unknown."

Whether or not you will ever suffer an A.D.R. depends on many factors — one authority has named 32. These include age, sex, race, nutritional and physical status, mood and expectation, and other medications you may be taking. A key but often unrecognized factor is body weight. All drug dosages are averages. The standard medication is prepared for the 150-pound person, so if you weigh 110 and you're taking the standard dosage, you might be getting a 40% overdose. If you're sitting on one side of a desk and the doctor is on the other, you could be dressed in such a way that he misses your weight by as much as 30 pounds. It wouldn't hurt to bring up the matter of dosage strength. You may say, from experience, "I don't need much medicine. My body's very sensitive to it. Can you just give me the lowest dose possible?" Or, mention your concern to the druggist and have him be your advocate. It's easy for him to phone the doctor and diplomatically remind him that you're only 105 pounds and the dosage may be too strong. Any pharmacist worth his salt substitute will do it, and doctors know a good pharmacist can save their necks. They sometimes forget that, at either end of the bell-shaped drug dosage curve, there are 15% who don't fit into it — big people, little people, youngs, olds, and in-betweens.

I recently found myself outside the curve when I underwent minor surgery to correct an old football injury, and was subsequently put on corticosteroids. I was feeling so jittery and apprehensive that I finally discontinued the drug.

Blurred vision, palpitations, dry mouth, jitters, insomnia — all these are warnings that although the dose is fine as far as the doctor is concerned, your body, in its infinite wisdom, just can't tolerate it.

Fortunately, today's drugs have a wide range of safety, and though unpleasant side effects do occur, there's always the consolation that the effect for which the medication was developed is taking place, too.

When side effects are experienced, too many patients passively assume that this is a penalty that must be paid. They endure, like "good soldiers," when they should be calling the doctor or, if he's away for the weekend, the pharmacist. Either may suggest cutting the dosage — to three-quarters or one-half tablet instead of a whole one. (If it's a factory-sealed capsule, the only thing to do is try a weaker strength, which requires the doctor phoning in a second prescription.) Another possibility is to take it after your meal instead of before. This will affect its absorption, giving you less blast for your buck. But in a side-effect situation, that's exactly what's needed. Some products are best absorbed and most effective in an acid setting — which is the condition of the stomach before meals. Others do best in a neutral environment — and eating first creates that milieu. Instructions for taking medications are not etched in bronze. Your doctor or pharmacist can help you adjust them.

There is, incidentally, something you can try if you find that your antibiotic makes you increasingly irritable and jittery as the days go by. Some people assume it's the illness, but it's just as likely to be the treatment. The antibiotic shotgun wipes out friends as well as foes in the gut — congenial bacterial flora as well as the specific pathogens that are its chief target. That can cause diarrhea. It can also irritate and unsettle. But you may find yourself smiling through if you ask your doctor to consider prescribing Bacid to supplement your antibiotic. Each Bacid capsule is a colony of the kind of amiable bacteria — actually *Lactobacillus acidophilus,* which you add to creams to make cheese — that repopulates your gut with the good guys again. You can often achieve the same desirable result without a prescription, simply by taking a cup of a good yogurt every time you take your antibiotic. Parents who've tried it with sick and cranky youngsters couldn't believe they were the same children.

Why drugs and drinking don't mix

Every now and then, we read in the newspaper about a celebrity's death involving barbiturates and drinking. We tend to think, "Well, that's the Beautiful People for you — one wild party too many." But it may not even have been a party. From a chemical point of view, barbiturates — and tranquilizers — break down into compounds similar to the end products of alcohol. The tricky thing is the cumulative effect — not one plus one equals two, but one plus one equals four. The body's ability to detoxify these poisons is overloaded.

Keep in mind that alcohol was once used as a surgical anesthetic. One reason it's been discarded is the narrow range between the dose needed to create a condition where the patient "feels no pain" and one where he slips over the line from "dead drunk" to dead. Other anesthetics with greater bands of safety have been developed. So the warning SHOULD NOT BE TAKEN WITH ALCOHOL is a serious one. But even without whiskey, barbiturates and tranquilizers have been known to combine synergistically to cause side effects and, in some cases, death.

Antibiotics and alcohol are not exactly meant for each other either. As anyone knows who has ever "chug-a-lugged" a couple of beers, in a situation where restroom facilities are limited, alcohol stimulates the kidneys. When a person drinks 8 ounces of beer, the kidneys, offended by the irritant, may expel 10 ounces of fluid. Some of the antibiotic in the system goes prematurely down the drain. And, since alcohol is an irritant to the gut as well as to the kidneys, it may also interfere with optimum absorption there, too. For my money, one of the best signs of a good pharmacy is that it has a supply of warning labels and uses them generously.

Should you refrigerate it?

Labels are not always helpful. I've known overcautious patients who shrug off the problem by putting *all* medications in the refrigerator. Powders, pills and tablets are much more stable than liquids — which is why antibiotic capsules like ampicillin or tetracycline tablets can sit on the shelf at normal temperatures. Their enemy is moisture, which is more likely to be picked up in the cooler. There are some capsules that require refrigeration for reasons of their own. Bacid, for example, is a medium for bacteria which would grow at room temperature. A cold environment inhibits that growth.

Antibiotics in solution are unstable. The first thing to do when you want to start a chemical reaction is add water, and when you pick up your prescription from the druggist, that step has already been taken. Oxidation has begun. It's the same process that rusts iron, and spoils milk. Refrigeration slows it down, but can't stop it, so in a week or two your once potent antibiotic will be as impotent as the water that transports it.

Down with sleeping pills?

In view of their well-known potential for addiction, you may wonder why both Dr. Berry and I included Seconal on our prescription drug list. My own feeling — as you'll discover in the chapter on yoga — is that there are better ways to fall asleep. But there's little chance for yoga exercising in a cramped space ship. And, in any given life, there are bound to be occasional special situations or emotional storms when sleep, though needed, won't come.

You're on an important business trip. You came all the way from Keokuk to New York City, only to find that your hotel room is over an Elk's convention. Next morning, you have to make the presentation on which your job, and maybe your company, depends. You need your sleep. No way to change your room? One night of Seconal isn't going to make you a drug addict. It's in my medicine cabinet. I don't think we've used it more than three or four times in that many years. But it's there if it's needed.

Are Rx drugs better than OTC drugs?

There's a story told about a celebrated 19th century Shakespearean actor named Macready, who was known both for his generosity in writing theatre passes for his friends, and for his abominable handwriting. Once, struck by the total illegibility of the pass Macready had written for him, one of his friends decided to take it to a nearby apothecary. The druggist accepted the slip of paper, glanced at it and retreated to his jars and vials. A moment later he handed a bottle to Macready's friend with the brisk comment, "A most excellent cough remedy, this. I certainly hope it helps you, sir."

I often get the impression from patients that prescription drugs are the best. The Rx is their ticket of admission to drugs that are taboo without them, and the doctor's notoriously illegible signature handwriting — like Macready's — is part of the mystique. Actually, many OTC compounds are every bit as good as their prescription opposite numbers. As a matter of fact, it's as a prescription drug that almost every OTC drug begins.

Consider a prescription product introduced to doctors by Smith, Kline and French representatives as a cold and allergy suppressant: Ornade. It was so successful that soon patients were asking their doctors to prescribe "that capsule with all the little pellets in it." S.K.F. created a whole new company to market a repackaged product that was renamed Contac. The good news for patients was that with mass marketing — potentially boosting sales 20 times or more — the price came down. The same was true of Di-Gel and dozens of other one-time Rx drugs that proved themselves as "ethical" drugs in doctors' offices and then went commercial.

Stability that will give it a long shelf life is a must for the OTC drug. It's got to sit in an unheated warehouse in Billings, Montana over the winter, and sit out the summer in another one in Biloxi, Mississippi. If it turns purple, a chemist checks it out, and a new formula is reached by trial and error. It may be on a druggist's shelf for a year, and in your bathroom cabinet for two or three.

What about generics?

Consumer advocates and the U.S. government through its Medicare-Medicaid programs are pushing hard for the use of less expensive generic drugs instead of the costlier trade-name brands. I'm for that, too — but with some reservations. Some of the generics being sold are produced by "bathtub manufacturers" with poor quality control, short shelf life, and even inferior ingredients. The Food and Drug Administration (FDA) has dried up most of them, but once in a while an unscrupulous chemist will drop out of a large company to do his own thing and begin underselling with a similar but second-rate product. In one documented case, a patient chose to purchase a cheaper antacid tablet than the brand his doctor had recommended. Two weeks later, his pain was so acute that exploratory abdominal surgery was performed. To the surgeon's surprise and the patient's consternation, the more than 100 antacid tablets the man had swallowed were discovered, lodged in his small intestine, totally undissolved.

The big companies are now producing generics themselves as part of their product line. Eli Lilly's is likely to be far superior to that compounded by, say, Unknown Drug Company of South Trenton, New Jersey. So if you want to save with a generic — and the savings in some, though not all, cases can be substantial — ask your doctor to suggest one he's found reliable. Or ask him to write the prescription in a way that allows your friendly neighborhood pharmacist to pick a winner for you.

Rx oneupsmanship

I hate to reveal these deep dark physician secrets, but since World War II, premed students haven't had to study Latin as a prerequisite for admission to med school. Most of us post W. W. II docs know about as much Latin as we do Sanskrit. We still use a handful of Latin abbreviations to write our prescriptions, so the pharmacists will believe

27

we are doctors. But I wouldn't have the mistiest idea of what Latin words the abbreviations represent if it weren't for the fact that I needed to know in order to explain them to you. So, good for a little oneupsmanship with your friends and neighbors — though not much more — here are the ones you'll find on most prescriptions:

SIG   (signetur) — let it be labeled.
PC   (post cibum) — after meals.
AC   (ante cibum) — before meals.
HS   (hora somni) — at the hour of sleep (at bedtime).
QID   (quater in die) — four times a day.
TID   (ter in die) — three times a day.
BID   (bis in die) — twice a day.

Now you can decipher a prescription — if your doctor writes more legibly than Macready.

PRESCRIPTION MEDICATIONS AND THEIR USAGE

Full instructions for the proper use of prescription medicines seldom appear on the labels, and doctors often give patients only the specifics — how much to take how many times a day. The next time you receive a prescription, ask your doctor to tell the pharmacist to label the medicine, then look it up here for additional instructions. The products are identified by their brand names.

Antibiotics

Take the following medications on an empty stomach or one (1) hour before meals: do not take with fruit juice unless specified below. If in liquid form, discard any unused portion after *two* weeks.

Ampicillin	Oxacillin
Cloxacillin	Penicillin G
Erythrocin	Penicillin VK
Erythromycin	Symycin*
Ilosone	Tegopen
Ledercillin VK	Tetracycline*
Nafcillin	Unipen

*May be taken with juice.

Take the following medication on an empty stomach or one (1) hour before meals. This medication should NOT be taken with milk or antacid preparations. The drug may either be taken with water or juice. Milk or antacid preparations may be used an hour after taking the medication.

Achromycin   Terramycin
Panmycin   Tetracycline
Sumycin

Antibiotic Drops and Ointments

Discard any unused portion of the medication after 10 days of use.

Chloromycetin Ophthalmic
Chloromycetin-Hydrocortisone Ophthalmic

The medication labeled:

Aureomycin Ointment

may stain clothing. Do not use in the eyes.

Sulfa and Urinary Tract Medicine

These medications should be taken with plenty of water:

Azulfidine   Sulfapyridine
Gantrisin   Sulfathalidine
Succinylsulfathiazole   Triple Sulfas
Sulfadiazine

The medication labeled:

Azo-Gantrisin   Pyridium

should be taken one-half (½) hour before meals, unless otherwise directed by your physician. This medication may color the urine orange-red.

Stomach and Bowel Medications and Laxatives

When taking the medication labeled:

Colace   Metamucil   PeriColace

you should NOT take mineral oil. Take medication with a full glass of water.

The medication below should be taken one-half (½) hour before meals.

Atropine sulfate   Phenobarbital and Bel-
                                 ladonna

Belladonna Tincture   Pro-Banthine

Blood Builders and Iron Medicines

The medication labeled:

Ferrous Gluconate   Iron Preparations
Ferrous Sulfate

should be taken just before, with, or after meals, but NOT with antacids.

Cortisone Products, Antihypertension and Diuretic Medicines

While taking the medication listed below, one or more of the following foods should be taken daily, especially if you are not supplied with a potassium supplement: apricots, bananas, cantaloupe, orange and grapefruit juice, peaches, prunes and raisins.

Cortisone Preparations   Lasix
Edecrin   Prednisolone
Hydrocortisone   Prednisone
Hydrodiuril   Thiazide Preparations

Nitroglycerin Tablets

Nitroglycerin tablets are to be dissolved under the tongue at the first appearance of pain, or as directed by your physician. The drug is unstable and will decompose if it is exposed to excessive heat. To prevent loss of potency, keep the tablets in the original container. Close tightly immediately after each use.

Blood Thinners (Anticoagulants)

You should carefully follow your physician's directions as to the dosage and frequency of this anticoagulant medication. Periodic determination of prothrombin time is essential. Do not stop taking the drug or begin taking any new drugs without consulting your physician.

Suppositories

Remove wrapper of suppository and insert the suppository as directed with gentle pressure, pointed end first. Do not handle suppositories excessively as they melt at body temperature. KEEP IN A COOL PLACE.

Medicines that May Cause Drowsiness

The following medication may cause drowsiness; AVOID taking other depressants (Example: alcohol); use care when operating an automobile or other machinery while taking the medication listed below.

Actifed	Librium
Ambodryl	Lomotil
Atarax	Meprobamate
Benadryl	Miltown
Bonine	Ornade
Chlor-Trimeton	Phenergan
Codeine	Phenobarbital
Codeine Cough Syrup	Pyribenzamine
Cogentin	Serax
CoPyronil	Stelazine
Darvon	Teldrin
Demerol	Temaril
Dilaudid	Thorazine
Dramamine	Triaminic
Empirin Compound	Valium
Equagesic	Vistaril
Equanil	

Medications with Which Alcohol Must Be Avoided

While taking these medications, NO ALCOHOL should be taken.

Amytal	Diabinese
Antabuse	Doriden
BetaChlor	Dymelor
Carbrital	Elavil
Chloral Hydrate	Flagyl
DBI	INH

Insulin
M.A.O.I.
Nembutal
Nitroglycerin
Noctec
Noludar
Nydrazid
Orinase
Phenergan

Phenobarbital
Placidyl
Quaalude
Seconal
Somnos
Thorazine
Tolinase
Tuinal

General Advice about Medicine and Meals

Take these medications either DIRECTLY before, with, or after meals.

Aminophylline
APC
Artane
Aspirin
Azulfidine
Butazolidin
Cortisone Preparations
Darvon
Diabinese
DBI
Furadantin
Griseofulvin
Hycodan
Hycomine
Hydrocortisone

Hydrodiuril
Indocin
INH
Macrodantin
NegGram
Nydrazid
Orinase
PAS
Percodan
Prednisolone
Prednisone
Reserpine
Theophylline
Thiazide Preparations
Tolserol

4 WHOEVER HEARD OF A COBRA WITH LOWER BACK PAIN?

THE NURSE WAS new, and she didn't knock before she walked in, so I can't really blame her for screaming and running for help.

It had been a typically busy morning for me at the Reston-Herndon Medical Center, and my morning office hours were over. As has been my custom for several months — a custom with which Mrs. Alldredge was unfortunately unfamiliar — I had sprawled gratefully on the floor, and assumed the position known in Hatha Yoga as the Corpse.

The idea is to gradually relax every nerve ending and muscle fiber in your body, starting with your toes and progressing slowly and serenely up to the *auricularis superior* above the ears. Apparently my performance was an Academy Award-winner. I ignored the sound of the door opening, keeping my eyes gently closed as often prescribed for yoga postures of this kind. The fact that I neither blinked an eye nor moved a muscle as she stared down at my prostrate figure was probably the clincher for Dottie. Convinced that I had expired of a sudden coronary, she sprinted down the hall to summon another doctor.

I still do the Corpse, the Cobra, the Locust, and assorted other yoga exercises on my noon break. But now I hang a DO NOT DISTURB sign on my office door before beginning.

Yoga as therapy is something no self-respecting doctor would even admit he knew about as recently as a couple of years ago. So you may well wonder, (a) Why do I use it? and (b) What does modern medicine think of this ancient art-science?

Well, it is no longer possible, much less sensible, to ignore yoga. People who once confused it with a cultured dairy food product now read about the benefits of yoga in their magazines and see it performed on television. Every major city has at least one daily yoga TV program, and sometimes as many as two or three. I'm told there are 3,000 yoga instructors in New England alone. Yoga courses are being taught in YMCAs and YMHAs all over the country, in community colleges, high school phys ed classes, and even elementary schools. The "far out" is no longer so far out. Maybe, like pizza and egg rolls, yoga started

33

elsewhere, but it's become as American as organic apple pie. It's part of the whole growing do-it-yourself health movement.

A good many physicians, including myself, have taken yoga courses. Although we don't understand exactly why and how it works, we find a lot of body wisdom in it. It's unlike exercise systems aimed at producing muscle strength or bulk — something not particularly needed by most of us today.

Such practices as cupping and leeching and scarifying the flesh to release evil spirits have faded away. But 3,000-year-old yoga has hung in there. Nothing survives that long unless there's something to it. People have tried yoga and it works for them. If something is therapeutic, it's foolish to dismiss it as without merit simply because it came out of a monastery instead of a medical laboratory.

YO-GA is a Sanskrit word meaning "re-union." In his book *Yoga & Medicine*, Stephen F. Brena, M.D. explains that yoga has religious implication but that it "stands first for the correction of human dysharmonies into a harmonious unity."

The philosophical system called yoga, one of the three great systems of Hindu philosophy, is said to seek glorification of God in man. Karma Yoga is the "yoga of action" and Mahatma Gandhi was its greatest modern disciple. Rāja Yoga, the "yoga of self-realization" involves superior psychophysical training. Hatha Yoga, the "yoga of health," is the most popular form of yoga in the western world.

My reasons for signing up for a Hatha Yoga course were twofold. Patients of mine who'd heard of yoga — or tried it — wanted my medical opinion, and it was embarrassing not to have one. They'd come to my office and say things like, "Doctor, when I do the Lotus position, I get a little pain in my back. Could yoga be bad for me, or am I just doing it wrong?" Or, "You know, ever since I started yoga, I don't have that nervous stomach I used to have."

I had a personal interest as well. Since falling off a 20-foot obstacle course wall while in the Navy in World War II, I've had back problems. I'd been close to surgery twice, but backed away because of possible bad results. So I considered taking the course not just to answer my patients' questions, but also to see if there was, in the time-honored phrase, "something in it for me." One day, after sitting there like a dummy once too often, I recklessly promised a patient, "In the great Sehnert tradition, I'll take the course. Check back with me next month, and I'll let you know what I think of it."

My timing couldn't have been better. It just so happened that my neighbor across the street, Gerta Goldberg, is a skilled yoga teacher who was giving a course at the Arlington Y. I arrived and looked around.

There we were — 35 women and me. I slipped into my gym togs and went to work. I arrived as a Doubting Thomas, I left as a Convinced Keith. For the last three years, I've found that if I do my yoga daily, I'm free of back pain.

Day after day, we Americans are assaulted in the media — which feed on the new, the novel, the trendy, the sensational — with up-to-the-moment reports on the latest with-it social, philosophical, or medical development or discovery, without knowledge of which our lives will be shortened, soured, unfulfilled, even terminated. After we've tried a dozen brand-new, guaranteed miracle diets (and find that the more we diet, the more we remain the same), a set of circulation-threatening rubber exercise underwear (that squeezes us of perspiration like a sponge and leaves us limp as a dish rag), and bought a lot in Florida for retirement living (that can be visited at high tide only by submarine), we tend to develop a healthy skepticism.

So you may well be suspicious of yoga. You may be repelled by its strange name. You may even feel that as a good Catholic — or even a poor Presbyterian — you ought to have nothing to do with this exotic foreign "religion." No problem. Yoga has two identities. One is the physical; the other is spiritual and philosophical. When people ask me about the latter, I steer a neutral course, and explain that that's another whole bag of macrobiotic rice that needn't concern them unless they feel the need to explore it further. But you definitely don't have to be Hindu to enjoy — and benefit from — Hatha Yoga. I know ministers, priests and rabbis who are into it. (The biggest problem the rabbi has is trying to keep his yarmulke on his head while he's doing the exercises.)

Don't let the names of the exercises put you off. What I might call a rocking exercise, they label the Locust. What I might describe as lying on your back — the exercise that caused such a commotion at my office — they identify as the Corpse. What I might call arching my back, they call the Cobra. The names are a bit dramatic, but they're darned useful. They paint images for people to lock onto and duplicate. What could be more fluid or graceful than the movements of a cobra? And, whoever heard of a cobra with lower back pain?

Right now, for example, what are you doing? You're sitting in a chair. Maybe your legs are crossed cutting off circulation. Your knees and elbows are bent. If you were in the office, or ironing, your back would be bent, too, over a desk or table. This is your position whether you're driving a car or working at a hobby. Though relaxing, you're not relaxed. Many yoga exercises are the anatomic opposites to these positions we live our lives in.

Yoga encourages spinal mobility. Now, people don't spend a lot of time writing praiseful letters to the editor about it, but our spine is unique. It's the only sliding joint in the body. It can slide in five different directions: to the front, to the back, to the left, to the right, and then twist like a corkscrew. But by our 20th birthday, most of us have stopped using the spine except to bend forward to tie our shoelaces. Many yoga exercises are designed to loosen up the ligaments and muscles in the back to give us greater mobility and to avoid the stiffness of middle age that is a result of lack of stretching and exercise. If children took up yoga in grade schools and used it all their lives, they'd be limber adults, not predestined to the stooped shoulders and pot bellies we automatically associate with the post middle-aged and elderly.

Breathing — the simplest, most natural process in the world — is another thing yoga focuses on that we've neglected. People don't really breathe very much anymore. That may just be an urban defense mechanism. But in my office I find that patients — particularly women, who tend to take little shallow breaths — have forgotten how to breathe. Yoga gets you to lie down on the floor and gradually elevate your arms until your hands are held over your head, while you do nothing more demanding than inhale slowly for, say, 30 seconds. By the time you're at the top of your breath, your belly is pushed out to look like you're six months pregnant. Then as you exhale, you slowly lower your arms sucking in your abdominal wall until it almost touches your spine. Ridiculously simple? Sure. Childishly fundamental? You bet. But it moves the diaphragm and whole respiratory system almost 100%. It blows out the old air and draws in the new. And air is about the cheapest, safest medicine I know — except at evening rush hour on outbound streets!

Is yoga medically sound? Well, we know, for instance, that if muscles are tense we not only get fatigued, but our blood vessels become constricted. Learn to relax them and your blood pressure goes down. The heart doesn't have to work hard pumping blood through narrowed tunnels, and with the whole vascular bed less tense, the pulse slows. Western physicians are beginning to see this light. There's a new book out called *Orthotherapy* in which orthopedic surgeon A. A. Michele recommends what are, in effect, yoga-like exercises, as one way of staying out of his office.

I've seen yoga help people relax tensions, tone up physiques, and turn off smoking and drinking. I find patients with gastrointestinal problems, nervous stomach, peptic ulcer, headaches and backaches getting dramatic relief. I know that sounds like a TV commercial and I know it's only anecdotal evidence with no clinical trials to cite to support it, but the results are there. There are, of course, no instant medical or metaphysical miracles. And if any yogi promises them, he's no yogi, but just an exploitive promoter. However, yoga has to be learned — like learning to swim or paint. You just don't take a yoga lesson or two, and find that, "Poof!", all your problems are gone. It takes weeks and months of learning to do yoga well.

Once my patients have learned to do the relaxing exercises, I prescribe yoga for convenient periods. I may instruct a businessman with a nervous stomach to take 15 or 20 minutes off his lunch hour for yoga at the office. And maybe later in the afternoon, say at 4 p.m., when he's all tight and tense and mad at the world, I tell him to turn off the lights, lie down on the floor, and do it again. Some of these patients have been able to get off their tranquilizers and get rid of their stomach and headache complaints.

I practice what I prescribe. So when an executive tells me how busy he is, I can look him right in the eye and say, "I'll match your schedule with mine any day for being busy. I find time at noon, and I set aside a half-hour before I go to bed, too." Then what can he say? Only, "Okay, doc, I'll give it a try."

Linda and her back problems are a good example of what yoga can accomplish. Linda moved to Washington from Ohio when she graduated from college. She'd been to family doctors, orthopedic surgeons, osteopaths, and chiropractors. Everyone but a Chippewa medicine man. She'd gotten all kinds of backyard advice, too. But she was getting persistent pain in the back, and nothing seemed to chase it away. That's bad enough for someone in their sixties. For a 21-year-old, it's a disaster.

Someone told Linda that I teach my patients to do yoga for their back conditions, and she came in to see me. I immediately put her through my regular medical tests to check her muscle strength and range of motion — things like bending to each side, toe touches, pushups, raising and lowering legs from the prone position. Linda was weak and tight on everything. I found that one of her legs was slightly shorter than the other — something that yoga people are acquainted with and refer to when discussing spinal health. So I ordered a quarter-inch heel lift for one shoe, and gave her some simple exercise instructions. Linda didn't get overnight results. But each week she came back feeling a little better. And, after 18 months of pain before coming to see me, in about 18 weeks she was well. She wrote me recently from her new job in Ohio that she's getting along fine, is doing yoga exercises for her back every night, and couldn't be happier.

Tension headaches can yield to yoga, too. Andrea is the busy wife of a foreign ambassador. She's been on the Washington social merry-go-round since her first week in town. It's her national obligation — almost a patriotic duty — to attend formal, often dull, diplomatic dinners and parties, and to entertain and small-talk no matter how badly she feels. At my suggestion, Andrea took a yoga course. Now, whenever she feels one of her headaches coming on, she lies down and breathes deeply to relax, then sits up and does neck exercises. Things like putting her chin on her right shoulder, then moving it to her left shoulder, then onto her chest, then arching it back to look at the ceiling. This is followed by a shoulder stand. Earlier, Andrea's only option was to take a very strong pain medication, grit her teeth, and smile painfully through. Now she is able to dominate her headaches before they dominate her.

Insomnia is another happy hunting ground for yoga. Edna is an elderly lady who was living on Sominex and other potions she'd picked up over the sleepless years. Part of her problem was that she didn't understand that the body loves ritual. After we evaluated her, we decided that, first, she didn't get enough exercise. Second, the longer she thought about going to bed, knowing she was just going to toss and turn, the tenser she got. So we gave her a different kind of medication. We got Edna to follow a strict yoga ritual, at a time of day when interruptions or phone calls were unlikely.

Her bedtime is usually 10:30 or so. She takes a relaxing bath around 9:30, and goes down to her front room around 10 for yoga exercises. TV and radio are turned off. There's a dim light in the next room. Edna lies down on a large clean towel on the rug and begins her ritual*: (1) the Corpse — lying on the floor with her mind turned off, just deep breathing, thinking of nothing; (2) straight leg raising; (3) the Twist; (4) the Cobra; and (5) a shoulder stand — which, by the way, even an older person like Edna can learn to do. By the time she's finished, she's relaxed, able to read 15 minutes and slide off to sleep. Edna hasn't touched her bottle of Sominex for more than a year.

Yoga's helped some of my hypertensive patients, too. I have one patient who has been on medication for high blood pressure for some time. Now, when he's really uptight — gritting his teeth, clenching his fists, muscles tightening in the back of his neck — he just breathes slowly, relaxes from his toes up to his ears, and gets that pressure down. He does yoga exercises regularly, has substantially reduced his salt intake, gets regular sleep. The combination of common sense and yoga has enabled him to cut way down on his hypertension medication.

*For additional details regarding this series of postures, see the Treatment Index exercises in the *Self-Help Medical Guide.*

Some enthusiasts — usually students who've taken yoga, rather than those who teach it — claim that yoga even prevents colds. One suggested method, kind of folk yoga, involves immersing your nose in a cupped palm filled with lukewarm salt water. The saline is brought up into the nostrils by inhaling and forced out by exhaling. A couple of my patients have tried it on their own, and found it less than enjoyable. I don't endorse that, but I do see some physiological common sense to shoulder stands that tip the body upside down and increase blood flow to the nose. Getting that rush of extra blood into your head not only cleans out all the "cobwebs," but improves the flow of healing white blood corpuscles to the tissues of the nose and throat. That's close to the roof of the house you live in, and you know that often people on the top floor don't get as much water pressure as those living in the cellar. With that white cell bonus, mucous membranes are going to be repaired more rapidly, and there are less likely to be gaps in the membrane for germs to penetrate.

Americans, beset with bad habits, insomnia, financial worries, physical neglect, complain "I don't have time to think." Yet we consistently deprive ourselves of that time when it's available — plugging ourselves into newspapers on commuter trains and TV sets in our living rooms. A recent study of business executives astounded me with the statistic that in his or her 50 weekly working hours the average busy manager spends only 19 minutes thinking. I'll bet chauffeuring, housekeeping, babysitting wives don't do much better. A session of yoga allows you time to think and provides another psychological plus as well. I'm convinced personally that some of the depression we see today is related to poor circulation. I'm persuaded that regular yoga exercises like shoulder stands, with their increase of blood flow to the brain, are likely to have some very positive therapeutic effects.

There's a lot more to yoga and other imports from the East than I've been able to say briefly here — a lot more than I, who only dabble in it, have taken the time to learn. There's the whole area of transcendental meditation (called TM by devotees), which induces a state of alert wakefulness that appears to be beneficial to the body. Studies exploring these positive benefits are now under way in several medical centers. Do-In, a Chinese system of self-massage, based on acupuncture points, seems to be growing in popularity.

A considerable amount of religious fervor can accompany an interest in yoga — serious study of the Yoga Sutra of Patanjali for the quest of the soul and the cultivation of maitri (friendliness) and sukha (virtue). I find I've gotten all I need from practical, healthful yoga. But open a book of yoga philosophy, and you will find it has a great deal ethically in common with our own Judeo-Christian ethics and morality. The heavily illustrated *Light on Yoga,* by B. K. S. Iyengar, is considered by many to be a thoughtful and comprehensive introductory text.

There are so many hardcover and pocket books available on yoga now that it's difficult to recommend any one in particular. Richard Hittleman, who produces a California TV series called *Yoga and Health,* has written a whole shelf of them. *Yoga & Medicine* by Stephen F. Brena, M.D. merges yoga concepts with modern medical knowledge. A short book written for the general public, it presents physiological concepts and everyday examples that can be used in yoga. Lilis Folan has written one called *Lilis, Yoga and You* that women seem to enjoy, with its recommended exercises for 30 minutes a day.

Expect no miracles, but don't be surprised if you feel a lot better for doing it — particularly if you've been on the tranquilizer track for years. Many people get into yoga as a last what-have-I-to-lose resort. They say, "What am I doing to myself? Going to psychiatrists, paying $50 an hour, spending $10 a week for medicine, and I still feel terrible." I've known several who have turned all of that around.

Yoga *is* something different. I heartily recommend it — after competent instruction. There are some hazards. Don't try any of the advanced positions before you are ready for them. And when you are ready for them, avoid distractions and other interruptions. It was a rare accident, but I know of one instructor who momentarily lost control while doing a headstand — with her head bearing all her weight — as she tried to explain it to her class. She toppled over and injured her neck.

Some of the early hippie yogi seemed quite far out — with unkempt shoulder-length hair, dirty fingernails, and you weren't quite sure if they were selling yoga or hash. But of late, yoga has stepped out of the counter-culture and been embraced by a middle America that is a lot more open minded than is generally realized — even to accepting the incense that yoga classes sometimes feature.

Incense may smack of strange and exotic regions and religions, but its pungent odor makes practical sense — helping to heighten the deep breathing awareness that's so important in yoga. Such utilitarian reasons are not, however, always satisfying to the American dabbler determinedly probing for deep meanings and symbolisms.

Gerta Goldberg tells the story of a celebrated teacher she studied with, who was worshipfully asked by an earnest matron at a lecture, "Swami, tell me please — what is the mystical, theological reason for the use of incense during yoga?" He smiled. "In India," he replied, "at religious festivals, there are often thousands of people crowded together in one room. At such times, we do not need a mystical theological reason. At such times, incense is a necessity."

5 DO YOU LISTEN WHEN YOUR BODY TALKS?

"DOCTOR, MY HEAD aches all the time. What does it mean?"

Illness makes itself known to you through feelings, sensations and reactions your doctor calls symptoms. When you say "My face feels hot," you are reporting a symptom. It is your body's way of talking to you. When the doctor looks at you and notes "The patient's face is flushed," it is called a sign. The "body talk" you report is pieced together by your doctor with his signs and findings to make a diagnosis.

Some symptoms are as familiar as coughing, vomiting, headache and sore throat. Others may be strange and frightening: sudden blindness, a sharp pain in the abdomen, localized paralysis.

Unusual combinations of symptoms, called syndromes, may be labeled with names based on their discoverers — Adams-Stokes Syndrome (slow heartbeat and spells of dizziness), or Guillain-Barre Syndrome (a viral infection of the brain with pain or tenderness in the muscles, weakness, loss of tendon reflexes, and unusual laboratory findings in the spinal fluid). A less dramatic collection of symptoms — runny nose, slight fever and sore throat — ended up as the nameless waif, the common cold.

But what good is body talk to you? In his book, *A Primer of Clinical Symptoms*, Dr. Robert B. Taylor defines a symptom as "the noticeable part of an iceberg that cautions of hidden danger." Dr. Karl Menninger, in *Whatever Became of Sin?*, adds that symptoms are "produced and occur in many ways — physiologically, chemically, neurally, hormonally and psychologically." A symptom then, is a signal that there is something wrong with the body's machinery or its processes. It is a red light that registers on your own personal computer, your consciousness. The signal says "Check me!" or "Help me!" If you don't pay attention to your body talk, you won't get the message — and that "iceberg" will come seemingly out of nowhere and threaten your clear sailing.

Symptoms are not limited, of course, to people. Who hasn't heard the squeaking of a bike wheel, the broken fanbelt flapping in the car, or seen steam geyser up from an auto radiator? These symptoms speak a familiar language: "grease the axle," "replace the fanbelt," "open the

42

hood and cool me off." By recognizing and handling these symptoms correctly, you protect yourself and help the world around you to run more efficiently.

Right now, body talk may seem like an intelligible foreign language. But it's possible to understand what your symptoms mean and learn to interpret them. And, until you can, skilled help is readily available.

Dr. Menninger uses a good analogy in his book. He says, ". . . in civilized countries the symptom is a ticket of admittance to the doctor's office, a ticket that today is usually promptly utilized and promptly honored." Once this "ticket of admission" is given at the front door of a doctor's office, clinic or hospital, it sets up a series of events, questions and procedures designed to translate this foreign language so that advice can be offered and medication and treatment begun.

In the centuries since Hippocrates first hung his shingle from the branch of an olive tree, doctors and nurses have learned a great deal about the patterns and probable paths of symptoms. Health professionals, who have watched symptoms evolve, have, in effect, learned the body's language.

They have learned that symptoms can speak for illness that is physical or emotional. That a flushed face can be related to the fever associated with a strep throat or to an emotional reaction of anger or guilt. That skipped heartbeats may be caused by rheumatic fever or by a chronic anxiety condition. If the symptom is the result of nervousness, the patient may not consciously know why he has the symptom. As the psychiatrists say, "The anxiety is repressed."

Sometimes body talk is simple. You're kicked in the foot by a horse. There is immediate pain, swelling and loss of function. Pain says, "Don't walk on me." When a loved one dies, loss of appetite and insomnia may be symptoms of the emotional injury.

What makes a sore throat sore? What is it saying? First, there is swelling of the mucous membrane in the throat, as cells are attacked by viral or bacterial invaders, and histamine is released into the surrounding tissue in an allergic-defensive reaction. The dilating effect of the histamine on the small arteries causes them to leak serum into the tissues. This stretches the mucosa, activating local pain fibers. Second, the postnasal drainage from an associated nasal infection causes irritating mucus to flow over and coat the already swollen and tender tissue. Bacteria flourishing in the tissue secrete irritating toxins. Third, there may be actual cracks in the mucous membrane where it has dried out because of abnormal breathing through the mouth. The nasal airway is plugged and its normal air conditioning and moisturizing functions are no longer working.

To understand this drying effect, stop reading for a minute for a quick demonstration.

(1) Open your mouth wide. Wider!
(2) Breathe in and out rapidly ten times.

Now, note how dry your throat feels? This demonstrates how quickly symptoms can develop when normal function is altered.

If we speak body language, these symptoms even tell us what to do for treatment. The body instructs us to: "Wash off that irritating mucus"; "Take the humidifier off the shelf and add some moisture to the air for my nose and throat"; "Squirt in some nose drops so the swelling will be decreased temporarily, and I can breathe normally for a while"; "I'm very thirsty from losing all those fluids by sneezing — give me lots of water"; and "Gargle with hot water so that the healing white cells in my blood will rush to my throat to fight off the invading bacteria and viruses."

This type of body back-talk shows the body's wisdom. It is constructive and helpful. When you're sick, you may tend to think only of the discomfort, the disruption of your schedule or your loss of income. But don't rush that healing process. Bear in mind that some symptoms are an attempted corrective process, a repair mechanism, a self-regulating system of maintenance worthy of your admiration and appreciation.

One hundred years ago Samuel Butler said, "All our lives long, every day and every hour, we are engaged in the process of accommodating our changed and unchanged selves to changed and unchanged surroundings." Symptoms are often body talk about these environmental changes. The throat feels dry because the air is drier; there's been a change in the weather. The humidifier on the furnace has conked out. Perhaps you've smoked too many cigarettes and the hot dry smoky air has dried out the normally moist throat surface.

The body is not complaining. It's simply reporting. Illness arrives after you have repeatedly ignored the trouble reports. If you had *fixed* the humidifier, *increased* your fluids for 24 hours, or *stopped* smoking at the first report of dry throat, the self-regulating repair system would have moistened the throat, toughened the normal mucous covering, and there might have been no strep throat or viral pharyngitis.

If you had properly understood your body, you might have gotten some extra sleep, increased vitamin C intake, and taken hot salt gargles. It is quite likely you would have stopped the trouble on the spot!

This early action is what doctors call preventive medicine. Unfortunately, through ignorance of this language of symptoms, the good advice that the body gives you is not accepted and disease continues to take its toll.

Health has been described as your body living in harmony with its environment. When internal and external events cause changes in this harmony, disease occurs. Symptoms then signal a change in harmony.

What Are Some More Examples of Body Talk?

Heat and redness of skin

It is likely that many readers of this book have at some time experienced a boil. This common skin infection causes redness and heat around a hair gland or oil follicle. It is warm and painful when you touch it. The heat is caused by an increased blood supply to the spot. A protective inflammatory response brings in white blood cells and antibodies to fight the bacteria, fungi, or parasites that invade the skin.

The symptom of pain tells you not to move that part of the body because movement might slow down the battle or spread the infection. The symptoms of heat and pain radiate a general sensation of aching that slows down your usual activity and helps conserve energy for the healing processes.

As the battle against the germs escalates, the area becomes swollen and aches. If the boil is on your hand, you will find some relief from the aching by elevating the hand. This helps drain away the extra fluids near the boil.

This body talk becomes part of the specific treatment your doctor recommends for a boil: rest and elevation. He orders hot compresses to rally your healing forces and shorten the infection's duration. He may also recommend antibiotics or surgical drainage to speed healing.

Palpitations and irregular heartbeats

This symptom is quite frightening. Fortunately, it is rarely serious, because it's one body bulletin that people rarely ignore.

Palpitations are painless and represent an extra beat of the heart that can be caused by too much coffee, tobacco, medication, or anxiety. The symptom is usually reported as a "fluttering" in the chest, or a feeling that the heart has "jumped." It may be accompanied by a sighing sensation or felt while inhaling slowly.

The patient may experience palpitations during times of stress: after several days with less sleep than usual, before a test or an important meeting or during a week of marital discord. This same period of stress may also be accompanied by excessive use of coffee or cigarettes.

Sometimes medications such as APC tablets, cold tablets, appetite-control medications, or thyroid tablets may be a factor in bringing on the attacks.

One triggering factor is quick position change, such as getting out of bed too quickly or shooting out of a chair to answer the phone or doorbell. The body talk says, "I'm lightheaded," or "I think I'm going to faint."

The heartbeat regulator (the pace maker) is having trouble adjusting to the quick switch from a circulatory system that is horizontal to one that is vertical — all in 5 seconds. It really is a complex series of events if you think about it. The pulse rate must be changed. Nearly every artery in the body must add some tone to its wall (constrict) if it's below the heart. Those above the heart must release some tone (dilate) to compensate for gravity. It's no wonder the heart may skip a few beats — like a car motor missing when it goes from a flat road into climbing a hill.

Here, your body may be saying, "Sit on the edge of the bed for a few moments to let me adjust." Or "Let's ease up from the chair and take 60 seconds to stand upright and go to the door. What's the hurry? It's probably just a door-to-door salesman." This is a symptom saying, "You're Okay — but *easy* does it. Slow down a bit."

Some types of heart disease may also lead to irregular heartbeats and must be considered as a possibility by all who experience palpitations. This cause is the exception rather than the rule, however, and should be evaluated by your doctor.

Palpitations are an example of lack of harmony between the body and its environment. It may mean that your body disapproves of the chemicals you are putting into it. It resents the caffeine, nicotine and amphetamine-like compounds being forced into the electrical circuits of your heart. It could also be telling you that you are working too hard — running a long distance race as though it were a 100-yard dash. The symptom warns, "Slow down before your motor burns a bearing."

The doctor treats the symptom by stopping the offending stimulants — with your cooperation — helping you identify offending day-to-day stresses, and recommending ways to live in harmony with your world. He also investigates possible heart disease and reassures you, relieving your understandable anxiety, if no evidence of serious heart or other disease is present.

Fatigue

One of the most common symptoms in today's medical world is fatigue. It appears in forms described as "tired homemaker syndrome," "executive exhaustion," or "tired blood." It may appear as a presenting complaint for poor physical fitness, anxiety, depression, chronic infections, anemia, thyroid deficiency (hypothyroidism), cancer, or leukemia.

The body talk associated with this complex group of diseases usually requires an expert interpreter: your doctor.

As he listens to a patient's report of symptoms he gets certain clues. The nervous, anxious patient says, "I wake up in the morning all worn out." The patient with a chronic disease may say, "I wake up refreshed but run out of steam by 11 a.m." The depressed woman says, "Why do I go on?"

A careful medical history is of prime importance in the interpretive process and is usually more helpful than a stack of lab reports. An old medical maxim that is sometimes overlooked says, "Listen to the patient, doctor, and he will tell you what is wrong with him!"

Once the cause of fatigue is determined, then *specific* treatment can be recommended. Generalized tonics or vitamin shots are seldom indicated. The odds are that the reasons for fatigue are such relatively innocuous conditions as poor physical fitness, chronic anxiety state, or iron deficiency anemia. But it is your doctor's responsibility to carefully screen your state of health and rule out the more serious problems.

The symptom of fatigue says, "Get off your weary duff and visit the doctor for evaluation."

Excessive thirst

One of the first symptoms we understand as children is thirst. "Wa-wa" usually enters The Baby Book a few weeks after the word "Ma-ma" brings smiles to the faces of proud parents. Later, the active teenager, after heavy exertion, learns the deep satisfaction of a big glass of cool water. Water lost from sweating is replaced in response to the symptom, thirst. We all understand this body talk, but what is the body saying if persistent and excessive thirst is felt?

Probably the classic example of this type of thirst is associated with diabetes mellitus. In this disease, a deficiency of insulin, a hormone manufactured by the pancreas, causes elevation of sugar in the blood. The high level results when blood sugar (glucose) stays in the arteries and veins after digestion instead of being transferred into the body's cells where it can be used for energy.

As the sugar circulates in the system, it is filtered out by the kidneys and excreted in the urine. Normally very little sugar "spills over" into the urine. But when blood sugar is elevated, a larger amount of sugar finds its way into the urine — where simple urinalysis can easily detect it.

Sugar has the chemical characteristic of binding water to it. As the kidneys try to filter out the sugar, an excessive amount of water is carried out with it. The patient becomes dehydrated and must then drink large amounts of fluids to replace the lost water.

You might want to try another demonstration to observe this type of thirst. Perhaps you've noticed it already. Eat a very sweet dessert or a large candy bar on an empty stomach. Within 30 minutes you'll experience a strong thirst, much like the diabetic's.

The body talk of thirst plus excessive amounts of urine are clues that diabetes may be present. Treatment includes regulation by a low carbohydrate diet (the source of sugar), the addition of insulin by injection in some cases, or medications.

Another cause of excessive thirst may be dehydration associated with fluid loss from vomiting, diarrhea, and fever. In all cases, this symptom is an alert that fluid levels are low and replacement is "requested" by the body. It is analogous to the red light on the dashboard of your car that signals low fuel supply, or trouble in the cooling system.

Loss of appetite

Too much appetite is a much more common symptom in doctors' offices today than too little appetite. However, when the body registers the latter symptom it usually signals serious trouble.

Alcoholism frequently is associated with loss of appetite. The alcoholic, by consuming 2,000 or more calories each day in alcohol, upsets the balance of the body and does not experience normal hunger. When people constantly "drink their meals" and burn alcohol instead of food, they soon suffer from lack of vitamins, minerals, proteins and other vital nourishment and develop weight loss, liver disease, and other disorders.

Another type of loss of appetite (anorexia) results from drug abuse. Whether the person is on drugs such as pot (marijuana), downers (barbiturates), uppers (amphetamines) or "hard" drugs like heroin or morphine, his awareness is altered and in the chemical fuzziness that results, appetite may disappear. The habitual user of chemicals soon develops the same signs of malnutrition and vitamin deficiencies as the alcoholic.

Impaired appetite is frequently an early sign of liver disease such as hepatitis, cirrhosis or cancer. It also accompanies stomach cancer and chronic kidney diseases. Loss of appetite, like fatigue, is a general symptom that requires a thorough history and work-up by your doctor. This body talk says, "I need help. Please listen to me!"

Hoarseness

Perhaps as we discuss "body talk," it is appropriate to discuss a symptom involving a difficulty in talking: hoarseness. Hoarseness is usually caused by viral laryngitis, but it is also frequently caused by abuse of the voice in speaking, singing, shouting, or excessive smoking. It can also indicate vocal nodules or a cancer of the larynx.

Hoarseness is your throat saying, "Stop irritating me. Rest me. If you don't, I'll quit on you."

If you could look at the voice box (larynx) as the ENT specialist does when you have laryngitis, you would see red, swollen vocal cords. If there is a secondary bacterial infection there could be white, green or yellow spots on the surface — even some streaks of blood. When your ankle is red and swollen, you rest it. A strained back is rested by lying in bed. The cardinal rule for laryngitis, too, is rest. "Don't talk," this symptom pleads hoarsely.

If your eyes become red and irritated from getting a face full of smoke while building a fire in the fireplace, you avoid more smoke. Your larynx is also saying "Don't smoke. Please stop that irritating habit. Give me a chance to recover!"

Feeling good — a sense of well-being

We've talked about what your body says when it is trying to protect you or report something. That sort of body talk is usually warning you about trouble, or scolding you for your bad health habits or life style.

There are many times, however, when you are being complimented by your body. The sense of well-being after a vigorous 30-minute walk or jog through the park is your body saying, "Good show. That extra oxygen I got from deep breathing really refreshed me." When you awaken from sound sleep without the headache you sometimes have on Sunday morning — because you had two glasses of orange juice while playing bridge at the neighbors instead of the usual two or three highballs — your body is saying appreciatively, "Thanks, pal, I feel better without the booze."

49

The title of that recent public television series on health was no accident. It emphasized the wise health practices that leave you "Feeling Good!"

Learn to listen for complimentary comments from your body. When your taste buds say, "Man, this food tastes so much better since I quit smoking"; when your back says, "I feel much better riding in George's Volvo than in Henry's Pinto"; and your nose complains, "Why must you make me sneeze by hanging around Aunt Tillie's cat?" — stop and think about the reasons for symptoms and the lack of them!

In *The Well Body Book,* authors Mike Samuels, M.D. and Hal Bennett declare, "Your body is a three-million-year-old healer. Over some three million years of evolution on this planet, it has developed many ways to protect and heal itself."

Right — but it can use some help from you. And it's getting it, whenever you eat just the right amount of a nourishing, well-balanced meal; whenever you take time out of a hectic work schedule to relax a bit with your children; whenever you breathe deeply of good fresh exhilarating country air. At those times, stop a moment and let that healing invigorating wave of well-being wash over you. Listen carefully. It's your body complimenting you. It's saying, "Now that's the way to live. Let's do this again soon!"

6 HEADACHE, HEARTBURN AND THOSE OTHER HELLISH TV ILLS

In THE SPECTRUM of ill health that ranges from the trivial to the traumatic, there sits a segment of bothersome but not disabling disorders that I think of as "the TV illnesses."

What a callous and indifferent world it would be if you did not hear each day on television the warm friendly voices offering you "dramatic," "remarkable" even "amazing" relief for headaches, heartburn, insomnia, burning eyes and — more discreetly — "itching hemorrhoidal tissues"?

The symptoms associated with these mini-ills are examples of more body talk.

Headaches

From the moment headache lightening strikes you, to the moment the "miracle ingredient" draws its own invisible dotted line of blessed relief through your brain, what is this sometimes agonizing symptom telling you? It may be warning that you are suffering from nervous tension, a product of today's harried hurried life-styles. But what is happening inside your head?

These headaches occur when tense head and neck muscles limit the normal flow of blood, reducing oxygen supply to the brain. It's much the same as what happens when your heart muscle reacts — in something we call a heart attack — to a coronary insufficiency. That's an oxygen shortage, too, but considerably more dangerous than a headache.

In the typical tension headache, your body — at the "gut" or subconscious level — is feeling stress. A situation is unresolved or frustrating. ("There's big trouble in Suzie's marriage, and I think I know why, but if I call, Tom's going to accuse me of meddling.")

A headache can also be saying, "Please, no more overtime this week!" (fatigue headache). Or, "I'm so hungry, I could eat a horse" (hunger headache). Or, "Stop hitting the books so hard — or, at least, get a better study lamp" (eyestrain headache). Or it could be signalling a minor or a serious physical ailment — such as fever, sinusitis, carbon

51

monoxide poisoning, stroke, concussion or other damage from a head injury, a neurological or brain disorder, glaucoma, or disease-caused oxygen shortage.

Headaches that are persistent, severe, come on suddenly, are accompanied by neurological symptoms like loss of coordination or double vision, follow a head injury, or can be pinpointed in the ear or eye or a localized part of the head, all shout, "See the doctor, immediately." So, incidentally, does any recurring headache in a child.

Heartburn

The talk involved in heartburn or acid indigestion is similarly quite blunt: "It always happens when I drink Charlie's coffee," or "Whenever I rush through lunch, my stomach hurts," or "I can't believe I ate the whole pizza!"

The doctors call it dyspepsia and the TV ad writers call it "gasid indigestion." It is a burning sensation in the upper abdomen. The symptom begins an hour or so after eating and is often related to coffee, cola drinks, alcohol, spicy foods, onion, garlic or other hard-to-digest food. The distress is usually relieved by milk, antacids, bicarbonate of soda or soda crackers.

What is your stomach growling about? Excessive acid. The acid is the result of stimulation of the acid glands in your stomach by emotional stress ("hurry, flurry, worry"), food (hot and spicy), or irritants (alcohol or caffeine). Once the glands have excreted the hydrochloric acid, irritation of the lining cells of the stomach occurs — unless it is promptly neutralized by food, milk or antacids.

If this body warning goes unheeded and the symptoms recur for many months, the ultimate result of repeated damage to the stomach lining is a peptic ulcer. The body not only tells you what not to do ("Don't touch that pepperoni pizza!") but what to do ("Man, does that glass of milk feel good"). It also hints that your life style leaves something to be desired ("I never have stomach trouble on weekends when I don't rush all the time" or "I feel so much better when I take a yoga break at the office").

Insomnia

Insomnia involves regular difficulty in falling asleep, restlessness and frequent awakening and an inability to return to sleep.

Anxiety states and depression are the most common causes of insomnia. These are frequently brought on by faulty family or other interpersonal relationships. Poor sleeping habits and lack of a bedtime ritual cause much insomnia. These are related to poor life-style habits such as frequent variations in the hour of sleep; coffee, tobacco and other stimulants prior to hour of sleep and insufficient physical exercise. They all disturb the body's normal cycle of activity and sleep.

Physical illness which causes coughing or shortness of breath while lying down can seriously interfere with sleep. Hiatal hernia of the stomach, backaches and urinary tract conditions, too, may lead to insomnia. Other secondary symptoms may then develop that include fatigue, headache, irritability, nervousness and depression.

Insomnia tells you that you are not in harmony with your environment, or that a part of your body is out of sync and needs treatment. Insomnia is itself not a disease or condition. It's a symptom offering advice: get more exercise; establish better sleeping habits; solve those personal problems; switch to Sanka; see the doctor.

Burning or Itching Eyes

When the television commercial shows smoke, glare, and irritants at work and the red sore-looking eyes that result, cause and effect are readily apparent. It is another example of one of your body's *protective* symptoms.

Your eyes are talking to you. The television ad writers would have you believe the eyes are saying, "Get me those El Perfecto Eye Drops," but they are really saying, "Help! Get those irritating car fumes, vile smelling cigarettes, and dry winds away from me!"

The fact is that when any mucous or skin surface dries out, it broadcasts a distress signal that we interpret as soreness, burning or itching. If you've been using paint remover in a project at home, and get some on your hands, it can remove the protective oil in your skin as well as the oil base paint from the chair. At the first burning symptom you head for the sink for a thorough washing with water and an application of hand lotion. The burning disappears as the skin returns to its normal, protected condition. Much the same applies to burning eyes. Wash them with cold water for a few moments and close them for a while. They'll quickly return to their normal moist state.

Another common cause of burning eyes is rubbing. Some people just can't seem to keep from picking nervously at their eyebrows, smoothing their eyelids, and unwittingly transferring the dirt, bacteria, viruses and irritating chemicals found on their hands to the sensitive eye tissues. Sometimes the problem is eyestrain, and recurring eye infections (conjunctivitis) are often the first clue that glasses or a new prescription are indicated. If you have any of these symptoms, the eyes

53

may be saying, "Take me downtown for an eye test," "Wash your hands," or, less politely, "Keep your dirty hands off me!"

Other possible disorders associated with sore eyes are: blocked tear duct, allergies, styes (chalazion), iritis and glaucoma. These should be seen by an eye specialist (ophthalmologist). All of these produce more severe frequently painful symptoms that urge, "Take me to a doctor."

Rectal Irritation

I've heard that the advertising budget for one of America's largest selling ointments, a product for hemorrhoids and rectal itching, is more than $20 million per year! That indicates how frequently this symptom speaks.

Most of the irritation is caused by hemorrhoids, also known as piles, and is expressed as itching, burning, and pain. Hemorrhoids are varicose veins of the rectum that bulge out of the mucous membrane. They may be either internal, well inside the anal passage or external, below the sphincter muscle. When cracked, hemorrhoids cause bleeding, discomfort and a variety of burning sensations. They can become engorged with blood and a clot can form causing severe pain. These blood clots (thrombosed hemorrhoid) within the vein are usually the size of a grape and are very tender when touched.

Other pain and irritation may come from an inflammation of small pockets in the mucous membrane in the lower rectum (cryptitis), cracks near the hemorrhoids (fissures) or skin inflammation around the anus (pruritus ani).

What does it mean to have varicose veins called hemorrhoids? All varicose veins have one thing in common. The wall of the veins is distended by blood under elevated hydrostatic pressure. The blood pools or congests in these veins as it tries to make its way back to the heart.

This demonstration will give you an idea of what I mean.

(1) Place your hand on a table in front of you at the level of your heart.
(2) Look at the veins on the back of your hand.
(3) Now drop your hand to your side at the level of your chair seat for 20 seconds.
(4) Examine your hand and the veins again. They have popped out because of increased hydrostatic pressure.

Even as you are performing this simple experiment, the veins in the rectal area are being "popped out" a bit by your sitting position. This is true as well of the veins in your feet and lower legs. It should, therefore, come as no surprise that hemorrhoids are common in truck drivers, elderly people, heavy equipment operators, typists, and others who sit in one place for long periods of time. Although they occur, too, as a result of obesity, the straining that follows constipation, and the pelvic vein congestion that occurs in pregnancy.

If the truck driver who eventually developed hemorrhoids had listened to his early symptoms of rectal aching (after that 8-hour non-stop drive from Chicago to Washington three years ago) he would have followed a more sensible plan. He would not have driven more than 2 hours without a rest stop and 10 minutes of walking about to relieve the pressure on his rectal veins. He would have learned to do rectal muscle "sets." (This involves squeezing the rectal muscles hard, as one does after a bowel movement. This should be done for 30 seconds each time, several times while walking around and every 15 minutes while driving.) He might also have learned to take a few minutes at a truck stop to lie *face down* on the cab seat to ease the hydrostatic pressure on the rectal veins. To prevent the development of hemorrhoids, the typist or others whose life style involves sitting for long intervals should go and do likewise.

What if the rectal symptoms are itching and irritation rather than aching and soreness? If the rectal and anal area are sore from diarrhea, constipation, or overzealous wiping of the skin and mucous surface, they are pleading, "Clean me more carefully."

It is not unusual for chemicals and bacteria normally found in the feces to cause the symptom of itching when in contact with the tender skin of the anal area. The symptom is similar to that caused by turpentine or other irritants on the hands and can be relieved by prompt, simple cleansing with water.

The way this is done depends on the hygienic preference of the individual. A simple way is to sit in a little water in a tub or bidet and carefully cleanse the anal area, drying it gently with paper tissue or a towel. Others may prefer a wet face cloth for cleansing or products such as Wet Ones.

Usually it is best *not* to use soap or other possible irritants such as rubbing alcohol, salves or ointments for cleansing. Keep the area clean with safe, inexpensive water.

Headache, heartburn, hemorrhoids and all those other hellish TV mini-ills preach the same sermon: "Listen to your body!"

7 EATING, AMERICAN STYLE

THE TROUBLE WITH preventive medicine is that, like peace and happy marriages, it isn't very dramatic. That's too bad. The perfect way to sell it to Americans would be through a good spell-binding TV series. Recently, educational television tried to go that route, but "Feeling Good" was welcomed by viewers and reviewers with the kind of enthusiasm usually reserved for rabid dogs and bill collectors.

Undaunted by its less than lukewarm reception, I've been toying with the idea of translating preventive medicine into television myself. Here's a sample scene from my first effort — a pilot for a series to be titled "Marcus Wellbeing, M.D." — which illustrates the difficulties of turning whole wheat bread into high drama.

The scene is the bedroom of pepper-tongued but lovable Mrs. Glenda Goodperson. Dr. Wellbeing and his handsome young associate, Dr. Smiley, are making a house call at her bedside. If you'll take your TV dinner out of the warming oven, we can get on with the show.

SMILEY: Mrs. Goodperson, frankly we're baffled by your case. We've run every lab test in the book. Brain scans. Liver biopsy. Lumbar tap . . .

MRS. GOODPERSON: Don't beat around the bush, young man. I've had a good full life. I've paid my dues to society, I'm not afraid of driving into that Great Parking Lot in the Sky. What you're saying is my case looks hopeless?

DR. WELLBEING: (Interrupting hastily) No, Mrs. Goodperson, we're not licked yet. In fact, I believe I have the answer for you right here in my little black bag.

MRS. GOODPERSON: (Gratefully and with renewed hope) Dr. Wellbeing, you don't mean — a new miracle drug!

DR. WELLBEING: No, better than that. (Opens bag) Here, Mrs. Goodperson. Use these things and I can promise you better health. No overnight miracles, mind you. But soon. And for the rest of your life. (Removes objects one at a time as Mrs. G. looks on.)

MRS. GOODPERSON: (Aghast) An empty saltshaker? A sugar bowl with-

56

out sugar? A carrot. An apple. A loaf of whole grain bread? A bottle of safflower oil? Dr. Wellbeing, have you lost all your marbles? I knew those long hours you put in and all those house calls you make were taxing your strength. But now you've gone too far. *(Picks up telephone)* Long Distance, get me Chicago. Yes. I want to speak to the President of the A.M.A. *(Dramatic drum roll as at execution — up and out.)*

No, preventive medicine probably wouldn't make very gripping television viewing. Catastrophes are dramatic: a multiple car crash on slick highways at 100 m.p.h., a plane ditched at sea, a towering skyscraper inferno. But the "medicine" that could have prevented them — driving at a safer speed on wet roads, better maintenance by the jet's ground crew, replacement of a frayed lamp cord — is dull as a reading of an automobile parts catalog.

In the same way, open chest massage for coronary arrest is theatrically impressive. But using skim milk and artificial sweetener in your coffee instead of cream and three spoonsful of sugar, jogging for a half-hour three times a week and cutting out cigarettes — all of which could have helped prevent the coronary — would not exactly keep television viewers on the edge of their couches. And surgery ("Retractors! Scalpel! Sponge! Good Lord, doctor, she's hemorrhaging!") for carcinoma of the colon ("Any metastasis yet, doctor?" "No, I think we've got the whole thing.") is considerably more suspenseful than a closeup of a radiantly healthy family chomping raw apples, carrots, bran and whole grain breads — roughage which the latest studies indicate may be remarkably effective in preventing abdominal cancers in the first place.

There's a lot of good sense to the words of Dr. Jean Mayer, Professor of Nutrition at Harvard University: "The main diseases we deal with and the main causes of death are influenced by nutrition — and they're more easily prevented than treated." Yet most physicians say little or nothing about the food you choose to eat, other than an occasional: "You've put on a little weight since last time, Mary — better go easy on the desserts."

There's good reason for that. Medical schools have traditionally paid little attention to nutrition, and have, in fact, probably helped to foster a kind of polite contempt for it in the physicians they train. Most doctors know less about nutrition than the counterperson in your local Burger King. They prefer instant successes — diseases that surrender cooperatively to antibiotics — to the thankless, well nigh impossible task of trying to change their patients' eating habits. As Darwin dramatically demonstrated with instant results when he introduced the Australian aborigines to sugar, it's easier to form bad habits than good ones.

Yet increasingly, it's becoming clear that what we eat influences our health and can shorten or lengthen our lifespans. The medical profession laughed at "food faddists." And we still do officially — at some, with good reason. But it is no longer possible to deny the correlations between poor nutrition and some of our toughest and ugliest enemies: cancer and coronaries, among them.

Here, then, is your finest opportunity in self-help medicine. You eat three meals a day, plus occasional snacks, and this goes on seven days a week for 52 weeks a year. That's more than 1,000 opportunities a year to do something positive for yourself in preventive medicine. Few areas offer that many occasions for self-improvement. I'm not recommending it, but you could do worse than choose your viands off the pet food shelves at your local supermarket. Ever read a label on dog food and see what's required to qualify the product as adequate for Rover's nutritional needs? Yeast. Soy grits. Supplements of Vitamins A, B-12 and E. Riboflavin. Niacin. Iron. Copper. Manganese. Cobalt. Phosphorus. Pantothenic acid. I don't know how the stuff tastes, and given a choice I guess I'd prefer a good steak myself. I know my dog Champ would, too. But from a nutritional viewpoint, it's clear that Friends-of-Fido is a more powerful lobby than Pals-of-People.

Short of applying for dog licenses, what can we do about improving our own nutrition? Quite a bit — and the things Dr. Wellbeing took out of his black bag are as good a place as any to begin.

The Saltshaker

For centuries it was a luxury, so valuable that in Tibet and Abyssinia salt cakes were a medium of exchange. In recent years, it's become a staple so omnipresent and inexpensive that the average American takes in 14.5 grams a day — four or five times as much as the American Heart Association believes appropriate. And that is many times the one gram a day that is all the body actually needs.

What's wrong with the tiny crystal that heightens the flavor of so much that we eat? Well, we know that the more salt consumed, the more likely you are to have hypertension and heart disease. Every time you tip your saltshaker hundreds of grains of salt are distributed over your food. Each grain you swallow seizes a certain amount of water and imprisons it in solution around it. This is particularly significant in the cells of the arteries and in the heart and kidneys. As each blood vessel and little capillary captures fluid in this way, they become increasingly boggy — narrower and less effective. The heart must pump harder to push the blood through these narrowed channels, and in order for all parts of the body to get their share of life-giving blood, blood pressure must increase. That, as you know, isn't good.

The Sugar Bowl

During the period of upsurging sugar prices in 1974, consumers hissed but nutritionists hurrahed. Once a costly delicacy, sprinkled sparingly, sugar now makes up an unprecedented one-fifth of our caloric intake, and has been termed by Dr. Jean Mayer "a new food . . . which the human system, at least in many people, is not equipped to live with."

Strong statement? Well, sugar is strong stuff in our diets. You'll not be surprised to read this statistic — that by his or her teen years, fully one-third of the typical American youngster's teeth have developed decay. And it's no news to you that sugar and the sweets you take it in are fiendishly fattening, and that the calories they provide are empty ones, cheating you of nutrition. But only recently have medical scientists joined the "food faddists" who for years have declaimed noisily against the health hazards of $C_{12}H_{22}O_{11}$ — alias table sugar or sucrose. Eminent University of London Emeritus Professor of Nutrition Dr. John Yudkin believes that sugar may be a greater cause of arteriosclerosis (hardening of the arteries) than saturated fats. He points, for example, to East African tribes on a high fat diet who have almost no heart disease — because, Dr. Yudkin theorizes, their diet is so low in sugar. He compares their diet to that of the inhabitants of St. Helena Island, who eat little fat, exercise a great deal, smoke very little — all excellent health habits — yet have a high incidence of heart disease, related, he suspects, to their high consumption of sugar.

Sugar may be sweet, but not innocent. We don't know for certain that it's the sugar in our food that elevates cholesterol in our blood — although we do believe it dangerously raises triglycerides. And we're not uncontestedly sure that those higher values should be blamed for coronary disease. But the evidence is mounting — and our suspicions should be, too — that sugar is at least a co-conspirator and that it's an active participant in illnesses such as ulcers and diabetes as well. Sugar is sneaky. It isn't only in our tea and coffee cups. It lurks everywhere in our processed foods — in the dressings we put on our salads, the ketchup and relish we daub on our burgers, the peanut butter and jellies in our sandwiches, our canned vegetables and fruits, the very bread we eat, as well as, more conspicuously, in our cakes, candy bars and ice cream, soft drinks and even our stews. Americans are now consuming a two-pound bag of sugar per person per week — and that's more than we take in of that eternal staple, flour. We worry a good deal about drug-pushers in our schools. Maybe we need to mount a companion campaign to rid the schools of the vending machines that so successfully push equally addictive candy bars, cupcakes, and highly sweetened soft drinks.

Whole Grain Bread

My father, grandfather and great-grandfather were bakers, and I remember their pride in the plump sacks of grain they hauled to the bakery from the local miller's, and the rows of robust and fragrant whole grain breads they drew from the oven. The supermarket chains and their soft white sandwich breads hurt the business a bit. The old German bakers knew bread should be baked tonight to be eaten fresh and crunchy tomorrow. But people bought the message of the radio hucksters that soft bread is the best bread — and, since it took two days for the packaged white breads to be trucked in from the big city bakeries, their added preservatives gave them a pantry shelf life homemakers appreciated. Forced by that competition to do so, my father reluctantly began to bake breads made of processed flour. But he never ever ate them.

Remember how Mrs. Goodperson scoffed at whole grain bread? Dr. Wellbeing should tell her that Africans on their native diets of unprocessed breads made from stone ground meals — millet, corn, potato, bean — rarely have intestinal cancers. But as soon as they become "civilized," picking up Western eating habits of soft, smooth, refined foods, those cancers become prevalent. Mrs. Goodperson might be impressed, too, by studies with rabbits. In their natural habitat, where bulky greens are available to them, stomach cancers are rare. Bring them into a lab and put them on manufactured animal feed pellets, and malignancies appear. A common missing ingredient when intestinal cancers are present — in rabbits or people — seems to be roughage: the good, coarse, fibrous parts of grains, fruits and vegetables that help to speed food down our digestive tracts.

We've long associated roughage with "regularity." But that old line about an apple a day keeping the doctor away now seems to be more than a rhyme. It's folk wisdom. *Medical World News* reported in September, 1974, that roughage has been shown to be effective in treatment of diverticular disease of the colon. There is experimental evidence that it plays a role in preventing cholesterol gallstones, in controlling obesity, and possibly reducing blood cholesterol levels. Epidemiological studies, showing that deaths from diverticular disease and ischemic heart disease have both risen as roughage consumption has dropped, tend to verify these findings.

The ways in which roughage does — if it does — prevent cancer and heart disease are complex or unknown, But researchers are accumulating data, and they believe that food with a high fiber content moves through the body's digestive system more than twice as fast as soft refined foods — thus cutting in half the time available for cancer-causing viruses and chemicals in the gut to burrow into vulnerable tissues in transit.

A low bulk diet, generally heavy in sugars and other processed carbohydrates, can also be a fattening diet. Dr. Kenneth Heaton of Bristol University in England points out in an article in *Lancet* that a high-bulk diet helps weight control three ways. First, roughage displaces other more fattening nutrients in the diet. Second, it requires chewing, which slows down the intake of food, and increases saliva and gastric juice production which, in turn, distend the stomach and make it report that it is "satisfied." Third, the roughage reduces the absorptive efficiency of the small intestine, so that a portion of the food eaten is not fully digested or burned by the body. So, aside from the vitamin and mineral content of that apple and carrot of Dr. Wellbeing, they — along with whole grains, and particularly bran — may perform a singular service in helping to prevent onset of our number two cancer enemy (after lung in men, and breast in women): carcinoma of the large bowel.

A Bottle of Safflower Oil

He might have used corn oil, or any polyunsaturated type, but what Dr. Wellbeing was saying here was, "Lay off the animal fats." Meat on the table used to be a Sunday treat for most families, but it's become a way of life. The stuff tastes good. No doubt about that. But the price appears high in health terms — most conspicuously, increases in atherosclerosis and heart disease. You're probably already familiar with the highly publicized epidemiological study comparing the health of a group of native Japanese with a matched group of Japanese families who emigrated to the United States. The stay-at-home Japanese on their traditional diet of fish, rice and vegetables enjoyed a low incidence of heart disease. The new Americans, switching enthusiastically to our high animal fat diet, suffered dramatic increases in coronary ailments.

Much more work is being done in an attempt to confirm correlations between heart disease and animal fats. Or, indeed, to disprove it, if the evidence should point that way. National Institutes of Health is funding a long-term study. In the meantime, most cardiologists and, indeed, the American Heart Association, recommend a prudent approach to diet, limiting the quantity of animal fat and increasing the proportion of polyunsaturated vegetable oils such as safflower and corn oil.

Pediatricians influenced by grim autopsies from both the Korean and Vietnamese wars — revealing alarming signs of arteriosclerosis in as many as 75% of 19- and 20-year-olds who should have been in the prime of health — have begun to recommend this prudent diet even in young children. They're telling mothers to limit them to three eggs a week, to use margarine instead of butter, to switch them to skim milk or the tasty "99" variety, to return the ice cream sundae to its original Sunday-only status, and to focus on lower fat ice-milk instead of butterfat-rich ice cream. A lowered animal fat diet automatically means fewer calories, too, and since overweight is associated with heart disease, going in that direction can't help but be helpful.

We don't need to give up dairy products. The dairy industry shows signs of recognizing that it must — and can — come up with more low-fat cheeses and similar lower cholesterol products. We don't need to give up steak and roast beef either. But with coronary heart disease striking about one million Americans each year, we certainly need to prudently cut down. As long ago as the 17th century, poet John Milton recognized the dangers of dinner table excess when he wrote in *Paradise Lost:* "But many shapes of death, and many are the ways that lead to his grim cave . . . Some . . . by violent stroke shall die, by fire, flood, famine, by intemperance more, in meats and drink which on the earth shall bring diseases dire." Milton was sightless, but there was nothing wrong with his vision.

DIETARY RULES

What kind of dietary program can you put your family on to keep each member as healthy as possible based on what we know today?

Rule one

Take the sugar bowl and saltshaker off the table. Use some salt in cooking, but cut down the amount the recipe calls for. None should be routinely added when the meal is served — consciously try to use less.

Highly salted foods like dehydrated soups and boullions, pretzels and potato chips should be less frequent visitors to your table.

Take even more drastic action with sugar. Don't just cut down — cut it out. Taper off gradually, or switch to granulated sugar substitutes for table and baking. Honey and dark brown sugar aren't quite as bad as white. Cakes and pastries or candies made with sugar should be special occasion items only. There are plenty of "diabetic" products on the market now to fully satisfy your sweet tooth. Or better yet, become a fruit-aholic, substituting fresh fruit snacks for the cake break. Some time back, when I did some work for an international pharmaceutical firm, I fondly remember visiting the company's director of research in Berne, Switzerland. At 10 a.m., in would come a little lady in a white apron with our coffee break — only instead of coffee and pastry, it was a big bowl of shiny fresh fruit. We'd sit there munching apples, feeling virtuous, and solving our problems.

That's certainly better both for adults and children. Arriving home from school shouldn't be the occasion for half a chocolate cake and milk, but rather a bowl of fresh fruit, or carrot and celery sticks, dates, nuts and raisins or other dried fruit, or occasionally some nutritious home-baked granola cookies.

Rule two

Don't settle for half a loaf. That is, don't eat a loaf of bread made from half the grain of the wheat — the poorer half. Modern commercial white breads use a 35-year-old "enrichment" formula, and are sorely lacking in bran and wheat germ. There has been a rich harvest of "natural foods" recently even among the big commercial bread bakers, so take advantage of it — shop for and enjoy the new multi-grain breads, wheat germ breads, oatmeal loaves, even granola breads. When you bake your own breads, follow the Sehnert Bakers traditions — use recipes calling for whole grains, rolled oats, bran and the rest.

Rule three

Eat something raw daily — preferably two somethings. Besides adding necessary vitamins and minerals, raw fruits and vegetables add valuable bulk to the diet.

Rule four

Check and balance your fat intake, dropping from the American average of 40% to 50% of your food calories down to 35% or less. Balance the intake between animal and vegetable varieties. Polyunsaturated vegetable fats like safflower and corn oil have the effect of controlling the saturated high-cholesterol fats like butter, lard and meat fat. Use margarine at the table, oil for cooking and baking, skim milk for a beverage, ice milk instead of ice cream, more cottage and part-skim cheeses, trim meat fat before cooking, limit eggs to three weekly per person.

Rule five

Eat more fish and fowl. Some people think fish is brain food. It's not, but serving it shows you've got brains to begin with. Fish and poultry meals — lower in calories and fat than beef, lamb or pork — should replace many meat meals. Veal is another good beef substitute. Beans, nuts, and new soya-meat extenders and substitutes are other good sources of protein.

Rule six

Learn to read labels, and to compare brands. Consumerism is forcing more detailed labeling. Ingredients in prepared foods are listed by law in order of quantity in the package. When sugar is the first or second ingredient in a long list, eater beware. In breakfast cereals, for example, if sugar is the first or second ingredient, your children are eating candy for breakfast.

Go easy on such additives as monosodium glutamate (MSG), nitrites and nitrates. MSG has been banned from baby food because it can be dangerous for infants, but we still haven't removed it from adult foods. It's a taste enhancer and tenderizer, but it isn't necessary and could be harmful. Nitrites and nitrates are found in smoked and preserved meats such as sausages, franks and spam. Sometimes the artificial red color gives them away — other times, you have to read the label to know it's there. We don't know for sure what happens in our bodies, but we have tentative evidence that they may be carcinogenic. So a bologna sandwich for lunch every day could be a carcinoma sandwich for your child. Not for sure. Just maybe. Peanut butter seems a lot safer.

Don't be sold by the word "natural." Almost anything can be called natural, including sugar and salt. True, there may be no preservatives added, but that doesn't mean the other ingredients are manna from heaven. "Organic" is another trick word. Everything that grows grows organically. So-called organic fertilizers haven't been proven superior to chemical fertilizers. Plants don't know the difference. They're happy so long as they get the nutrients they need.

Rule seven

Nobel Prize winner Linus Pauling says it works. Others say it doesn't. Vitamin C does seem to work for some people in preventing colds, or stopping them early. No one seems to know why, and there are many medical skeptics and conflicting studies. If you don't enjoy colds, you might want to run a clinical trial in your own family. When someone feels a cold coming on, give them 1000 to 1500 mg of C every 3 or 4 hours until the cold has either run up a white flag or conquered the patient completely. You may be one of the fortunate people C works for, in at least shortening your cold. For best results, stay away from sugar during the test. There is some tentative evidence that it may inhibit the action of the vitamin.

Rule eight

Expect no miracles from foods. Any claim that a diet of grapes, or yogurt and blackstrap molasses, or a diet of rice, can cure a disease or make you healthier is nonsense. The miracle of nutrition lies in variety. Our bodies require a great many nutrients, all of which must work in concert. There is no single food or even small group of foods that contains every nutritional element we know is necessary for good health — much less those nutrients still undiscovered.

Yogurt is a nourishing milk food, usually low in fat, and the content of *Lactobacillus acidophilus* in it is particularly valuable when our bodies are depleted by antibiotics of these friendly bacteria. But normally, it's no better for us than milk. Molasses is relatively rich in iron, but so are a lot of other foods. Wheat germ, the rich heart of the wheat grain, is an excellent food, rich in vitamins and minerals, and a fine addition to home-baked goods and for ice cream topping. But it's no magic powder. Granolas may provide good roughage and be a big improvement over other breakfast "sugar frosted" or chocolate cereals "enriched" with minuscule vitamin traces, but some are heavier on sugar than they should be. Your own home-made granola with nuts and fruits may be better than anything you can buy in the supermarket or health food store, and costs less, too.

Rule nine

This rule is Chinese — an old proverb that says that when you eat, the first eight parts are for you, and the last two for the doctor. It's a maxim that all of us, but especially that 30% of Americans who are overweight, should take to heart. It's especially true if that "last two parts" are made up of sugar, salt, animal fats or processed foods without bulk. Many of us can blame being overweight on our mothers, who believed fat babies were healthy babies, and may have caused our bodies to manufacture as many as 20% to 30% extra fat cells we must carry around for life. But it's a honeycomb of cells beneath the skin that can flatten out and collapse. We can keep them that way and be a lot healthier if, when they send out a message that says, "Fill me!" we learn to ignore the command.

We're lucky to be able to eat American style. Half the world's people don't get to eat very much at all. But let's not push our luck.

8 HERE'S HOPING YOU'RE COPING!

*"I don't know why I'm paying that psychiatrist
$50 an hour. All he ever does is turn my
questions around and ask me what I think. If
I knew, I wouldn't be there."*

IN MY OVER 20 years in medicine I've had many patients tell me that. In retrospect, I'm discouraged when I count how few have been helped by psychiatrists. This is not meant to be vindictive. Psychiatrists have done the best they could given their traditions and teachings, but I feel they've had an empty medical bag — for many kinds of cases — for many years.

The emotional problems that most people have not only don't require a psychiatrist's services to begin with, maybe they shouldn't even be classified as mental illness. Dr. E. Fuller Torrey of Washington, D.C., author of *The Death of Psychiatry*, says it all, and, since he's a psychiatrist himself, I'd say rather courageously, in a recent *Washington Post*.

"The reality is that psychiatry is an exceedingly dispensable profession . . . in the process of being dispensed with . . . (by) the onslaught of psychologists, specially trained social workers, nurses and others into territory which psychiatrists had considered their exclusive preserve. What these non-medical practitioners have been doing simply is helping people solve problems of unpleasant and unwanted human behavior, and have been doing a good job of it at that."

Continued the turncouch psychiatrist: "All the research today indicates they get just as good results as psychiatrists in treating those patients who merely have problems of living — floundering marriages, trouble raising children, difficulty finding meaning in life, problems getting along with others and themselves . . . This should come as no great surprise. These were never psychiatric problems to begin with, though psychiatrists have long found it convenient to lump them together with true brain diseases and treat them both under the mantle of medicine."

67

These problems of unwanted behavior have been given many names — anxiety neurosis, hypochondriasis, hysterical personality, alcoholism, drug addiction — but they're really stress diseases: an inability to cope. Not mental illness, just difficulty in handling pressure-cooker environments. That's why social workers, other counselors and group therapy have been so successful in helping these people. You can get a lot of insight from listening to a neighbor who's had a similar problem.

Self-help groups — people being their own doctors — can be tremendously beneficial. (I'm personally opposed to encounter groups — too many angry people there, at advanced stages of coping breakdown.) National self-help groups like Recovery, Inc. can do a good job. (There are chapters in most major cities.) A survey of people participating in that group's group sessions showed that 20% were referred there by psychiatrists, and another 17% by other professional counselors.

That kind of growing professional acceptance is seconded by patients themselves, who affirm the benefits of mutual support — support which even a loving wife or husband, with the best intentions in the world, sometimes cannot provide. One young mother of four who, after two years of psychiatric treatment that started with a post-partum depression, finally took part in group therapy, said, "A few of these sessions were better than months with my psychiatrist. It must be that misery loves company, because just to find out there are other people with the same problems, who felt just as unable to cope as I, was a tremendous boost." Psychological self-help is an exciting new area, and that's why we've included it in this book.

If we're going to learn how to cope with stress, we've got to understand a bit about it. Stress is, of course, part of life. The individual who hasn't been stressed hasn't lived. We're stressed when we accelerate onto the parkway at rush hour to join a line of speeding cars we hope will part enough to let us slip in. That's mild, momentary stress. We get it when we play Bank Teller Roulette — choosing the line that doesn't move because a man five people ahead is picking up his payroll. Or at the supermarket when we play Checkout Bingo — selecting a line where the cash register tape gets stuck, a man forgot to get bananas, and a woman's check needs verification but the manager is in back signing in a produce shipment.

We're stressed when half the family comes down with the flu one week, and the other half the next. That's a longer term, moderate stress.

And we're stressed when our business fails, when we lose a loved one or when our marriage becomes one battle after another. This is severe stress, stress that can last weeks, months, even years.

Stress causes anxiety. But if we don't react to stress with anxiety, we may not act at all. And, that may not be good. For example, if a lump in the breast appears and we aren't made anxious by it, we may ignore it. That could be a fatal lack of action. On the other hand, if we panic, and allow ourselves to be immobilized, then again, we may not act. The best response is a moderate amount of anxiety — enough to get us to take thoughtful action.

Anxiety is your body talking, telling you it's got problems. We understand when our skin turns bright red that it's saying, "Whoa! That's too much sun!" We get under a tree. When our brain talks to us in the form of anxiety at being unable to cope, we've got to find ways to reduce that heat, too.

There have always been ways people have responded to stress and anxiety. Over the years, psychiatrists have assigned names to these "defense mechanisms." You're angry at your boss, and you yell at your wife — that's substitution. You blame someone else for your difficulties — that's projection, or scapegoating. You pretend the problem doesn't exist — that's repression, or denial.

There's been no shortage of less than ideal coping styles either. You may recognize yourself in one or more of the following categories:

• Do you feel overworked? Do work pressures interfere with your family or other interests in life? Do you feel that when you've met one challenge, another immediately appears? Do you feel pressured by responsibilities and inadequate to do all the things you must do? Do others often irritate you by their slowness? Are you proud that you've never missed a day of work because of sickness? Do you feel you could accomplish great things if only you could work harder and longer? Do you keep putting off taking your vacation?

If you've answered yes to most of these questions, you're a coronary-prone personality, sometimes called Type A. Type A people are men or women from LaMancha, pursuing the impossible dream. No matter how hard they work, it escapes them. They're over-achievers, often from a family tradition where the child proudly shows her mother a B on her report card and Mom sniffs,

"It should have been an A." Or Junior happily reports to dad that he was one for three in the school baseball game, and his father says, "Son, you're not keeping your eye on that ball — you should have been three for four." These over-achievers often do well in business, but at the expense of their families, and with the final achievement frequently hypertension, a coronary or both.

● Do you feel periods of illness are a relief — opportunities to relax that you don't often get? Do you welcome the care and concern of others when you're sick? Do you worry about your health? Do you feel that when you're sick, troublesome situations sometimes seem to resolve themselves without your having to do much?

This is the hypochondriac, who copes by copping out. Typically, this is the youngest child in the family. When Baby Jane or John had an illness he or she stayed home an extra day from school at mother's insistence. Often the hypochondriac is the third child of the family. There are lots of studies showing, incidentally, that the oldest child is the leader. In wartime, first-borns were most likely to volunteer for hazardous missions. You could ask for 12 volunteers, and 11 would be eldest children.

● Do you drive a car to let off tensions? Does the world of adult authority and requirements excite your contempt? Do you get angry when people tell you what to do? Do you tend to drive away your troubles — at high speed?

This is the accident-prone coping style, most often seen in young men — which is why their second leading cause of death is the auto accident. I can recall many of such patients. Away they go at 75 m.p.h. thinking about how they were overlooked at school for the lead in the play, or turned down for a Saturday night date. Pretty soon — BAM!

I think we're going to be seeing more accident-prone coping in women, because they're being stressed in new, larger career responsibilities and jobs they're fighting for and winning. They're smoking and drinking more, becoming more subject to stress diseases, and they're going to be involved in more auto accidents, too — to the point where, I suspect, insurance companies in another four or five years will be setting the same high rates for young women they've already got for young men.

● Do you feel you often confront situations out of your control which you must nevertheless force yourself to manage effectively?

Do you feel a lot of anger you can't express for fear of the consequences? Do you feel you just push on against difficulty after difficulty, slowly losing but never giving up? This is the ulcer-prone coper, whose problems may have begun with, "Big boys don't cry."

The manager who finds himself pushed into daily personnel situations in which he would like to scream with anger or weep at disappointments learned, as a boy to cope by "locking his feelings inside." He was taught "don't show your emotions. Don't cry." Eventually he's rewarded with an ulcer — if stressed enough.

• Do you experience times when you feel supremely happy, confident, good, powerful, and other times worthless, guilty, poor, miserable, weak? Do you feel the first way when drinking, the second when sober? Do you feel confident, capable, alert when you've consumed coffee or smoked cigarettes? Down, fuzzy, uncertain, confused, depressed when you've missed a cigarette or coffee at the regular time? Do you drink coffee or smoke when you anticipate a situation in which you'll feel the need to be alert or on guard? Do you drink when you get angry? Are your goals in life so unreachably high you're constantly drinking from frustration. Have you had arguments with your family because of alcohol? Have you lost time from work because of drinking? Do you drink alone? To escape from problems?

The adult alcoholic (or anyone who is "chemically dependent") frequently learned his coping habits from watching his father come home from work angry at his foreman or boss. He watched and listened as Dad told him about the confrontation on the job — and how he had stopped at the Corner Tavern to have "two or three beers to cool me down." In reality, the father was "running away" from a stressful situation with the help of alcohol.

• Do you feel like running away? When things in school or at home don't go right, would you like to pack up and leave?

One faulty and immature way of coping with many stressful situations is to run. Psychologists tell us that there are two basic solutions to a difficult or threatening situation: fight or flight. Others suggest a third solution, peaceful co-existence — otherwise known as adaptation or adjustment.

The wife or husband who deserts the family "cops out" by flight. The soldier frightened in battle deserts.

• Do you resent others for not taking care of you enough? Feel worthless? Feel a failure? Feel joy gone out of life? These are the depressive-suicidal copers. Women do have a tendency toward depression because of cultural and hormonal-chemical factors and premenstrual tensions. There's an annual Worry-In that's given for women in northern Virginia and sponsored by the Arlington County Medical Auxiliary, with assorted guest speakers in the mental health field. When it's over the consensus generally is that many of the anxieties are not so much a matter of hormones as a matter of overloaded life-styles and social calendars.

Anxiety occurs when your decision-making reaches a fork in the road: Do you quit the part-time job or not? Do you tell your husband he must stop his drinking so much (and risk a show-down), or say nothing? The damage of anxiety is not so much which decision you make — but hanging in between. Soon the anxiety can lead to depression because you have lost sleep, eaten poorly and not been in harmony with your world. Often when you make the decision (and it may be right or wrong) the anxiety disappears. But if you get too busy and have to make too many decisions each day, you become a victim of anxiety.

● Are you easily annoyed or often irritated? Have temper outbursts you can't control? Feel like striking somebody instead of saying something to them?

This is the angry-homicidal coping style. When they're unable to cope, out comes knife or gun. Push one more button and they become enraged bulls. Recently in Falls Church, a 16-year-old boy was with two of his friends. They kidded him a little too much. He said, "Just you wait!", got his dad's revolver out of the house, and killed one of the boys.

● Do you have periods — days, weeks, months — where you couldn't take care of yourself because you just couldn't cope with things? One more decision and you'd flip? Do you continually defer decisions? Does decision-making make you feel tired? Do you feel nervous and shaky inside, over such decisions as what tie or skirt to wear? Or when someone says something that hurts your feelings?

This is the Age of Anxiety, and that's the anxious style of coping. Of all the styles mentioned, it's the most common. All of us have high levels of anxiety — a job unfinished, a deadline to meet, a floor to scrub or freezer to defrost, a French test you didn't study for. Life used to be simpler. Your major decision for the day would be whether to chop wood or pick corn. And if it was cold, that decided it for you. Today, in any given day, we have to make hundreds of decisions. As Future Shock closes in on us, there'll be even more.

● Do you have regular set times to completely relax? Do you concentrate on finding and developing open interesting relationships? Do you know which friends you feel most comfortable and relaxed with? Do you see them as often as you should? When someone is angry with you, can you sympathize with them? Do you find yourself at ease in situations others consider to be fearful? Do you often risk opening yourself up to others, so as to have the pleasures of intimacy and honesty with them? When coping with a difficult problem, do you characteristically look for the interest and pleasure you can gain from the change? Do you feel comfortable enough with yourself to deal with many new demands calmly and practically? When you are upset, do you allow your feelings to work themselves out completely? Do you enjoy sleeping and dreaming? Do you feel that the universe is completely whole and that you are part of it? Are you plugged in? This is normal coping style, and about 70% of us fall into this category.

Anyone can learn to cope. The astronauts worked out every possible or predictable stressful situation in advance, and were prepared to handle each. Soldiers today are prepared for the stress of P.O.W. camps. Knowing what to expect helps to plan in advance what your appropriate responses ought to be.

What influences coping styles initially? Our families are crucially involved. Children grow up devoid of coping experiences if mom and dad never learned to cope. The child learns early in life that when dad is upset he goes to the bar and pours himself a drink, followed by two more quick ones. He's saying, "That sonovabitch sure screwed me, but I'll get even with him." But he's tranquilized by his booze. Pretty soon, his 15-year-old son copes with that test he flunked by having three or four beers on Friday night. He's coping, but he's on his way to alcoholism.

Our coping styles are influenced by the cultures we live in. In the old west, the six-gun was a coping tool. In today's inner city ghetto, it may be a knife or tire chain. Some of our responses to coping may be genetic. Tall, lanky ectomorphic types tend to respond to pressure with their stomachs, and end up with ulcers. The heavy muscled mesomorph body type takes his troubles to heart — he's coronary-prone. Stress seems to search out the flaw in the balloon, wherever it may be.

Self-respect is an important element in being able to cope. Individuals with low self-esteem always rate low on coping tests. That's not surprising. It takes a certain amount of faith in yourself to be able to solve a difficult problem. On the other hand, successful coping helps build self-respect. Even small successes can build confidence and prepare us for bigger challenges ahead. Volunteer work in the community, helping to win your neighbors' esteem, can help build your own.

When your body shows signs of anxiety — butterflies in the stomach, lump in the throat, rising sense of panic — seek the cause and do something about it. Something positive. Something realistic. Dr. Hans Selye, author of *Stress Without Distress*, points out that overambitious goals and objectives, beyond our experience and skills, are a frequent cause of stress. If, unlike the little locomotive in the children's story, we-think-we-can't-we-think-we-can't, then we probably won't pull our train to the top of that steep unrealistic hill.

Dr. Selye suggests you be really sure that a stress is worth it. Do the do-able, and avoid the undo-able. In effect, don't waste your time trying to befriend a mad dog. I have a patient who had to make that decision. Rosemary and her husband had lived in a small community in Texas in a very close family, with a strong Catholic and paternalistic structure. He worked hard, was promoted to his company's Washington office. Suddenly Rosemary, who'd been in a protected secure environment all her life had to start coping with a variety of uncertainties, without her family and church to back her up. Or her husband, whose hours were now longer and less flexible. Soon this happy marriage began to crack like the Liberty Bell. Fights. Tears. Visits to the psychiatrist. Finally, I suggested that she go back to her family in Texas for a month or so — for a rest. Meanwhile, her husband had a chance to rethink what was happening to their lives. Was this what he really wanted? He decided it just wasn't worth it. He went back to Texas where, according to a recent letter from Rosemary, the fracture in their marriage has been mended.

We need to take time out to think about stress, to plan stratagems to deal with it. Studies have shown that the average executive working 50 hours a week allots less than 19 minutes per week for thinking. Just 19 minutes a day — or better, three times that — would help wipe out a lot of stress. That incredible thinking machine, the brain, can solve a lot of problems if we give it time to set up options. Often we don't. Limit stress to a scheduled time when possible. The office manager who keeps her door open all the time, proud of the fact that anyone can drop in with a problem any time, is under constant stress. If that door remains closed except between 4 and 5 p.m., she'll be in much better shape to cope. Other adjustments are possible. Stuck in traffic? It's clear you're going to be a half-hour late to work? Relax, slip in a tape deck, and plan to work a half-hour late, or cut your lunch hour in half.

Selye recommends regular diversions — outside interests, time set aside for rest and relaxation. A few years back, the Ten Commandments recommended something called the Sabbath. Too few of us take advantage of the restful visit to church or synagogue once a week, and the setting aside of the whole day for relaxed non-pursuits. According to one medical study in Israel several years back, there are surprising dividends. Synagogue-attending Sabbath observers were found to have significantly fewer coronaries than nonobservers. Selye recommends keeping an eye on the silver lining. When you've failed, take stock of what you've achieved. In effect, count your blessings. Old trite phrases those may be, but they're synthesized folk wisdom as well.

How can you know if you're coping well? Is there some do-it-yourself quiz that you can take periodically? Many similar personality tests have been written but none more practical than the following quiz, prepared by Frank S. Caprio, M.D., which appeared in the November 1974 issue of *Harper's Bazaar*.

Answer *yes* or *no* to each of the following 20 questions.

(1) Do you have a feeling of continuous anxiety and sometimes of panic?

(2) Do you feel tired all the time and find that you complain more and more often that you are not getting enough sleep?

(3) Are you always worrying about your health? Do you feel your work is suffering on account of it?

(4) Do you often feel depressed for no good reason?

(5) Are you tense and restless and unable to relax?

(6) Do you get sudden tremors — "the shakes"?

(7) Are you afraid of being alone?

(8) Do you ever want to end it all?

(9) Do you sometimes wonder if you are losing your mind?

(10) Do you take other people's criticisms as personal threats or rejections?

(11) Do you lose your temper more often and find it harder to get along with people?

(12) Do you find it hard to concentrate these days?

(13) Do you feel remote from people who were close to you and things you used to like — your family, friends, sports, books?

(14) Have you started to let your appearance run down — are you careless about cleanliness, your hair, your clothes?

(15) Are you worrying a great deal, taking life more seriously, enjoying it less?

(16) Are you dependent on tranquilizers to carry you through the day?

(17) Is it becoming harder for you to make small decisions — such as what to wear, what to have for dinner, what to do next?

(18) Do you dread ordinary everyday situations — caring for your children or playing with them, going to parties, or even to the store?

(19) Has your attitude toward food changed — do you find it tasteless, hard to swallow, so that you don't care if you eat or not?

(20) Do you find yourself living more and more in the past?

If you answered yes to six or more questions, you would be wise to check with a doctor, minister, or psychiatrist without delay, or visit your local mental health clinic.

If you answered yes to three or four questions, you are not coping as well as you should and may be headed for trouble. What can you do for yourself before you look for outside help? Here are some treatment tips.

- Get enough sleep and rest. Take a daily nap. One at noon is best or if that isn't possible get one right after work. Set up a ritual that gives you a regular hour of bedtime. Avoid sleeping pills except for special situations.

- Get regular exercise. Relaxed muscles mean relaxed nerves. Choose whatever exercise is realistic for your age and living conditions: hiking, biking, walking, golf, tennis, home calisthenics — but do it on a daily basis.

- Avoid hurry, flurry, worry. These far too common life styles alter your patterns of eating, sleeping, working and recreation. They are *learned* habits and can be *unlearned*.

- Love more. Most people need to learn to love people and use things instead of loving things and using people. The Living Bible says "Love your neighbor. . . . Do for others what you want them to do for you. This is the teaching of the law of Moses in a nutshell." Matthew 7, 12.

- Listen to your body. When you are under stress you get symptoms called anxiety. Coping with anxiety is like reading a barometer: there is little you can do about changes in the weather but we can learn to observe the warning signals. Examples are "Tension in my neck muscles"; "Gnawing feeling in pit of my stomach" etc. When stress gives these signals — back off, ease up.

- Don't be afraid of compromise. In a stressful situation you can either fight, back off or compromise. Seldom is the ideal situation available.

- Avoid coping solutions that involve alcohol. A little relaxation is fine, but drinking each time you are faced with a problem soon leads to alcoholism. (This is also true of addiction to marijuana, and drugs in general.)

- Identify your fears, even *list* them. Talk your problems over with yourself and others who will listen. Try to think of ways to cope with them. Seek information about the things you fear. Knowledge can bring runaway fears down to earth. Make a decision, right or wrong, and then act on it. Anxiety results when you sit in the middle and let your fears tug at you from opposite directions.

- Avoid disruption. Try to maintain a balance in the face of disruptive elements. Reestablish calm after unavoidable upsets by following comfortable pre-set routines. Get yourself together. Disorganization produces anxiety, confusion and anger.

- Laugh more. Laughter is a good tension breaker. Laugh at yourself so that you don't take yourself too seriously.

- Avoid self-pity. Self-pity is an immature and selfish response to situations and usually a waste of time and energy.

- Avoid loneliness. Reach out, take the initiative in friendship. Treat people as though they were already your friends. Seek out compatible people.

Now, with that insight and some treatment tips you can prevent trouble and maintain good mental health. Here's hoping you're coping!

9 *YOUR* HEALTH HISTORY AT *YOUR* FINGERTIPS

YOU'RE ON A quickie holiday tour of Europe. It's Wednesday, so this must be Paris. It's a sticky August day, with your clothes adhering to you like Saran Wrap. You've just entered the Louvre Museum with your group. There's an obligatory pause to admire the graceful Winged Victory. Slowly, you continue up the majestic curved staircase.

You feel faint, and grope for the handrail. In unreal slow motion you topple backward. The lights go out.

Blacking out in your home town, only a phone call away from family, friends and personal physician is frightening enough. To faint and collapse thousands of miles from home with no one to speak for you, to explain your condition to the internist hovering over your insensible body in the Emergency Room of a Paris hospital is even worse.

It could easily have been the end of the tour and the line for the U.S. tourist to whom it actually happened. Two sympathetic American travelers had accompanied her to the hospital in the hastily summoned ambulance. But there was little that they could tell the doctor. Their acquaintance with his patient had begun on a chartered jet only a few days before. Her health history? They knew nothing of it.

Dr. Renoir was puzzled. There were no signs of trauma. No blow to the head. The coma could be caused by any of a half-dozen conditions. With his patient's respiration weakening, he needed vital clues.

Then — "Oh, yes!" — the women remembered something. "A small thing perhaps, but . . ." Ms. Jones carried a small jeweled box with her at all times. Sometimes she took pills at mealtimes.

The pillbox, unfortunately, told the doctor nothing. It contained three different kinds of pills, but no hint of prescription or pharmacy identification. Shrugging his shoulders, he tucked the small container back into Ms. Jones' pocketbook. As he did, he noticed a billfold in which was — "Zut, alors!" never before had he seen anything like this — a document marked "Medical Passport."

In its pages, he found what he urgently needed to know — a concise description of his patient's past and present illnesses, the significant notation that she was a diabetic, and the exact dosage of Orinase she'd been taking. He immediately ran a blood sugar test, confirmed that she was in diabetic shock, and reestablished chemical equilibrium in her body with an emergency injection of insulin.

Under the stress of travel, possibly with a bit of cheating on her diet in French restaurants, Ms. Jones' diabetes had run wild. Her Medical Passport had cost her only $6. It had saved her life.

There are only 40,000 Medical Passports now in use in the United States. There should be 1,000 times that many. There are adult and children's editions of the Passport. I believe the time is not far off when children will learn to keep their own health records, similar to these Passports, in the 5th or 6th grade — an excellent time for learning and forming sound lifetime habits.

It's not generally known, but a half-dozen companies already produce portable personal health records. One of the finest is the pocket-sized, nonprofit product of the Florida-based Medical Passport Foundation, so fortuitously discovered in the purse of that American tourist. Internist Claude E. Forkner developed it some 20 years ago, when this long-time medical innovator was a clinical professor of medicine of Cornell University Medical Center. His Medical Passport is used by the U.S. State Department for its overseas personnel, by Pan-Am executives, and a number of clinics and hospitals, private doctors as well as by tens of thousands of others like the Families Sehnert and Eisenberg.

I recently had surgery and found an unexpected personal bonus from my use of the Passport. As part of the routine workup, a blood test called the hematocrit was taken. The result was "higher than normal." There was some concern as to whether further studies might be needed — perhaps even delaying the surgery for a day. When I was able to show the surgeon past similar "high readings" dating back nearly 20 years — but all "normal" for me — everyone was reassured and the surgery went off as scheduled.

Few of us will star in so dramatically life-threatening an episode in our lifetime as did the diabetic tourist. So why should we bother to acquire and keep current Passports of our own? Here are some reasons that occur to me:

To give us mobile records

Ours is a floating, highly mobile society. You move to a new town and start with a new doctor. Even if you get your records from your last doctor — and many people don't — there may be information missing. It is vital for both medical and economic reasons that your doctor know your history, lab results and past medication use. Only then can you have a good continuity of medical care.

To overcome emergency room memory block

A woman writing to Dr. Forkner to request a Medical Passport told him about her brother-in-law's several severe illnesses, and added, "Last month, he had an attack, and we had considerable difficulty in the hospital remembering his illnesses and medications. In the excitement of the emergency room, we couldn't think clearly."

To clock x-ray exposure

Science has come to realize that yesterday's x-rays were not without hazard. The Medical Passport allows the building of a lifetime record of cumulative exposure from every likely source, including your dentist's office. Ten years from now, we may have something definitive — for example, that anyone who has had more than 15 x-ray studies over a period of five years should be checked for signs of a particular cancer. The sum total of your exposure, and whether you need or need not worry will be clearly recorded on the proper page.

To forestall memory fade

Even my most intelligent patients sometimes draw a blank when trying to remember things like the last time they had a tetanus shot. One PhD told me with cool aplomb that he'd had his last booster only two years earlier. He phoned next day to report that his wife's memory was more accurate on the matter, and he'd been five years off — enough, if the rusty nail he'd gotten in his foot had carried tetanus spores, to have made him a very sick professor, if not a dead one.

Weight changes, too, can be documented over long periods, as can such things as cholesterol levels, and a climbing pattern may be just alarming enough to convince you it's time you did something about the fact that you've let yourself go to pot. On the other hand, you can draw comfort and consolation from it — as I have from the fact that I weigh only 166 today, as compared to the 165 I weighed in 1955.

To provide easy accessibility

Contrast these two cases. A man found himself in need of surgery while on a trip to San Francisco. His ECGs showed abnormalities, and doctors hesitated to operate without knowing more about his medical history. It was three weeks before his records arrived — three very expensive and anxious weeks. A woman was stricken with pneumonia while visiting Phoenix, Arizona. Serious complications developed.

Here, too, records were urgently needed. But there were no frantic telegrams to her New York physician. No need to disturb the patient in an oxygen tent with lengthy questions in an attempt to put together some kind of history. The nine doctors involved in her care had all the data they needed. When she was admitted to the hospital, she'd simply presented her Medical Passport.

To control crazy-quilt records

You'll see many different doctors and different kinds of doctors in many places in your lifetime. Each will have a piece of your medical record. But you're the only one who can put it altogether into a total health biography, and only you can have it available whenever and wherever you need it, whether you're 1,000 miles away from your physician, or he's away from you on vacation. The best lab studies, the best examinations — even regular visits each year to the Mayo Clinic for its annual $500 three-day physical — aren't going to mean a thing, unless those records are instantly on call. With your Medical Passport, you *can* take it with you.

To avoid duplicating costly tests

Any time you take a test, the results go into your Passport. That can be useful for someone like the Air Force retiree who wrote to request one because he was moving to an area without military medical facilities, and felt a Passport would give him "a great amount of reassurance." At a time in his life when income was at its lowest point, he wanted to avoid the repetition of expensive, perhaps unnecessary tests.

To make traveling safer

A Chicago woman, "afraid to travel because of several allergies, asthma and a heart condition," had regretted many missed holiday experiences, but stayed at home until she learned of the Passport. With security in pocket, she was able to travel without fear. Requests have come from as far away as Africa, where a medical missionary came across a Passport carried by another traveller and immediately wrote for one of his own.

To establish family disease patterns

Knowing what common problems and illnesses predominate on a family tree — and they'd be recorded in the Medical Passport's complete family history — can help the physician recognize a hereditary problem. Tay-Sachs disease, or Huntington's chorea, for example. Grandfather may have died of something as vague as "the fits," but fitting that in with other incidents can establish a familial pattern that's important to bring to your doctor's attention. It could lead a daughter to genetic counseling, help to track potential dangers to future offspring, and make it possible to anticipate and avoid them.

To prevent loss of records

It's riskier than you think to say, "I trust you, Dr. Johnston," or "I know I can count on the Reston-Georgetown Medical Center." What happens when the doctor dies, or there's a fire in the group's record room? You're protected against misfortunes great and small, and against incompetence as well. Records transfer requests should take high priority in a doctor's office. There ought to be a quick clearing-house arrangement — as fast a turnaround as checks at a bank. But the doctor's aide has lots of work to do, bills to get out, insurance forms up to her collarbone, and so records requests somehow sink to the bottom of the pile, waiting for that quiet week when the doctor's at a convention. *Result:* Often in the best of offices and clinics, you can request a transfer of records when you move, and then wait four to six weeks for them. Sometimes they don't arrive at all.

Your Medical Passport is you at a well-organized glance. Anything significant in your life is noted there: results of ECGs, urinalyses, blood chemistries, x-ray tests, lab tests of all kinds, reports of annual checkups, proctoscopies. If you move, your new personal physician has a running start on diagnosing and treating any problems that may come up. He'll know when immunizations are due, what followup studies need to be done. If you break your eyeglasses, not to worry — your prescription's right there for the optician. So are — along with hypersensitivities to penicillin or other drugs and allergies — your Blue Shield-Blue Cross membership numbers.

But the Medical Passport doesn't contain every possible piece of information. Confidential matters — psychiatric treatment, VD episodes, sexual behavior and personality problems — are omitted to protect the patient in case of loss.

Where can you acquire a medical record of your own? There are two sources I can recommend — the first, since I use it for every member of my family, I suggest most enthusiastically:

(1) Medical Passport Foundation, P.O. Box 820, Deland, Fla. 32720. Cost, $6, includes passport, protective cover, history.

(2) Systemedics, Inc., Box 2000, Princeton Air Research Park, Princeton, N.J. 08540. Systemedics makes a billfold-sized, microfilmed Health Tag, in which they'll enter from 14 to 40 pages of history, drug registry, findings, ongoing illnesses needed for evaluation, etc., at a cost of $14.

Once you've got your history, you need to keep it up-to-date. Your doctor and his aides can help you there. First step ought to be setting up a regular 15 or 20 minute appointment with your doctor for the express purpose of reviewing your files and deciding what's wheat and what's chaff, recording only the former. Once that major chore is done, you'll need special attention only to incorporate major findings — like the result of an annual checkup, tests and all. An aide does that at my office for a small charge, about $10. If that sounds like a lot, think how much the man in San Francisco would have saved if he hadn't had to wait around three weeks for his records to catch up to him. Most of the time, the doctor will enter episodic visit results of significance at the time of treatment, and some of it you can do yourself— recording height, weight, blood pressure and the like on the spot as he calls them off. Ordinarily, when one of my State Department patients returns from Asia or Africa, I sit down with him and ask, "OK, anything we ought to fill in here?" Often the answer will be, "Oh, yes, I almost forgot — I had a touch of cholera in Rangoon." Into the permanent record it goes.

There may be a few physicians who'll be less than delighted at the idea of your having a set of records of your own. What's progress in health partnership to me may seem like infringing on prerogatives to them. But I believe most doctors will welcome the Medical Passport's coming of age, and, in an emergency, any doctor would be eager to have it in hand.

And why not? When the Internal Revenue Service comes knocking at your door, you wouldn't dream of being unprepared for a tax audit. Shouldn't you be just as ready for the emergency that demands a body audit?

10 IN PURSUIT OF MARCUS WELBY

EVERY AMERICAN FAMILY would love to have its own Marcus Welby, M.D. Chances are if you asked Robert Young, who plays Welby on TV, he'd tell you that he wishes he could find a doctor for his *own* family who's as understanding, compassionate, skillful, sympathetic *and* ready any time of the day or night to speed to a patient in distress.

But the idea of Welby wasn't born in a scriptwriter's typewriter. He represents the kind of complete caring physician many Americans still fondly remember and some are still lucky enough to have — men like the late Dr. Lonnie Coffin of Farmington, Iowa, who practiced medicine 365 days and nights a year, holidays, too.

Could any Welby script match the real-life drama of Doc Coffin's matter-of-fact New Year's Eve journey to deliver a baby? Doc rode a mule team (the only transportation able to make it on snow-covered roads) a dozen miles through a raging blizzard to the railroad tracks, then tirelessly pumped a hand-car five miles into town to get the job done. "That was," he said later, "one helluva New Year's Eve party."

Could Welby act with greater wisdom than Doc Coffin when called to the side of a deeply depressed widow? The last of her seven kids had grown up and left her. Her husband was long gone. She felt alone, unneeded and unloved. Doc Coffin wrote no prescription for a tranquilizer or a mood elevator. He just walked her across the street to the dry-goods store, and treated her with a new pink gingham house dress.

Or what about the husband who called frantically one midnight to report that his wife's leg was paralyzed, and she couldn't put it down? Doc knew the young woman well. He'd delivered her. He dressed, drove to her home, spanked her on the bottom, and said firmly, "There's nothing wrong with you but a temper tantrum, and we both know it. Now, young lady, get that leg down!" Down it went — suddenly and miraculously cured.

Doc's last house call was on the way to the hospital, after he'd suffered a massive third coronary — one year after the American Medical Association honored him as "General Practitioner of the Year" in 1958. As his daughter and son-in-law were about to drive him to Keokuk Hospital for what he knew was going to be a one-way trip, the phone rang. Doc insisted on stopping off at the home of his ailing patient. He pulled him through a mild coronary. Only then did he set down his black bag and let his daughter drive him to the hospital where, shortly thereafter, he died.

Today, there are times and places where one not only cannot find a Lon Coffin or a Marcus Welby, but, indeed, any doctor at all. A half-dozen years ago, when I first moved to the Washington, D.C. area, a doctor friend of mine argued that point with me. Bill Nye is from my old home town of Lincoln, Nebraska, and during the course of the evening, the talk got around to the problem of finding a doctor.

Bill, who lives in a stable, established community, said I greatly exaggerated the problem. I offered to wager some money on a small clinical trial to prove I did not.

"Pick up the phone," I challenged, "and say you're a newcomer in town with a sick 4-year-old. I'll bet you can spend the entire evening on the telephone and not get a firm commitment from a doctor to see your child — not just tonight, but tomorrow."

To Bill, that sounded like easy money. He riffled through the Yellow Pages and began calling. He spoke to private physicians. He argued with answering services. He called hospital Emergency Rooms. At the end of the evening, he opened his billfold and reluctantly handed me a well-earned $10 bill.

I'm told that at any given time in this country, one family in every five is on the move. That's a lot of newcomers to a lot of communities, a lot of people going through transition shock. Making changes, adjustments, decisions, and often winding up in a doctor's office with what in my area we called — naming it for the community with a very high population turnover — the Reston Syndrome.

A man from Little Rock wins a promotion to Washington. Pretty soon, Sam and Betty Lou realize that what with the higher cost of living, the bigger salary that lured them to the nation's capital doesn't really amount to much. The status they enjoyed as community leaders in clubs and church work back home is just something else they left behind them. Suddenly, they're friendless and anonymous — migrant workers in a hardtop sedan. Sam has to be gone a lot more than he used to be. Betty Lou used to shop at a set of food and clothing stores where she was known and appreciated, and her credit was always good. She had a doctor she relied on, and a dentist who never filled a tooth that didn't need it.

She comes in to see me with tension headaches from all those adjustments and decisions. Sam comes in because he can't sleep nights, and he's drinking too much. Next thing that happens is the kids, who were top of the class in L.R., are doing poorly in school. Pieced together, the Reston Syndrome is a genuine social disease.

Of all the decisions that Sam and Betty Lou — or you, when it's your turn to move — ever have to make, choosing a new physician or a whole set of new ones may be the most difficult and crucial. Consumer Reports helps you select your new refrigerator and vacuum cleaner. Newspaper ads help you pinpoint your kind of supermarkets and department stores. But it may take days or weeks of exploration to find yourself a family Marcus Welby. I strongly urge you to face that problem early on — as soon as possible after the moving van unloads. It helps to have a plan even if, for your present purposes, it's only in reserve.

Put your old doctor to work

Enlist his aid before you leave town. He may have an old med school buddy, someone he respects, in practice in your new home town. He may be willing to phone an acquaintance — a former nurse, a hospital administrator, an officer in the county medical society — to solicit off-the-record recommendations. At the very least, he can scan his A.M.A. Directory for someone whose qualifications seem particularly solid to him.

Find your new doctor before you need him

You may need a family physician, an obstetrician, a pediatrician, or all three. Make connections with these primary physicians before that old illness lightning strikes. You'll have more freedom of choice and movement. You'll be more relaxed and less pressured than if you wait until you find yourself on the phone at midnight, possibly enjoying no better luck than my friend Dr. Bill Nye.

Run your own private poll

This is not only a doctor-finder, it's an ice-breaker. Neighbors, being only human, appreciate the opportunity to share and showcase their wisdom with humble seekers after truth beating a path to their portals. Making new friends over a cup of coffee (as a doctor, naturally I earnestly recommend the decaffeinated kind) is as good an immunization as I know against the Reston Syndrome. It gives your neighbor a chance to satisfy some natural curiosity about the new folks on the block, while offering you recommendations and assessments of doctors they have known and loved — or wished they'd never known at all. But don't stop with one opinion. Phone or visit a half-dozen neighbors. It's a great excuse to meet them. And while you're at it, ask about favorite dentists and drugstores as well. If you're lucky enough to have relatives in the area, contact them for counsel. Co-workers on the new job can be helpful, too. By the time your first week's Sanka-klatsches are done, you should have a good idea of which doctor to try first. And you'll have taken the first giant steps toward acquiring some new friends as well.

Pluck the medical grapevine

Friends and neighbors are likely to judge physicians as much on charm as on knowledge and skills. Not so medical insiders. So recommendations from someone in the medical field — a nurse, a medical social worker, or another physician — should carry some extra weight. The strongest recommendation is one you can get from a hospital staff nurse, intern or resident who has seen the doctor in action, and judge him on his ability to make good decisions, not small talk.

The medical grapevine hears all, knows all. It may not tell all. But when Nurse Nancy warmly commends you to the care of Dr. Hearst, you can be sure she knows that he is not the fastest scalpel in town, ready to operate at the drop of a blood count, and that he isn't up to his stethoscope in malpractice suits. If you don't know anyone in the medical field, try to find someone who does. One indirect but effective route would be to do yourself and your new community a favor by joining a hospital auxiliary or the volunteer ambulance corps. Or, get on the finest indoor track of all, join a bridge club. Chances are you'll meet some doctors' wives, who really know the score.

Let your fingers do the hiking

On a trip to South America, I found the Yellow Pages listings under MEDICO a fascinating source of information about local physicians. In fact, they came startlingly close to being unvarnished commercials. Dr. Gomez not only lists the medical school he attended and hospitals he trained at, but also the fact that he "studied at the Mayo Clinic." Now, this may only mean that he attended a two-day seminar there 20 years ago, but the unwary patient may be a long time finding that out. Because of medical association ethical restrictions on advertising in the United States, consumers are spared that kind of misinformation. But alas, they get precious little information of any kind. If you're lucky, your Yellow Pages categorize doctors by specialty, under headings like PSYCHIATRY or SURGERY. If not — and it all depends on how conser-

vative the local medical society is — you're stuck with bare alphabetical listings of physicians, often without the slightest clue as to what
type of medicine they practice, and the possibility of having to dial a
dozen before hitting the kind you need. When you need one in a hurry,
that's a lot of calling. Given a choice, I'm not sure but what patients
aren't better off the South American way.

Medical societies: well meaning but not much help

Your county medical society lists its number in the phone directory,
too. Call it to ask for a recommendation on "a good doctor," and you'll
be awarded three names, plucked in careful, painfully objective rota-
tion off the society's membership roster. Some may not even be taking
on new patients, but you've usually no way of knowing that until you
call. No way of knowing anything else either. Your questions about a
doctor's training, age, experience, or anything else will be deftly par-
ried with polite, but firm, "We're not permitted to give out that information." The medical society beats the Yellow Pages anyway. At
least, it breaks its members down by specialty.

The doctors' own Yellow Pages

Though a bit harder to get your hands on, professional directories are
used by physicians themselves to check on one another's credentials.
They can be just as useful to you. A set, alphabetically and geographically indexed, would cost you a stiff $150 from the American
Medical Association. But it costs you nothing but time to look the
listings over in a medium-to-large public library, or in a hospital or
medical society library. Often they're a few years old, but doctors don't
move around much once they equip and furnish an office.

Year of birth will help you weigh a younger, presumably more up-
to-date physician against an older, ostensibly more experienced one.
All med schools are supposed to be equal in quality, but some are
harder to get into than others. A Harvard med trainee, for example, is
assumed to have something extra going for him. Other tough-to-get-
into schools include Stanford, Tufts, Rochester, Chicago, Georgetown
and Case Western Reserve. It's important to remember at the same time
that less prestigious schools (and hospitals) have turned out some of
our finest doctors. It's the man — or woman — who matters, not the
academic suit of clothes he wears.

Your doctor's listing will tell you some other significant things about
him — the year he was licensed to practice, if and when he was cer-

tified in his specialty, both his primary and secondary specialties (family practice and geriatrics, for instance), and his type of practice (active, administrative, etc.).

If it's a specialist you're after, you'll find them by the thousands in the *Directory of Medical Specialties* which should be available for your scrutiny in many community hospital libraries and county medical society offices. These listings, too, are broken down geographically, within each specialty. So, for example, if you want to find an orthopod in Kalamazoo, Michigan, you'd look first under orthopedic surgery and then in the pages covering Michigan. The information here is similar to that in the A.M.A. directories, but it's more detailed — where he trained, for example. If the doctor you're looking up was accepted for internship or residency by the Mayo Clinic, Massachusetts General Hospital, Pennsylvania Hospital, Johns Hopkins, New York's Mount Sinai, Boston's Beth Israel or other prestigious "Blue Chips" unfortunately too numerous to mention, it's fair to conclude his medical school performance and later training were top drawer. You'll learn what his special interests are through the societies he belongs to (Society for Pediatric Research, American Thyroid Association, or Electroshock Research Association). You will find, too, his appointment to medical schools and hospital accreditations — about which considerably more will be said in the next chapter.

What do Nader's Raiders have to say?

The first ever "Consumer's Directory of Doctors" became available last year in Prince George's County, Md., and the Health Research Group that put it together performed a distinct service to the community — which, I must unhappily report, the county medical society did not seem to appreciate. The product of a questionnaire put to the county's 560 doctors in a one-week telephone blitz by volunteers, the survey gathered answers to such key questions as average waiting time to see the doctor, time allotted for seeing each patient, whether the doctor makes house calls, cost of visits, whether money is required at the time of the visit and much more. Unfortunately, only 115 physicians were completely open in their responses, with 263 refusing to cooperate and 84 failing to respond. Many gave fear of punitive action by the medical society as their reason. Theoretically, at least, censure for unethical advertising was a possibility since the society urged its members not to answer researchers' questions.

Other consumer groups are in the process of producing similar directories in their own areas, but it will be a long time, if ever, before this kind of information becomes available everywhere, unless doctors accept what Nader's group called "a challenge to the medical profession." As the directory puts it, "Medical societies can choose to retreat behind their advertising statutes and ethics to attack this consumer action, or they can recognize their responsibility to the public and themselves publish directories such as this one as a public service." What a fine idea! Medical societies are likely to resent the suggestion. But, indeed, given the present difficulty patients have in finding the right doctor, they should have come up with it themselves.

If there's no consumer directory in your area — and this is most likely the case — you might want to contact, or even form, a local committee to try to get one underway. Or, less ambitious, but personally useful, you might call several doctors you think might be right for you and ask them some or all the key questions the Nader task force used.

Set up an appointment

Okay. You've picked the man or woman you think is your kind of doctor. The next step is to make an appointment — 10 or 15 minutes, for which, most likely, you'll have to pay his regular visit fee. It's a worthwhile investment. Make it clear that you're a new patient and you'd like to get acquainted. Oftentimes the prospective patient will be given an introductory presentation by the nurse first. If you haven't asked questions on the phone earlier, it's a good idea to have your list ready. And don't — repeat *don't* — be shy about asking about the doctor's policies any more than you'd be embarrassed to ask a restaurant whether it's sanitary certificate is up-to-date.

Ask the nurse as many of the easy factual questions as you can to get them out of the way. Her candor and general attitude in replying will tell you a lot about the office and her boss. Here are some of the questions you might consider covering.

> Who covers for him on weekends, or when he's on vacation?
> Are patients seen first-come-first-served, or by appointment only?
> How long is allotted for a patient visit?
> What are his fees? Charges for such things as office urinalysis? X-rays? ECGs?
> Does he take phone call questions, or must you make an appointment to talk to him?
> Does he make house calls? If so, what does he charge?
> Does he bill at the end of the month, or insist on spot cash each time?

Get into controversial matters of practice philosophy, too:

How does he feel about vitamins and nutrition?
Preventive medicine?
Tranquilizers? Antibiotics? Diet pills? Breast-feeding?
Does he do any formal or informal patient education? If so, how?

If he thinks the way you do, this could be an excellent marriage. But don't have a closed mind. Where he differs from you, ask him why. He just might convince you. And, you may — at long last — be sitting across the desk from a Marcus Welby of your own.

11 HOW DOES YOUR DOCTOR RATE?

You've FOUND YOUR Welby. Now, how do you evaluate him?

Knowing what fellow patients think of him certainly helps. But opinions often collide head-on. The neighbor on your right tells you Dr. Charles is "marvelous . . . up on the latest medical developments . . . compassionate, dedicated, brilliant." You're sure that if there were a Nobel Prize for family doctors, he'd win it — until you speak to your neighbor on the left.

"Oh, Dr. Charles? I never use him! You wait an hour in his outer office, and then he pokes you in the chest, looks at your ears and throat, hands you a prescription, and mumbles something about seeing his nurse on the way out. And try to get him on Wednesdays or weekends — hah!"

So whom do you believe? A more objective approach to rating your physician would be to do what doctors do when they're evaluating a physician they don't know. They look at his practice style, his credentials, his affiliations. They judge him by the kind of office he runs and the staff he's hired to run it.

To help you at that task, I sat down with an expert, Dr. Arthur Hoyte[1] to work out a useful, usable doctor rating system. Many approaches were suggested, debated, dropped. The ones that survived were incorporated into the questionnaire and scoring sheets at the end of this chapter.

But before I go on, I must make it clear that this relatively simple report card cannot fully and fairly evaluate the person charged with the responsibility of getting and keeping you well. There are no doctors, no matter how poorly trained or how low they ranked in their graduating classes, who have not saved lives. And there are those who attended the finest medical schools and achieved the finest grades, who have won the most prestigious university medical center teaching posts and secured the most coveted hospital affiliations, who are cold, impersonal and even poor physicians.

[1]Director, Office of Programs for Student Development and Community Affairs, Office of the Chancellor, Georgetown University Medical Center, Washington, D.C.

So these suggestions form only a guideline for decisions. Use your common sense to make your own exceptions. Some doctors are rugged individualists who just don't fit the molds. If you like your doctor, his health philosophy and approach, get along well with him, find he's there when you need him, and your ills respond to his pills, that's more important than any of the points to the chart. Here, then, with that caveat, are the questions you should be asking.

Is your doctor a Lone Ranger, or an Organization Man or Woman?

Solo doctors will be incensed at the suggestion that they are not the best there is. As individuals, many of them are. They are often dedicated men who relate well to and are beloved by their patients. Many of them chose that practice style for the personal freedom it gives them — they want to be beholden to no one. Others have no choice — their partners may have died or moved on, leaving them to carry the practice load alone in a one-doctor town they won't abandon.

A substantial share of health care in this country is still handled by solo doctors — possibly as much as 40% of it. But, professionally, they've got to get a low rating for a number of reasons. They may be limited in the exchange of ideas on new methods and modalities. There may be little formal evaluation of their practices — no one to say, "If you'd tried this therapy instead of that, your patient might have made it." Or, "Was that tonsillectomy really necessary?" They're more likely to be overworked and overtired. Their patients are less likely to have adequate coverage on weekends, at night, or when Good Old Doc finally takes off on that oft-postponed trip to Europe.

An informal, loose association of solo physicians practicing in the same building is something of an improvement over the strictly solo situation. Four or five doctors may have a common receptionist, which is a saving in overhead that may be passed on to patients. Since they're all under the same roof, they frequently pitch in and help the other guy with scheduling and emergency problems. There may be a greater cross-pollination of ideas. ("Harry, could you come into my office and take a look at this growth on Mrs. Monsey's cheek?") They may discuss medical problems together at lunch, as well.

Sometimes they may be joint owners of the building, share costly equipment such as the x-ray machine and laboratory equipment and rotate calls at night and on weekends and holidays.

A variation of this type of association is solo practitioners at different locations who share emergency and off-hour call duties.

The doctor who is part of a single-specialty group practice offers you a number of added pluses — and a few minuses. Such a group might be made up of two obstetrician-gynecologists (OBGs), or perhaps three pediatricians, or five family practitioners, etc. Since they generally rotate days and hours, and the receptionist schedules you to see whoever is on duty, you get three or four doctors for the price of one. That can be a disadvantage, too, if you happen to like Dr. Green and are stuck in an emergency with Dr. Brown. But if your OBG man is out on a delivery, you don't have to wait until he returns to the office. A partner can see you this time. And, of course, the same is true when your doctor is ill or on vacation. Furthermore, when there's any special problem, the man who's treating you can conveniently huddle with one or more of his partners in a corridor consultation. Of course, your total health care may be a bit fragmented. When you require treatment outside their specialty, you'll have to be referred outside the group.

That's one reason I feel you're best off with a good multi-specialty group practice. It doesn't have to be a huge one. The roster of such a group usually includes a minimum of a family practitioner, a pediatrician, and an internist (possibly specializing in cardiology or gastroenterology), but it's likely to include a general surgeon, and OBG man, and perhaps a radiologist. There are some really big groups. Mayo Clinic, with over 1,000 doctors, is the General Motors of the profession, and groups like the Ross-Loos Clinic in California and the Kaiser Groups have several hundred. But according to the American Group Practice Association, the typical affiliate has about 10 physician members.

I've always practiced in small multi-specialty groups, and I guess my bias shows. But, if there is such a thing, it's an objective bias. It comes from knowing the great potential for evaluating — and improving — the quality of medical care in an atmosphere conducive to the exchange of ideas among doctors. A poor doctor won't last long in a group of this kind, and, indeed, the careful screening that goes on prior to taking him in makes it unlikely a poor one will become a member of the group in the first place. I like the potential for integration of medical information into one patient record, and the likelihood there'll be enough staff to have a good medical records librarian or secretary and thus higher quality records. There's easy referral to other doctors. They're right there in the building.

Patients of such a group are not likely to endure the ordeal one young mother faced recently when her 8-year-old son skidded on a rock while coasting his bike, and was thrown into the road. She bundled him and her two younger children into the car and rushed him to her pediatrician. He cleaned his bruises, but advised her to take the boy to a plastic surgeon to have his chin stitched and to the orthopedist to check what appeared to be a broken arm. So she piled the children back into the car — they were already cranky and upset — and headed across town to the plastic surgeon. He sutured the chin.

The baby was now crying for something to eat. The injured boy was in pain and crying, too. The middle boy, aged five, was just plain tired. But off they cruised to the orthopedic surgeon, who took a quick look and said, "We've got to have x-rays." Where? Back in the plastic surgeon's building. So it was back in the car for the x-ray lab, and then turnabout to the orthopod again to have the arm set. It was, the mother later said, the best argument for one-stop group practice she'd ever encountered.

In the multi-specialty group, and to some extent in the single-specialty group as well, there's more efficient use of paraprofessionals. A nurse-practitioner for routine care, or a physician's assistant to remove casts, do minor surgery and run lab tests makes it possible to hold down the high costs of medical care. It's like the shopping advantage of the supermarket vs. the Ma-and-Pa store. You get a little more, with more convenience, in large groups — with some loss of the personal touch.

Patient education facilities are likely to be better, too. The American Group Practice Association has been a leader in developing patient education materials, and encouraging the creation of patient ed departments, with aides especially trained to teach breast examination, nutrition for diabetics, and the like. If all of this sounds good, and you're wondering if there's a multi-specialty group in your area, a letter to the A.G.P.A., P.O. Box 948, Alexandria, Va. 22313 might help turn one up for you.

For those who'd rather select a group than a doctor, there's another option. It's too soon to fully and fairly evaluate them, but Health Maintenance Organizations (H.M.O.s) offering prepaid health care are rapidly increasing around the U.S. The Federal government has been cultivating them assiduously on the theory — which may or may not prove correct — that large multi-specialty groups modeled after Kaiser-Permanente will be able to hold down health costs by delivering care more efficiently and economically than "corner store" fee-for-service doctors. Most people don't yet have an H.M.O. option, but some 200 are already functioning, and proponents — who, naturally, have been issuing optimistic statements — predict they'll provide as much as 20% or more of all care by the mid-1980s.

In buying prepaid medicine, you pay a fixed monthly fee for your family's care — averaging $60 per month for a family of five. This is probably more than you'd be likely to spend in a year in which your family proved reasonably healthy. But it generally includes annual health screening and preventive programs you'd otherwise be unlikely to participate in. And, it insures you against the unexpected serious illness requiring costly hospitalization, and provides lab tests, medications at cost, and almost unlimited out-patient care. Prepaid groups can be a good deal, particularly if, as is often the case, your employer picks up about half of the tab. But big isn't necessarily better, and everyone's heard complaints about the impersonality of some of the large groups servicing labor union memberships and corporate employees. In most H.M.O.s, you can choose a family doctor and he serves as manager of your health care. In general, an H.M.O. should give you a good health buy. But all the things we've talked about boil down to one fact: Good doctors make good H.M.O.s and poor doctors make poor ones.

What kind of "shop" does your doctor work in?

The kind of hospitals your prospective physician is affiliated with tells you something, too. If it's a university teaching hospital — like Columbia-Presbyterian in New York City or the University of Nebraska Medical Center in Omaha — requirements for attendings (a doctor who has staff privileges and can admit patients of his own) are stiff. It's a plum appointment, and he must earn it, often with teaching responsibilities for doctors and nurses training. He's likely to be involved with up-to-date techniques and therapies, and that's important at a time when discoveries are coming in like jets at Dulles International Airport — too fast for the average practitioner to keep track of them, let alone develop expertise. The cure rates for certain cancers, for example, are three to five times higher at some university medical centers where highly sophisticated team treatment methods have been perfected than they are in community hospitals where older methods are still being used.

There are pitfalls everywhere, however. The national reputation of a physician is not always your moneyback guarantee of satisfaction. The more in demand he is, the harder he is to reach with a nagging question — like the distinguished fertility expert whose aide wouldn't put through a phone call, insisting that the patient make an appointment and drive the 60 minutes to his office two weeks later to ask her one simple question. When she arrived, he couldn't even examine her. She was in mid-period.

Think twice, too, about the surgeon who operates at three or more hospitals. The fact that he's an attending at a half-dozen might tend to impress you, but making rounds when your patients are all over town can be a real time-killer. What's worse, the doctor could be in surgery at Hospital C when you're in post-surgical shock at Hospital A — which is why one surgeon wrote in a recent medical journal that he personally preferred an average, competent surgeon with a decent reputation to the "hotshot chief surgeon" known world-wide who spreads himself thinner than cream cheese on a diet lunch sandwich.

Every community, of course, doesn't have a university hospital center. But the larger the hospital — 200 beds or more — the more likely it is to have specialized equipment, intensive and coronary care units, and the like. And the more restricted the staff privileges, the more likely some form of peer review functions to keep "bad apples" off the staff.

Smaller hospitals are often proprietary — that is, they're owned by one or even a dozen or more physicians. Sometimes they're called Your City Doctors' Hospital. The physicians who practice there are usually part-owners, who have, in effect, bought their way in. They may be very good doctors, practicing conscientious medicine, taking continuing education courses. And, if you're in a rural area, it may be the only show in town. But their standards are generally not as high as community hospitals. Controls are looser, and doctors practicing in them often do so with the knowledge that no one is looking over their shoulders. Experience has proven that that is simply not the best way to practice medicine.

It used to be that if a doctor had no attending privileges, you could assume he just wasn't much of a doctor. But I know several perfectly able men who've chosen to confine themselves to pure office practice. They're 45 minutes from the nearest hospital in a heavy traffic area, and they've decided they can do more for their patients by using that extra 90 minutes a day at the office. Too, they save the time the hospital would demand from them in participation in hospital committee meetings. When a patient has to be hospitalized, they make arrangements with someone they feel has all the right skills. They're not second-class doctors by any means, but simply responding to modern problems and needs.

What about your doctor's credentials?

The *American Medical Directory* and the *Directory of Medical Specialties* available at some public and most hospital and med society libraries will again be helpful. If that's inconvenient, the doctor's nurse or assistant should be willing and proud to tell you during a quiet moment. Does he have a teaching appointment at a medical school-affiliated hospital? (Clinical instructor, or assistant clinical professor?) Is he a consultant — to a Veterans Hospital, for example? Is he board-certified? (If he's been board-eligible for 10 years, but never passed the two-part exam that makes him officially "boarded," it's fair to wonder why.) Board certification helps doctors in so many ways that the doctor who remains only eligible (meaning he's finished his required specialty residency) risks becoming a second-class medical citizen, unable to get the more prestigious hospital appointments, losing out on referrals, perhaps even getting lower fees from insurance companies. There are, of course, many doctors who "just never get around to it." It's just that the rigorous preparation required to pass is a sign that they're well-disciplined and want to be the best.

One rung higher than board certification on the specialty ladder is the Fellow. Thus, Rex Smith, M.D., F.A.C.S. is a Fellow of the American College of Surgery, and Charles Thorne, M.D., F.A.C.O.G. is a Fellow of the American College of Obstetrics and Gynecology. They are members of the college (an honorary group) dedicated to improving the state of the art of their specialty, with the privilege of wearing surplice, robe and mortarboard at ceremonies, and the responsibility of teaching residents in training, writing and publishing papers (to earn, though not to retain the honor) in medical journals. If your doctor's a Fellow, he is no slouch at his specialty, and has won the esteem of his peers. Don't, however, be impressed by the letters P.C. after his M.D. They just mean that he's a member of a Professional Corporation — which is nothing but a legal and business entity having to do with the way he conducts his financial affairs.

If he's a family physician — what kind?

A half-dozen years ago, the family doctor seemed destined for early extinction. In general, only a few med students were opting to become General Practitioners. "My son, the neurosurgeon" was the wave of the future. Now, all that has changed. Today, many of my medical students are telling me as sophomores that they plan to go into family practice. Thanks to the determined efforts of the American Academy of Family Practice and its push to create residencies in that new "specialty," the financial rewards are no longer dramatically skewed toward the surgical and other specialties, and there's no longer the problem of obtaining hospital appointments either. G.P.s, now called F.P.s, are becoming first-class citizens after 20 years of riding in the rear of the medical bus.

The new F.P. undergoes three years of residency now — active, supervised patient-care training. He's learning obstetrics, pediatrics, minor surgery and psychotherapy. So he comes on the scene as more highly trained than the old G.P. he succeeds, and better qualified to manage more of your problems and refer prudently those he feels require other skills.

The thing the A.A.F.P. is proudest of is that, unique among specialists, in order to remain board-certified, the F.P. must pass a certification reexamination every three years. That means he can't loaf along on his laurels. He's got to take continuing education seminars and courses steadily. These are high standards, and they've put pressure on other specialties to consider doing the same. The sooner the better for patients.

Does your doctor run an assembly line?

If he sees more than four patients an hour — giving you less than 15 minutes for a typical visit — he's practicing assembly line medicine. If he's got six or eight appointments an hour, he's approaching cash register medicine. We've done studies at Georgetown that show that four patients an hour is about right in terms of care, and that a doctor can still have good support, pretty good recordkeeping, and a respectable income. It's possible to double that, but the equation balances out badly for the patient — the higher the volume, the lower the quality of medicine.

Is he a medical V.I.P.?

If your doctor-to-be is, or has been, president of his hospital medical staff or his county medical society, that usually speaks well for him. You have to put up with an awful lot of brickbats and extra work on those jobs, and the man who accepts them — many doctors duck them — probably has a higher than average sense of civic responsibility and humanitarianism. That bodes well for patient care. It means, too, that he has the respect of his colleagues, and he's not likely to have any skeletons in his closet — other than the one he uses to point things out to his patients. Of course, if he should develop a taste for power, and move on to be a ranking state or national officer, he risks cutting sharply into practice time, and what starts as a hobby can seriously detract from healing time and availability in time of your need. He's not going to do your gallstone much good from the podium of an A.M.A. convention in New York City.

How many societies does he belong to?

Medical knowledge is expanding at an awesome rate, so special interest society memberships — in the doctor's primary specialty, a

99

secondary specialty and several others — are essential if he's to have access to the medical meetings and journals that are an important part of his continuing education and your continued good health. To stand still is to move backward on the escalator. You'll find the societies a doctor belongs to in his or her paragraph in the *Directory of Medical Specialties* — with code numbers to look up in the front of the book. There are groups for every disease and situation — societies dealing with muscular dystrophy, cancer, TB, psychotherapy, computer medicine, infants and the elderly, *ad infinitum*. Every physician should belong to three or four, but if you find 15 after his name, you've got to wonder if he isn't either a politician or a professional joiner.

What kind of staff does he have?

Does he have trained "extra hands" — a physician's assistant or nurse-practitioner? There aren't enough of these to go around yet, and the doctor who has one shows he's right up on the latest trends and practices modern medicine at its best. He knows how to delegate, turning over minor and routine care to well-trained assistants so that he can be available for the major ones. Likely the same can be said for the doctor who trains his own paramedics. You don't have to worry about getting second-class care either. He's fully responsible medically and legally for anything a member of his staff does, and he never forgets it. They've got to be good before he turns them loose on you. Another thing about his staff: Is it friendly, pleasant, or give you the feeling of real interest in you only at the moment that you hand your $10 bill across the desk? You can learn a lot about a doctor from the staff he keeps.

Does he run a school for patients?

An OBG man of my acquaintance has a remarkably lifelike pair of breasts in his office. They're made of a yielding plastic material that startlingly simulates the feel of natural flesh. Patients watch an audio-visual presentation on breast self-examination in a special patient education booth — in which educational slides on Pap checkups, breast-feeding and other subjects are also available. Then a nurse-educator takes the patient into a consultation room to test her skills. She's given the pair of breasts — which have within them three faintly discernible lumps. No patient leaves the office until she has learned to locate all three. That's patient education at its finest.

Doctors who use trained aides, educational cassettes and films, and make available well thought out brochures on care and prevention of various diseases are innovative, and expressing a philosophy that tells the patient, "You're my partner." I'd rate a doctor even higher who takes the trouble to write and have printed patient information aids of his own, answering most-asked questions, and expressing his own particular views of how to manage a particular ailment.

Does he practice "scrapbook medicine?"

I have in my office a set of records forwarded to me by a doctor whose patient had moved to my community. It's a squirrel's nest of lab, ECG and consultant reports, illegible, incomprehensible episodic notes on lined yellow Woolworth pads that not even James Bond could decode, 5 × 7 in. index cards, correspondence — everything but the lady's wedding portrait. That's scrapbook record-keeping — full of memories of visits past, but so disorganized as to be of little practical value. But this high-chaff nonsystem is the way 70% of American health records are kept.

You can judge a doctor by the records he keeps. In fact, if a group or individual is known for quality care in a community, you can bet there's a careful record system backing them up. If you're lucky enough to land in the hands of a doctor who takes a thorough baseline history at your first visit — not just a cursory yes–no questionnaire, but one that really jogs your memory of symptoms, problems and life-style — and who asks probing followup questions, you're probably in good hands.

Sitting across the desk from the doctor, you may not be able to tell if he's using one of the new, carefully organized and indexed, problem-oriented records systems, with a place for everything. But you'll know that everything's in its place if he doesn't have to fumble, hunt for the last visit, and finally give up and start a fresh page, or, worse yet, index card.

How's his deskside manner?

I say deskside because, with the house call just about dead, you won't learn anything about your doctor's bedside manner until you're hospitalized. I've saved this for last because it's still the most important item of all. His warmth, communication skills, and whether you instinctively like and relate to him count for a great deal.

Dr. T. Hale Hamm, one of my teachers at Case Western Reserve medical school and now retired but still an esteemed educator, once told me, when I asked him "How do I develop the best bedside manner?" "Be yourself, and people will come to you who like you. Those who don't like you won't come to you." As time goes by, doctors establish a panel of patients who like and are like them. Some like the explain-everything-doctor, like myself. Some like the doctor who is so dominant they don't have to do anything but show up when he orders them to. So the doctor's deskside manner should reflect your own style and personality.

What I'm saying is that even if a doctor flunks out on most of the points we've noted here, if he's a warm interested person, the kind of man or woman you can relate to — well, your instincts count for a lot of points in this rating game. The converse applies equally. A man may have all the good qualities and characteristics that I can imagine or itemize. If your gut reaction is negative, then find yourself another doctor.

Here, then, is one approach to rating a physician. I cannot claim perfection for my scheme. It should, however, be useful, and it's better than starting from zero. A score of 36 or more means you've found your Marcus Welby — at any rate, a doctor to whose care you can comfortably commend your body. Below 10, you'd probably do well to take your business elsewhere.

NEW DOCTOR QUESTIONNAIRE

1. What is your specialty? _____

2. Do you have? ____Boards ____Board-eligible
   ____Was board eligible but not now

3. Do you have a sub-specialty? ____No ____Yes (describe)

_____

4. What type of practice are you engaged in?
   ____Solo practice   ____Group (multi-specialty)
   ____Group (nonspecialty)   ____Partnership
   ____Formal association   ____Loose association with
       with physicians in   physicians in same area
       same area or building   or building

5. What is your postgraduate education?
   Internship _____ University affiliation
            Hospital & Place   ____Yes____No

Residency _____ University affiliation___Yes___No
           Hospital & Place

Fellowship _____

6. What are your hospital affiliations? (List in frequency of use)
   (a)_____ ____Under 250 beds ____250 beds or more
   (b)_____ ____Under 250 beds ____250 beds or more
   (c)_____ ____Under 250 beds ____250 beds or more

7. Do you have teaching appointments?___No___Yes (describe)
   _____

8. Professional membership? ____AMA____State medical society
                             ____Local medical society

9. Continuing medical education
   ____AMA "Physician's Recognition Award"
   ____AAFP continuing education program
   ____Other (describe) _____

10. Will make house calls under some conditions
    ____No
    ____Yes (describe) _____

11. Accepts Medicare and Medicaid patients
    ____No   ____Yes

12. Is your office or medical arts building equipped to do these (please
    check)?
    ____Chest x-ray   ____Pap smear
    ____Complete blood count   ____Throat culture
    ____Electrocardiogram   ____Urinalysis

13. Do you have after-hours coverage?
    ____No
    ____Yes (describe) _____

14. Medical record system:
    (a) Problem-oriented medical records____Yes ____No
    (b) Automated or special medical histories ____Yes ____No

BASIC SCORE SHEET

Practice	Hospital	Boards	Recommendations	Points
—— Multi-specialty group practice	—— Full-time staff of a university affiliated hospital	—— Board certified in a specialty that requires periodic recertification	—— Recommended by intern, resident, and/ or staff nurse	—— (5 ea.)
—— Uni-specialty group practice	—— Part-time staff of a university affiliated hospital	—— Board certified in a specialty that does not require periodic recertification	—— Recommended by other physician(s)	—— (4 ea.)
—— Formal association of physicians practicing in separate locations	—— Staff member of a large community hospital (over 250 beds), not affiliated with a university	—— Board eligible to become certified in a specialty	—— Recommended by other patient(s)	—— (3 ea.)
—— Loose association of physicians practicing in one location	—— Staff member of a small community hospital (under 250 beds), not affiliated with a university	—— Board eligible at one time (no longer eligible for certification)	—— Recommended by Medical Society	—— (2 ea.)
—— Solo practice physician	—— No hospital privileges	—— Practicing physician never board eligible	—— No recommendations (selected from phone book)	—— (1 ea.)
				—— subtotal

Under each of the four categories, check the one entry appropriate for your doctor (or doctor under consideration). If you are not sure of any specific information, call your doctor's office for clarification (the receptionist should have all such information available). Allot points as marked in the right-hand column for checkmarks given, and add for subtotal.

BONUS SCORE SHEET

University affiliated internship and/or residency (score 4 points)

University sponsored training programs tend to not only better supervise the performance of their trainees but to expose each trainee to a greater variety and volume of clinical circumstances than programs sponsored by nonuniversity affiliated hospitals.

Points _____

Good medical records (score 4 points)

The "glue" that holds good health care together is good medical records. If your doctor takes a complete medical history (automated or some other method) and uses the new problem-oriented medical record systems that are now available, he deserves extra credit for it.

Points _____

Participation in continuing education programs sponsored by national, state and/or county medical societies (score 4 points)

In face of the trend in medicine toward greater specialization, more complex technology and an ever-increasing amount of information, the public desires reassurance that their doctors have kept current and are cognizant of the new advances in medicine. The American Medical Association (Physician's Recognition Award) and many state, county medical societies and medical journals now offer special awards and/or certification for continuing education activities.

It must be kept in mind that continuing education is for the most part a voluntary endeavor and it is up to the individual physician to remain current and informed. Some physicians choose to do so by reading and by doing so may not be given satisfactory acknowledgment of credit by medical societies.

Points _____

Personable and efficient office personnel (score 3 points)

Many feel that the attitudes and behavior of employees are reflective of those of the employer. Office staff can do much to enhance accessibility to care as well as give you the appropriate reassurance that your doctor is concerned about you as a person and not primarily your finances or an isolated part of your body.

Points _____

105

Makes house calls (score 2 points)

In general the patient's home is a poor place to conduct an examination. Not only are examining conditions such as privacy and light often inadequate, but instruments and office laboratory procedures that can be of help in making a diagnosis or in managing a patient are not available to the physician.

However, the truly bedfast or homebound patient of any age (e.g., certain cancer or stroke patients) and certain patients with acute infectious illnesses can and often should be treated at their homes.

Points _____

Accepts Medicare and Medicaid patients (score 2 points)

Suggests a concern that medical care be available even to those in our society who have always had the greatest difficulty in obtaining care.

Points _____

Member of the local medical society (score 1 point)

Indicates acceptance by peers and that potential educational support and exposure is available.

Points _____

"Deskside" manner

(a) Personality warm, rapport good with patients (score 3 points)
(b) Average personality, helpful attitude (score 1 point)

Allot bonus points as instructed
for appropriate items and enter
subtotal at right.   Bonus Sheet Subtotal_____

Final Score

Basic Score Subtotal_____
Bonus Score Subtotal_____
Rating Total_____

Scoring interpretation:
Outstanding 36–43
Excellent   31–35
Good   21–30
Fair   11–20
Poor   1–10

12 THE REHABILITATION OF MRS. MEEK

Day one: 2 p.m.

DOCTOR: You'll be just fine, Mrs. Meek. Fill this prescription, and make another appointment with the nurse for four weeks from today.

PATIENT: Thank you, doctor.

Day two: 10 a.m.

PATIENT: (On phone) Sorry to bother you, Dr. Bowman. But those blue tablets you prescribed . . . am I supposed to take them before or after meals?

DOCTOR: Before meals — to help relax your stomach.

PATIENT: Oh, thank you, doctor.

Day two: 3 p.m.

PATIENT: Logan's Pharmacy? I got some blue tablets from you yesterday. The prescription number is 74-10977. My eyes are blurring a lot. I was wondering . . . could the pills do that?

PHARMACIST: Yes, they could.

PATIENT: Should I stop them?

PHARMACIST: You'll have to ask Dr. Bowman.

PATIENT: But he's so busy. And I already called him once.

PHARMACIST: Well then, I suggest you telephone his nurse.

Day three: 9:30 a.m.

NURSE: Dr. Bowman's office. Nurse Jenkins speaking. May I help you?

PATIENT: This is Mrs. Meek. Doctor prescribed some blue tablets for me on Tuesday that are giving me a kind of blurring in my eyes. And my mouth feels like it's full of cotton. Should I stop the pills?

NURSE: Hold the line, please. I'll ask the doctor. (Long pause) Sorry, the doctor was busy with a fussy baby. He said to cut the dose to one-half tablet four times daily, and call back if you have any more trouble.

You've just witnessed a dandy example of how not to communicate with your doctor. A brief visit to Dr. Bowman's office in this painfully familiar scenario stretched into three days of discomfort, frustration and alarm for Mildred Meek.

Whose fault was it? Some would say, with some justification, the doctor's. He was in a hurry. Other patients were waiting. But he should have spent more time with Mrs. Meek — explaining, educating, anticipating problems — or, as more and more doctors are beginning to do, trained a nurse to do the patient education for him.

But Mrs. Meek must shoulder some of the blame. She played the role of the Passive Patient, totally dependent upon what a busy physician decided to tell or not tell her. She asked no questions in the office, partly because she believed the doctor would brook none, partly because she didn't know what questions to ask. She, I suppose, would have agreed with Webster's definition of the word "patient" as a person or even a "thing" to whom something is done. Its root: the Greek "pati — to suffer." Further definition, unfortunately fitting for too many pliant patients, "having the quality of enduring evils without murmuring or fretfulness . . . submission to the divine will."

Now divine seems to me a pretty strong word to use in respect to doctors. Some of us have been accused at times of playing God. Some of us have egos that inflate to the size of a dirigible. But it is a mistake to act — as too many patients do — as if, because we have some small control over life and death, we are the Lord's representatives on earth.

Patients like Mrs. Meek don't question, don't challenge, don't doubt. They are sometimes passive to an extreme — like the patient Dr. A. Russell Lee of Palo Alto, Calif. used to tell about. She had, as he spun the story, telephoned a doctor to hurry out and visit her long invalided husband, Henry. "He's taken a turn for the worse," she reported urgently. "Can you come right out and see him?"

The doctor drove out immediately, was ushered into Henry's presence, found him flat on his back and apparently no longer breathing. He felt his pulse, found none, and said sadly to the new widow, "You're right, Sarah. Henry took a turn for the worse alright. He's dead." At which Henry sat bolt upright in bed and exclaimed in dismay, "I am not!" His wife pushed him back onto the pillow. "Lie down on that bed, Henry," she exclaimed. "The doctor knows best!"

There are, of course, a lot of patients who don't heed *anything* the doctor says. Studies show that one-third of all patients seldom follow their physicians' advice — for a variety of reasons, some of them not unreasonable. Sometimes they don't understand the doctor's orders or the seriousness of the illness. Sometimes — like a motorcyclist patient of mine with asthma who just doesn't want to believe that dust is bad for him — they deny the disease. They're afraid a medication will have side effects. They emerge complaining "the doctor doesn't listen." They're dissatisfied with a prescription — which was all the physician took the time to give them. These patients still fall into the Passive Patient category, if only because they are too passive about their health to do anything about it. They don't let the doctor manage their problems, nor do they manage them themselves. Nobody's minding the store.

However, if you're reading this book, you're interested in your health. Perhaps you're a Passive Patient who is ready to be activated. Ready to take on greater responsibility for your own health — to develop a partnership with your doctor, knowing that he can do a lot for you, but that much of what he does depends on you. The Activated Patient doesn't leave the doctor's office saying, "Gosh, what a doctor! He didn't explain anything to me." The Activated Patient asks questions — lots of them. If he or she doesn't get answers, or even worse is put down, the Activated Patient considers finding another doctor.

Nothing is more important in becoming activated than learning how to communicate with your doctor, and it starts *before* you go in for your appointment. Many people freeze when they're alone with the doctor in the examining room, somehow forgetting all the little things they wanted to discuss with him, remembering only the major complaint — and maybe even forgetting some of the details of that. Do your homework. Write down the questions on an index card beforehand, and bring that "grocery list" along. Often when I see something like that, I'll just take it from the patient and go down the list one item at a time. My job is made easier, and I know that patient won't leave muttering, "I'm just as worried now as before I went in."

Use the other side of the card to record the doctor's recommendations. People have a way of forgetting them before they've left the doctor's office. Said one quite intelligent woman, "I'm no dumb-dumb. But when I'm at the doctor's, I'm so uptight about what he's going to say that once I've heard that I'm not going to keel over and die to-morrow, everything else just washes out of my head. I recall he said something about fluids and salt water. But how much and when I don't remember." She's solved her problem by taking notes in the office. The doctor appreciates that, because he knows she's going to make an attempt to carry out his instructions. It's nice to know somebody is.

I have frequently reached over and taken the index card — a piece of paper on which may also be written such items as ½ gal. milk, lettuce, tunafish, dinner rolls, O.J. — and looked at the ask-the-doctor list. In order to improve such lists, I have prepared one that I have used in my lectures and course. Try my version on your next doctor visit.

THE ASK-THE-DOCTOR LIST

Before the visit (complete this part yourself)

1. Why am I going to the doctor? (the *main* reason)   _____
_____

2. Is there anything else that worries me about my health?
____ No
____ Yes (please list) _____

3. What do I expect the doctor to do for me today? (in 10 words or less)
_____

During the visit (complete with help of doctor)

1. What is the diagnosis? _____
2. Why did I get it and how can I prevent it next time? _____
_____

3. Are there any helpful patient education materials available for the condition? (describe)   _____
_____

4. Are there any medicines for me to take?
____ No
____ Yes (describe) _____

5. Are there any special instructions, concerns, or possible side effects I need to know about the medicine?
____ No
____ Yes (describe) _____

After the visit (complete with help of doctor)

1. Am I to return for another visit?
   ____ No
   ____ Yes (when) _____

2. What should I do at home?
   ____ Activity _____
   ____ Treatments _____
   ____ Precautions _____

3. Am I to phone in for lab reports?
   ____ No
   ____ Yes (when) _____

4. Should I report back to doctor by phone for any reason?
   ____ No
   ____ Yes (when) _____

But you can't even get that far without properly explaining your complaints, and she who hesitates may be lost. One mother of three came into her doctor's office apologetically. "I strained my leg gardening, and it's been bothering me for a couple of weeks. It's really nothing, but my husband insisted I have you look at it." Well, it's a good thing he did, because an hour later she was in the hospital receiving treatment for thrombophlebitis which conceivably could have threatened her life.

Absolute honesty is important in the patient–doctor relationship. Sometimes the patient's wish to please the doctor can interfere — like that of the diabetic girl who handed her physician her week's urine test chart, and then pulled it back in dismay saying, "Oh, no, that's next week's results. Here are this week's." Withholding information can make matters equally difficult, as it did with the single woman who talked vaguely about "female troubles" and "menstrual difficulties." The gynecologist, realizing finally that she'd even lied about where she lived, decided she must have had an affair and was embarrassed to discuss her fear of pregnancy. She enthusiastically agreed to his suggestion of a lab test, but when that proved negative still seemed unrelieved. The OBG man finally got her to admit to vaginal discharges that she feared might be VD. That test was positive for gonorrhea — which fortunately was still at an early enough stage for effective treatment and cure.

111

Mention little things that bother you even if they seem unrelated to your major complaint. It's often the last words a patient utters as he rises from his chair to leave — "It's probably not important, doctor, but ..." — that give the doctor his best clues. If during the examination, your physician fails to check what you're nervous about, mention that to him. Perhaps a phone call interruption caused him to forget. Or it simply slipped his mind. Either the doctor will explain why he hasn't done it, or he'll do it. Either way, you're ahead.

Doctor's exams vary in comprehensiveness. But if you're visiting a doctor who doesn't know you or your family well and his exam seems cursory, there may be cause for question. One young mother told us how she took her 3-year-old to see a orthopedist: "He examined her, said she had a hip deformity, but that she'd probably outgrow it. He put her in corrective shoes, and told me to bring her back in six months. Then he said the shoes weren't helping and put her in sneakers. It bothered me, so I took her to another doctor. He gave her a really thorough examination, and said there was absolutely nothing wrong with her. It was in his office that I realized what had bothered me about the first doctor. He hadn't even taken Corey's slacks off — just rolled them up past the knees and asked her to walk!"

After the examination, most doctors will volunteer what's wrong — or that nothing is. If not, ask. What's the problem? What caused it? How can you prevent its recurring? Is there any reading material he can recommend to help you understand it better? If the explanation is in words of too many medical syllables, don't just nod and go home to worry. A simple plea — "I don't understand a word you're saying" — can bring him back to earth. If it's only a word or two that escapes you, ask for a definition, and for the significance of the problem. Otherwise you could wind up like the man hospitalized for hypertension and placed on a salt-free diet, who, never having had the hazards of salt properly explained to him, got all he wanted by filching salt packets from the trays of other patients.

If the doctor prescribes a medication, be sure to ask how it's to be taken. One man, who hadn't asked, nearly carved an eternal niche for himself in the annals of medicine by taking an anal suppository by mouth. Fortunately, he complained to the doctor about the taste of "that terrible medicine." If you miss a dose, should you take a double one next time? If you're allergic to any medications, don't waffle about it with, "I think I'm allergic to penicillin, but I'm not sure." Be as specific as you can. A Medical Passport (see Chapter 9) will certainly help. If you're taking another medication prescribed by another doctor, don't wait to be asked — tell him about it. Medications, like people, sometimes are incompatible.

A good question to ask is, "Are there any other things besides this prescription that will help me get better?" Mrs. Martin took home only a cough medicine prescription for her bronchitis. That question might have prompted the doctor to suggest steam, heavy fluid intake, bed rest and something to help her sleep at night — all of which would have been far more important in helping her body heal itself than the cough medicine that only suppressed symptoms.

If the doctor recommends gargles or soaks and you're not quite sure of how to go about it, ask him — or his nurse — to give you a step-by-step rundown. Or, now that you have it, refer to the *Self-Help Medical Guide* in this book. If he recommends a course of action that just won't work for you, tell him so. Many a young mother has complained to friends, "Boy, that doctor sure lives on a mountaintop. He said I've got to stay in bed for three days. But he didn't say who'd feed and dress the kids and do the dishes and the laundry." In her physician's presence though, she just nodded agreement. So he never did get to suggest alternatives to help her get that essential bed rest. He might have been able to arrange for a visiting homemaker, or spoken to her husband about taking a few days off from work, or persuading grandma to come and stay.

Ask about restrictions on activity, or other precautions, and how long they're to be enforced. One timid patient was told by a specialist not to walk on his injured foot too much. He didn't — for a year, long after it had healed. Don't be shy about financial matters either. The prescription you hesitate to fill because it may be expensive isn't going to do you much good. Ask if it's a high-cost item, and if the answer is yes, ask if he can substitute something similar — maybe a quality generic — in a lower price range.

Questions, questions and still more questions. Before you leave the doctor's office, there are these: Should I call if my condition doesn't improve? When? Do I need to come back for a followup? If you've had lab tests, ask when to call for results. If they're negative, he may not feel his office needs to call you — while you're sitting there worrying about which dread disease you're incubating. If there's an unspoken fear in your head, ventilate it. We're not there just to cure what ails you, but to cure the fears that ail you as well.

There are three legs to the physician's treatment stool: (1) the prescription; (2) instructions; (3) followup. Properly given instructions save the doctor's time by 50% or 60%. I've done studies showing this, and the patient who's been properly instructed may need only one call, while the poorly instructed patient may make three or four. When the doctor complains that his phone rings and rings and rings, it's usually because he or his nurse have not been preparing the patients well enough to be on their own.

Whether what you've experienced is an office or a hospital procedure — or even if it's only that the children have had immunizations — you need to know what *sequelae*, or aftereffects, you should expect. If the doctor doesn't warn you, ask. One young wife underwent insufflation, in which gas is bubbled through the fallopian tubes in an effort to clear them so that pregnancy may take place. The procedure went smoothly. Her doctor had told her that one day in the hospital was all that was needed. Thus reassured, though feeling awful, she left for home. "My family almost had to carry me out," she recalls. "I was a wreck, and when I got home I could feel air bubbles throughout my body. I was terrified, afraid they were emboli and that one would go to my brain and kill me. I had no medication to ease the pain. My mother dialed the doctor's office every five minutes. Finally, his nurse tracked him down. He told me what was happening was perfectly normal, and I could expect it to go on for three days. I love that man. He gave me my two children. But he should have been more thoughtful. I would still go back to him, but he needs to learn something about communication." So did the patient. Now, she asks questions.

Leaving the doctor's office with a prescription shouldn't mean the end of contact until the next visit. If there are side effects, he'll want to know. People assume they must suffer to get well. And sometimes they do, but often medication can be changed. I want to know, "Is there any yellow sputum when you cough? Has your fever persisted?" These things give a doctor feedback, signal disease changes, tell him that it's time now for the patient to start having activity.

Even physicians, when they become patients, can forget the importance of followup. One, being treated for hypertension with a combination of drugs, later recalled his despair — two years of it — in *Medical Economics* magazine in an article reminding physicians to solicit feedback from patients. Finally, the doctor went to *his* doctor, saying: "I can't stand this treatment! My life is upside down. I've abdicated as a father and flunked out as a husband. I don't do surgery . . . I'm a vegetable. I eat, I sleep, I work, and that's all." He was suffering from personality changes, impotence, constant diarrhea, dizziness. And, he'd never told his doctor — who had just not realized the misery being inflicted on his doctor-patient by the prescribed treatment. With an adjusted course of treatment, his ordeal ended.

Not only should you inform your physician of side effects — which may, incidentally, give him pause before he inflicts your medication on another patient — but you ought to record them in your own health record or Medical Passport. Next time the drug is suggested, you'll be prepared with a quick and inexpensive no. The longer a drug is taken, the more likely you are to suffer side effects, and they — or any diminishing effectiveness — should be reported posthaste to your doctor. A dose adjustment or a change of Rx may be all that's necessary to straighten you out again. That's a lot better than doing what too many patients, troubled by side effects do — chuck the medication in the toilet.

If you get home from the doctor's and your sympathetic best friend vigorously shakes her head and says, "Oh, that's not what you've got at all!" or "That stuff he prescribed for you never works!", you've got to choose between friend and physician. If your faith wavers, you ought to go to someone else for a consultation — but that someone else shouldn't be your friend Daisy, unless she's picked up her M.D. recently.

There'll be times when it'll be your doctor himself who wants another opinion on what's ailing you, and he'll refer you to a specialist he trusts. It makes sense to report back to him after he's had time to go over the other doctor's report, because he's still your primary physician and the coordinator or captain of your care. If you're unhappy with the treatment you got at the consultant's, by all means let him know. Author-surgeon Bill Nolen tells of a radiologist he sent a woman to for a series of treatments. After one visit, she asked to be referred elsewhere. "He was rude, wouldn't answer any of my questions, and acted as if I were an imbecile," she stormed. Said Dr. Nolen, "This wasn't the first complaint I'd had about him. I just don't send my patients to him anymore."

I have no desire to practice in ancient Babylon, where Hammurabi's Code decreed that the surgeon who failed to save a nobleman's sight paid for his malpractice with a hand. That, it seems to me, was carrying the Activated Patient concept a bit too far. But doctors do need to be challenged, to be questioned, and patients must not be shrinking violets in matters that involve their children, their lives, their bodies. It's possible to be a pest in a friendly way. Become an Activated Patient — in which case your conversations with your doctor should sound something like this encounter between Dr. Bowman and a thoroughly rehabilitated Mrs. Meek.

DOCTOR: Here, Mrs. Meek, take these blue tablets as directed.

PATIENT: What are they for?

DOCTOR: To help relieve the spasms in your digestive tract that you feel as cramps.

PATIENT: When do I take them? And, for how long?

DOCTOR: Take them before meals — one tablet three times daily until I see you next month. If you become free of cramps, discontinue them. Take them, though, whenever you have symptoms.

PATIENT: Any side effects, or anything else I ought to know?

DOCTOR: If you get blurred vision or dry mouth, don't be alarmed. Just cut down the dose to one-half tablet before meals. You'll know within a few days if you're going to have unpleasant side effects.

PATIENT: Anything special about my diet? And, any printed material I can take home to look at?

DOCTOR: Before you go, stop at my nurse's desk. She'll give you some instruction sheets about your diet and some general advice.

PATIENT: Thanks, doctor. I'll go see Nurse Jenkins now.

NURSE: Here's an instruction sheet about the medication routine, Mrs. Meek, and a booklet about your condition. Please look them over now before you go, while I'm setting up your appointment for next month. I'll answer any questions you may have.

TEN MINUTES LATER

PATIENT: I've read the material now and I believe it's all clear. Thanks for your help.

13 HOW TO SPEAK YOUR DOCTOR'S LANGUAGE

PHYSICIANS ARE NO different than other professionals (lawyers, computer programmers, scientists, etc.) who use highly technical terms or a specialized jargon when they talk to each other. And there are certain virtues to such professional language.

Such language is, for one, compact. Instead of saying "surgical removal of the tonsils," the surgeon says simply "tonsillectomy." Instead of saying "Your husband has an inflammation of the lining of his stomach," he says "It's gastritis." The doctor's language is also medically precise: duodenal ulcer and gastric ulcer may both result in what you call a stomachache, but to the doctor the difference is very important. That is why such specific concise professional communication is used in medical journals, reports and clinical records.

Unfortunately, when a doctor unthinkingly lapses into professional jargon at the office, or wrongly assumes that the patient understands all his instructions, problems can result. Ear drops put into the nose do not help swimmer's ear — and they smell awful!

So here is a small but important chapter on medical lingo. Words that may slip unnoticed into a doctor's instructions or conversation with you until, hours later, you wonder whether he said "diuretic" or "dietetic."

I don't suggest that you go through and memorize all these terms just in case your doctor happens to use them, but a simple read-through should help to put you more at ease with medical terminology — and the person who uses it. It's a painless way to "Enrich Your Medical Word Power," as we've come to call that portion (patterned after the regular "Reader's Digest" feature) in our Course for the Activated Patient. It is popular because medical language is to many a mysterious language. Our students are thus given "keys" to the hitherto "secret recesses" of the medical world when they increase their knowledge of medical words.

This chapter is not meant to be a dictionary. If you want more word power than we are supplying here, you could consider purchasing a medical dictionary for your reference shelf. My favorite over the years has been *Dorland's Illustrated Medical Dictionary*, but there are many others on the market.

And now on to A.

Abrasion — When a child "skins his knee" it is an abrasion. This is a very common injury, as most parents know, and it is not dangerous when carefully cleaned and bandaged. The skin is scraped away and the surface oozes blood. (The Medieval Latin word *abrasio* means "scraped off.") The blood quickly coagulates — and becomes a scab, which drops off when the new skin is formed underneath.

Angiograms — These are special x-ray studies which allow a doctor to follow the route that injected radiopaque dyes take through the blood vessels of the heart enabling him to detect any narrowing of the passages and generally assess its condition. Except for the injection, the process is relatively painless. An angiogram can be done by your doctor in his office, if he has the proper equipment, but it is usually done at a clinic or hospital. Movies or photographs, that can be referred to later, are taken and become part of your medical file.

Aspiration — A doctor who removes fluid from your elbow (in bursitis) or chest cavity (after a chest injury) with a hollow needle and suction device is doing an *aspiration*. (The Latin word *aspiratio* means draw away or remove.) As an Activated Patient, you may be called upon in an emergency to aspirate blood or mucus from an unconscious victim's mouth in order to enable him to breathe easily.

Atrophy — If the calf muscle of the patient's lower leg, the "gastrocs," has shrunken in size while the leg was in a cast, it has undergone *atrophy*. Other parts of the body can also become atrophied naturally. Compare the large tonsils seen in 6-year-olds to the shriveled ones generally seen in adults.

Antibiotic sensitivity — This laboratory test is done to determine which antibiotic medications will inhibit the growth of bacteria found in a throat or wound. After mucous material is removed and smeared on a culture plate, tiny paper disks, each previously soaked in a different antibiotic solution are placed on the surface. When incubation is completed, in 24 or 48 hours, rings without bacterial growth will be found around the disks of certain antibiotics. This will mean that the germ is sensitive to that medication and is destroyed by it when given in sufficient doses.

Barium enema — An x-ray test of the colon and rectum is taken after radiopaque barium has been introduced, via the good old-fashioned enema bag, into the lower bowel. It is used to detect cancer and other diseases of the colon and rectum — or to determine that they are *not* present.

Biopsy — When the surgeon removes a section of a woman's breast tissue, often a "lump," for laboratory studies, he is performing a *biopsy*. If your doctor says, "I recommend we take a portion of that cyst on your skin for testing," he is recommending a biopsy. The biopsied material will be tested by a pathologist, an M.D. trained to analyze tissues, etc.

Carcinoma — This type of cancer originates on the skin or mucous membranes that line the organs and cavities of the body. One example is the *carcinoma* of the lip found in pipe smokers who have irritated that area by heavy smoking for many years.

Cartilage — The firm white elastic connective tissue that covers the surface of bones at a joint. When the sports page of your newspaper reports that a star athlete has knee trouble, it usually means that a twisting injury has torn the *cartilage* off the bone. Since cartilage does not have a blood supply, it cannot heal and surgical removal is often required.

Cauterize — When the doctor says, "Nurse, hand me the electric needle, I have to *cauterize* the wound to control the bleeding," he is practicing a modern version of one of medicine's oldest arts. "Cauterize" comes from the Greek word *kauter* meaning branding iron. In ancient times a red hot iron was applied to wounds to stop bleeding and infection.

CCU — The initials *CCU* stand for the Coronary Care Unit (or Cardiac Care Unit) at the hospital. Special equipment and staff there monitor and care for patients who have had recent heart attacks or heart disease. Computerized equipment makes it possible to check the heart constantly, and the staff can catch and correct trouble at an early stage. (The ICU — Intensive Care Unit — is similarly manned by highly trained personnel to provide care for seriously ill patients at critical periods.)

Chronic — This word comes from the Greek chronikos which refers to time. A woman who has a chronic illness, unfortunately has an illness that is constantly bothering her or keeps recurring over a long period of time. Examples may be chronic bronchitis, arthritis or sinusitis. An injury (acute health problem) such as a broken ankle or bad sprain can also lead to a chronic condition, weak ankle.

Congenital — When an illness or handicap is referred to as being congenital, it is a health problem that has been with the person since his or her birth. The word congenital comes from the Latin congenitus meaning born together. Some congenital defects, such as hairlip, cleft palate and leaking heart valve, can be surgically corrected shortly after birth.

Contusion — A type of bruise that comes from an injury in which the tissue below the skin is damaged and blood seeps into it but the skin is not broken. The girl who has a "black and blue mark" is sporting a contusion from her bicycle accident.

Curettage — A surgical procedure in which diseased or injured tissue is scraped out of body cavities such as the uterus, brain, etc. (See D & C.)

Cystoscopy — This procedure allows a doctor to inspect the lining of the urinary bladder for the presence of cysts and other problems through a viewing tube (scope) inserted through the urethra. The test is done if a patient has had repeated urinary tract infections or unexplained bleeding associated with urination.

D & C — A common gynecologic surgical procedure, dilatation and curettage, is frequently abbreviated D & C. It involves dilating or stretching the opening of the uterus with a series of blunt, round instruments called sounds and then scraping the inner, mucous surface of the uterus with a spoon-shaped device, the curette. The procedure, done in a hospital under anesthesia, is used as a diagnostic tool for possible cancer and other conditions, and for endometriosis, abnormal bleeding and incomplete spontaneous abortion.

Dialysis — When a man goes to a medical center for treatment with the artificial kidney, his blood undergoes a cleansing process called dialysis. This involves passing the blood through a porous membrane which separates and filters out crystalloid particles (left in the blood by the failing kidneys) from the serum. The Greek word *dialysis* means a separation.

Diathermy — "Take the football player down for a *diathermy* treatment," orders the doctor. This type of physical treatment involves heating body tissue by passing high frequency electric currents through the injured muscle. It usually shortens the healing time if properly applied by an experienced nurse, aide or physical therapist.

Differential count — A specialized count of white blood cells done with aid of microscope after the blood has been smeared on a slide and stained. The stain helps identify the various kinds of white cells such as monocytes, lymphocytes, basophils, eosinophils, and so on. Each kind has patterns and counts that give clues to identifying infections, leukemia and other blood disorders.

Diuretic — A medicine or substance that increases the output of urine. *Diuretic* medicines are used, for example, in the treatment of congestive heart failure, high blood pressure, premenstrual tension.

Dyslexia — The inability to "see" letters in the proper order, causing reading problems. The word *dyslexia* comes from the Greek *dys* meaning disorder and *lexis* meaning word. Although sometimes mistakingly dubbed "retarded," 90% of dyslexia-afflicted children have normal or superior intelligence. The difficulty may be emotional, educational, or physical, such as a brain defect or eye muscle imbalance.

Edema — When the doctor says "Your grandmother has *edema* of the ankles," he means the lower legs are puffy, swollen and waterlogged. Edema results from a disturbance in fluid balance. Serious types come most commonly from heart or kidney disease. Less serious types may result from allergies or premenstrual tension. A diuretic is often prescribed for some forms of edema.

EEG — An electroencephalograph (EEG) is an instrument that amplifies the minute electric currents made by the brain (received by metal electrodes attached to the scalp) and transcribes them onto a moving strip of paper. This record, the electroencephalogram, shows the various patterns or rhythms called "brain waves." When analyzed, these waves give information about sleep, disease and functions of the brain. Biofeedback exponents use a simplified type of EEG while attempting to regulate their alpha (relaxation) brain waves.

121

EKG (or ECG) — The electrocardiograph (the EKG abbreviation comes from the German spelling elektrokardiograf) is an instrument that amplifies the tiny electric charges made by the contracting heart muscle and records them on a strip of paper. The patterns are then interpreted by a physician or computer to diagnose heart disease, irregular rhythm, rate and so on.

Embolism — The doctors predicted that the President would have an embolism (obstruction of a major blood vessel) in the lungs if they didn't tie off the diseased vein in his leg. An embolism results if an embolus or clot breaks off and is swept along in the bloodstream until it lodges in a vessel and blocks the flow of blood beyond that point.

Emetic — The doctor instructed the mother to give the little girl syrup of ipecac. This emetic was ordered because it would induce vomiting and get rid of the overdose of aspirin she had been given by her 5-year-old sister when they played "hospital." An emetic is a medicinal substance that causes vomiting.

GI series — When an order goes to the x-ray department for a gastrointestinal (usually shortened to GI) series, the technician prepares a barium solution or "meal" for the patient. After the chalky fluid that looks but unfortunately does not taste like a milkshake has been drunk, x-ray films and fluoroscopic observations are made to look for evidence of stomach ulcers, hiatal hernia, cancer and other abnormalities of the upper digestive system.

Glaucoma — This eye disease is marked by increased pressure inside the eyeball which can cause blindness. The pressure disorder results from the failure of fluids to leave the eye properly while continuing to enter at the usual rate. It may begin with sudden and intense pain (acute form) or with no symptoms and slow loss of vision (chronic form). An instrument called a tonometer tests the internal pressure of the eye and can be used to detect glaucoma. It should be a part of regular eye exams.

Glucose tolerance test — This test is frequently used to detect early diabetes and other metabolic disorders. After fasting (no breakfast on the test day) since the previous day, a blood sugar level is taken as a baseline. Then, a measured amount of sugar is dissolved in water (or in a citrous flavored drink) and given to the subject. Blood sugar levels and urine tests are then taken at prescribed intervals for three to five hours. Patterns of blood sugar and urine sugar can indicate certain disorders. Suspected diabetes mellitus is the most common reason the test is ordered.

Hemorrhage — The act of bleeding briskly or the discharge of blood from a broken vessel. It can be an arterial break (bright red oxygen-filled blood) or venous bleeding (flow of dark blood). Hemorrhaging can be internal or external. A severe blow, accident or fall can cause internal bleeding with injury of the spleen or liver. It can also occur with diseases such as peptic ulcer.

Hysterectomy — The surgical removal of the uterus or womb. The method can be done through an abdominal incision, or through the vaginal opening, from below, without leaving a scar. The Greek word *hysterikos* means womb.

Laceration — A wound caused by tearing or cutting tissue. It usually refers to cuts of the skin and scalp, but is also found, for example, in the perineum of a woman after childbirth. Deep or long lacerations may need stitches.

Lavage — The medical procedure of washing out the stomach or a body cavity. It is most dramatically seen when an overdose of drugs (for example aspirin) endangers a patient and a tube is inserted to wash the medicine out of the stomach. The word originates from the French word *lav* meaning wash.

Lesion — A word used to indicate any injury, hurt or wound. Also, a localized abnormal structural change in the body. A lesion can be a problem as minor as a pimple or wart or as serious as a fracture or a bullet wound, so your doctor's use of this medical jargon alone shouldn't cause alarm.

Mastectomy — The surgical removal of all or part of the breast. The most common reason for the procedure is cancer, but it may also be done for chronic cystitis and other breast diseases. There are several kinds of mastectomy operations. The most complete is called the radical, followed in turn by the modified radical, the simple and "lumpectomy." The kind chosen depends on the kind of cancer, extent of growth, its location, the history (both family and personal) and other individual factors. Many women have gone through this emotionally traumatic ordeal. The organization Reach for Recovery, a program sponsored by the American Cancer Society and made up of women who have gone through mastectomies themselves, has helped in preparing women for the operation and hastening their acceptance of it and healing afterward.

Menarche — The beginning of menstrual periods in adolescent girls. The periods may be irregular in time and amount at first until the menstrual cycle is established. The word's two parts come from the Greek *men* for month and *arche* for beginning.

Metastasis — The spreading of cancer cells via blood and lymph channels from the original site to other parts of the body. Early cancer detection emphasizes catching the cancer before *metastasis* takes place. That is why thorough periodic physicals and monthly breast self-examination are important.

NPN — This is the abbreviation for the laboratory test, nonprotein nitrogen. It provides a test of kidney function that can be done on the blood. Elevated levels of NPN commonly indicate kidney disease.

Palpation — One of the methods used in physical examination to obtain information about a patient's condition by feeling a part of the body with the hand. For example, a doctor can usually tell by *palpation* if the thyroid gland is enlarged. The process is painless.

Pap test — The testing of the cervix and the uterus developed by Dr. Papanicolaou. Cell scrapings are obtained painlessly from the surface of the cervix, then are smeared on glass slides, fixed with a spray, stained and examined under a microscope. This cytologic diagnosis may indicate cancer or other disorders of the uterus or cervix. The process is painless, and early discovery of such problems and prompt treatment — even in the case of cancer — promise a high rate of cure.

Thrombosis — When the doctor tells a woman, "Your husband has had a coronary *thrombosis*" he means that a clot formed in one of the coronary arteries of his heart. Thrombosis may also form in other vessels of the body such as those supplying the leg or veins of the rectum (thrombosed hemorrhoid).

Tumor — A swollen gland or diseased part of the body that becomes protuberant. It can be benign (not cancerous) or malignant. Common tumors are those associated with infected oil glands or fatty skin deposits, called "fatty tumors" or lipomas. The treatment is frequently surgical removal which, in minor cases, may be done in an office or clinic and requires no hospitalization.

Uric acid — This chemical test is done on the blood as a screening and diagnostic test for gout. High levels indicate presence of gout and improper metabolism of uric acid.

VDRL — This is a screening test of the blood for syphilis. It is the abbreviation for Venereal Disease Research Laboratory. Most states require this test as a premarital examination. If the test is positive, additional followup tests are done to see if there is evidence of present or past syphilis. Some other infections and conditions will give a "false positive" VDRL and additional testing is at times required.

14 ARE YOU OLDER THAN YOUR BIRTH CERTIFICATE?

JUST BEFORE STUNTMAN Evel Knievel blasted off on his celebrated $6 million jet-propelled skycycle flight across the Snake River Canyon in the summer of 1974, a reporter challenged him. "If you're so tough," he said, "how come your cycle's equipped with parachutes?"

"Because, I'm tough," Knievel reportedly retorted, "not crazy!"

We can't take all the risks out of life. Sleeping Beauty's royal dad found that out when his daughter pricked her finger on the only spinning wheel in the whole kingdom he hadn't managed to destroy. But even a daredevil like Knievel, whose business is selling tickets to his own funeral, eliminates as many hazards as he can. You may prefer watching Knievel to imitating him, but you can learn at least one thing from him: You'll live longer if you cut your risks.

Of course, knowing about health hazards doesn't always stop people from avoiding them. If it did, this country's multi-billion dollar tobacco industry would have gone up in smoke the year the Surgeon-General issued the famous smoking-and-cancer report. And people wouldn't need red lights on dashboards to tell them to fasten their auto seat belts. They'd put them on as automatically as they put keys into ignitions.

That's why the new science of Health Hazard Appraisal, developed by Dr. Lewis C. Robbins and his associates at Methodist Hospital of Indiana in Indianapolis is so important for you to know about. It's gotten 20-year-olds to wear auto seat belts. It's persuaded 30-year-olds to cut down on their drinking, and 40-year-olds to get into exercise programs. It has convinced 50-year-olds to change the over-eating habits of a lifetime. Like the parachute on Evel Knievel's skycycle, it helps you to cut your risks.

Health Hazard Appraisal — let's just call it H.H.A. from here on — is a kind of scientific fortune-telling that opens a window to your future by telling you how old you *really* are, compared to how old your birth certificate says you are. It does this by superimposing your life-style, family history and medical examination data on insurance actuarial tables for your age, sex and race. If the facts are unpleasant, it tells you what to do to modify and vastly improve them. It makes you your own best doctor.

The initial shock of learning that your body is going downhill faster than you are can be unnerving. It was to Nancy Phillips as she sat opposite me in my office, calmly composed and waiting for my summing up after her check-up.

I scanned her health history and looked up. "According to this, Nancy," I said, "you're 39 years old."

She lost her self-assurance: "Oh, there must be some mistake. I'm only 34."

"There's no mistake," I said, "Your chronological age is 34. What I'm talking about is your real age, based on your life-style and body condition. Your body is aging faster than you are."

Nancy couldn't have been more upset if a fireman had walked in at that moment to say her house had just burned down. But when I explained that she could turn those numbers around — that if she followed the suggestions I was about to make she could be 30 again — she felt a whole lot better.

Medicine Man magic in a doctor's office? No, just H.H.A. in the process of transforming a woman's life-style into something akin to that of my next-door neighbor, Colonel Alfonse Kloss, an Austrian Army officer. The colonel has a clean, well-tuned Volvo which he adjusts on a weekly basis, and it runs perfectly. He is a dynamic man who keeps himself very fit — and as well-tuned, he says, as his Volvo. That's what prospective medicine is all about: anticipating system breakdown and preventing it from happening.

H.H.A. is a byproduct of the U.S. Census, whose vital statistics tell us how many people died at what ages of which injuries or diseases. Insurance actuaries were quick to see the value of that kind of data, and seized the Geller-Gesner tables,[1] with their breakdowns by age, sex and race to help them rate the theoretical life expectancies of persons their companies were about to insure. Dr. Robbins and his colleagues go one step further. They feed in information on body condition, family history and life-style, and then suggest risk-modifiers that can turn the bad news to good.

Nancy Phillips, for example, falls into the white female, 30 to 34 years slice of the population pie. (Black female would be somewhat different because, for example, blacks in urban areas are more at risk for hypertension and as potential victims of violent crime.) She is evaluated in terms of risk for the 19 leading ills and injuries that ac-

[1]An abbreviated simplified version appears at the end of Chapter 15.

count for the majority of deaths in her particular category. Motor vehicle accidents (119 chances in 100,000) is the No. 1 killer hazard for her in that 5-year period. The next four risks in order of probability are breast cancer (100 chances), suicide (94), vascular lesions such as stroke (73) and arteriosclerotic heart disease (62).

Since Nancy is a moderate-to-heavy social drinker, she's rated higher than average on the possibility of a motor vehicle accident. But — and here is where the health hazard modifiers come in — cutting back on alcohol reduces that hazard. Regular use of her seat belt cuts the risk factor number even lower. Since Nancy had a sister with breast cancer, her risk factor doubles there. Again, regular breast self-examination and annual mammography will cut that number way down. Depression has been a problem for her, and that increases suicide risk. Therapy will reduce it. She's been smoking too much — which has special significance because of a family history of pneumonia. She's been dimly aware of all these things. It's only when they're down in black and white in a Health Hazard Appraisal that she is motivated to do something about them. The real vs. chronological age helps to dramatize it for her.

The H.H.A. does something about so-called failures to quit smoking and drinking, which I look upon as failures of physician-patient communication — failure to outline the ramifications in terms that have real meaning to the individual. H.H.A. establishes a health partnership. It works in many cases because, as Dr. Robbins has said, quoting Spinoza: "The chief desire of man is to preserve his own being."

I've seen it work even with teenagers, who are often tougher to motivate than a frog in a jumping contest. Jeff was 18 years old and an obese 260 pounds. He was too clumsy to play football, not popular with the girls, but on the surface seemed to have adjusted well enough. People, including doctors, had worked on him fitfully for years, but nobody's message had gotten through that armor of adipose tissue.

He'd been urged and exhorted with generalities: fatness is bad, it's dangerous to your health, you're making your heart work too hard. As any minister, preaching to a two-thirds empty church about the necessity to attend services regularly, can tell you, exhortation is not exactly the most successful behavioral tool known to man. Jeff continued to put away milk by the bucketful and ice cream by the half-gallon.

I took a history, gave him the usual tests, and then, like an accountant evaluating an income tax form, making deductions and noting penalties, I drew up an H.H.A. Maybe what scared Jeff was the teen-age wisdom current at the time, "Never trust anyone over 30." In any case, when I showed him that he was not 18 years old, but 30, Jeff finally got the message. Last I heard before his father was transferred to Japan, Jeff had lost 50 pounds, his blood pressure and blood lipids were way down, and I could confidently assure him that, in all probability, he'd added years to his life.

H.H.A. creates the Teachable Moment. All the American Cancer Society brochures and warnings meant nothing to most women, who preferred to look away rather than under their bras at dire warnings of breast cancer. Then headlines announced the breast surgery of the wives of the President of the United States and the Vice-President-to-be, and suddenly long lines appeared at mammography centers. The Teachable Moment — and that's what Dr. Robbins and his colleagues have given us with H.H.A. — may prove to be the best idea in preventive medicine since the Salk vaccine.

Two recent issues of *Patient Care* magazine, a publication for the family physician, dedicated almost 100 pages to explaining H.H.A. and how it works. That will undoubtedly expand considerably the number of physicians in the U.S. — now about 1,000 — using it. It's catching on in family practice residency training, too, and when I taught H.H.A. to a group of my students at Georgetown recently, their reactions were enthusiastic. Dr. Robbins has wisely set up a network of cooperating physicians around the country, with staffs that handle the computations for a small fee. If your doctor is willing to run an H.H.A. on you, he can find out more about it from those Oct. 1 and Oct. 15, 1974 articles in *Patient Care,* or by contacting Lewis C. Robbins, M.D., Health Hazard Appraisal Director, Methodist Hospital of Indiana, Inc., 1604 N. Capitol Ave., Indianapolis, Ind. 46202.

If you'd like to try your own appraisal, you'd better be good at math, and pretty strong on general medical knowledge. Furthermore, you'll have to know your blood pressure, cholesterol, and a lot more. It is possible, though, and the manual that tells all, called *How to Practice Prospective Medicine* — really intended for physicians — is available for $7.50 from Dr. Robbins. Running H.H.A.s on the whole family might be an interesting project for a long winter's evening — assuming you've got all the medical data you need.

You'll need a much shorter evening — really only a matter of minutes — to run the modification of the appraisal that I've devised for you, in consultation with an actuary and chief medical officer of a national life insurance company. Using the same philosophical approach, it will tell you your "medical age" based on the factors in your life that you can and cannot control. It follows, accompanied by explanations of things that are likely to lengthen or shorten your life, and recommendations on how you can change them.

But let me warn you. Statistics are only extrapolations from known data, and there are always exceptions — like the 100-year-olds we occasionally read about in the newspapers who claim the secret of their longevity is strong cigars and stronger drink.

I've used a somewhat less polished version of the following score card on my students. I find an interesting and expected spectrum of life spans as we circle the classroom, asking people their results after they've finished the calculations. Mr. A. will live to 63 — his wife to 71. Mr. B. is black and his prognosis — he has hypertension — is a distressing 52. On one night, I got to Raymond Smith, but when I called his name, Ray was silent.

I asked again. Still no reply.

After repeated prodding, Ray spoke up. "I shouldn't really say anything," he said. "I'm already dead."

The class roared with laughter, but Ray didn't really think it was too funny. Ray comes from a family of diabetics. His parents died young. His brother died early. The age Ray arrived at was 43 — according to which, as he explained, he should have already been dead three years.

So, again, remember that there are exceptions to every statistic. Even more important to remember is this: the purpose of a Health Hazard Appraisal is not to part the curtains on your future and scare you to death. Rather, it's intended to part them and, as your own best doctor, allow you to effectively change your future by modifying your health hazards, and adding years to your life.

MEDICAL VS. CURRENT AGE SCORE CARD

This three-part score card has been developed to allow you to compare your current age with your medical age, and stimulate your thinking about self-help and preventive medicine. It is designed to emphasize preventive measures and is not appropriate for those under 25 years of age or persons known to have coronary heart disease, cancer, emphysema, cirrhosis of the liver or any similar established disease. Some of the scores are arbitrary. The results should not be considered a medical crystal ball. (There are people like motorcyclist Evel Knievel who defy statistics and should by the usual odds have been dead years ago.) You will, however, find the Score Card to be challenging and educational. And if for you it is upsetting, hopefully it will be upsetting enough to motivate you to change your life-styles for the better.

Rules

If uncertain, leave blank.

Place scores (given in parenthesis) on lines provided in the + or − columns.

Total the + and − columns and subtract the lower number from the higher to find the total (+ or −) for each section.

Follow the instructions for calculating your medical age at the end of the Score Card.

Part I. Personal History

	+	−
(a) Weight. "Ideal" weight at age 20 was ___. If current weight is more than 20 pounds over that, score (+6) for each 20 pounds. If same as age 20, or less gain than 10 pounds (−3)	___	___
(b) Blood pressure. *Under 40 yrs.*, if above 130/80 (+12); *over 40 yrs.*, if above 140/90 (+12)	___	___
(c) Cholesterol. *Under 40 yrs.*, if above 220 (+6); *over 40 yrs.*, if above 250 (+6)	___	___
(d) Heart murmur. Not an "innocent" type (+24)	___	___
(e) Heart murmur with history of rheumatic fever (+48)	___	___
(f) Pneumonia. If bacterial pneumonia more than three times in life (+6)	___	___
(g) Asthma (+6)	___	___
(h) Rectal polyps (+6)	___	___
(i) Diabetes. Adult onset type (+18)	___	___
(j) Depressions. Severe, frequent (+12)	___	___
(k) Regular[2] medical checkup. Complete (−12); partial (−6)	___	___
(l) Regular[2] dental checkup (−3)	___	___

Subtotals ___ ___

Part I Total (+ or −) ___ ___

[2]"Regular" refers to *well people* who have thorough medical exams at a minimum according to this age/frequency: 60 and up, every year; 50–60, every 2 years; 40–50, every 3 years; 30–40, every 5 years; 25–30, as required for jobs, insurance, military, college, etc. More frequent medical checkups are recommended by other authorities. Dental exams: twice yearly.

Part II. Life-style and Family or Social History

	+	−
(a) Life-style		
Disposition. Exceptionally good natured, easy going (−3); average (0); extremely tense and nervous most of time (+6)	___	___
Exercise. Physically active employment or sedentary job with well-planned exercise program (−12); sedentary with moderate regular exercise (0); sedentary work, no exercise program (+12)	___	___
Home environment. Unusually pleasant, better than average family life (−6); average (0); unusual tension, family strife common (+9)	___	___
Job satisfaction. Above average (−3); average (0); discontented (+6)	___	___
Exposure to air pollution. Substantial (+9)	___	___
Smoking habits. Nonsmoker (−6); occasional (0); moderate, regular smoking 20 cigarettes, 5 cigars or 5 pipefuls (+12); heavy smoking 40 or more cigarettes daily (+24); marijuana frequent (+24)	___	___
Alcohol habits. None or seldom (−6); moderate with less than 2 beers or 8 oz. wine or 2 oz. whiskey or hard liquor daily (+6); heavy, with more than above (+24)	___	___
Eating habits. Drink skim or low fat milk only (−3); eat much bulky food (−3); heavy meat (3 times a day) eater (+6); over 2 pats butter daily (+6); over 4 cups coffee/tea/cola daily (+6); usually add salt at table (+6)	___	___
Auto driving. Regularly less than 20,000 miles annually and always wear seat belt (−3); regularly less than 20,000 but belt not always worn (0); more than 20,000 (+12)	___	___
Drug habits. Use of street drugs (+36)	___	___
Subtotals	___	___
Part IIa Total (+ or −)	___	___

(b) Family social history

Father. If alive and over 68 yrs; for each 5 yrs. above 68 (−3); if alive and under 68 or dead after age 68 (0); if dead of medical causes (not accident) before 68 (+3)   —— ——

Mother. If alive and over 73 yrs., for each 5 yrs. above 73 (−3); if alive under 68 or dead after age 68 (0); if dead of medical causes (not accident) before 73 (+3)   —— ——

Marital status. If married (0); unmarried and over 40 (+6)   —— ——

Home location. Large city (+6); suburb (0); farm or small town (−3)   —— ——

Subtotals —— ——

Part IIb Total (+ or −) ══ ══

Part III. For Women Only

(a) Family history of breast cancer in mother or sisters (+6)   —— ——
(b) Examines breasts monthly (−6)   —— ——
(c) Yearly breast exam by physician (−6)   —— ——
(d) Pap smear yearly (−6)   —— ——

Subtotals —— ——

Part III Total (+ or −) ══ ══

Calculations

           +   −

Enter totals from Part I   —— ——
                     Part IIa   —— ——
                     Part IIb   —— ——
                     Part III   —— ——
                     Totals   ══ ══
                 Chart Total (+ or −)   ——

Enter current age here   ——

Divide chart total by 12, and enter + or − figure here   ——

Add or subtract above figure from your current age to find ... YOUR MEDICAL AGE ══

HEALTH HAZARDS EXPLAINED

Now that you have completed the Score Card, you may want to know more about some of the conditions and hazards. Why does your doctor get worried about them? Some of his medical concerns are reviewed here. If you have other questions, please direct them to him.

Part I. Personal History

Weight — Obesity is generally recognized as a major health hazard, both physical and emotional. The problem is one of *overload*. Each pound of fat requires about three-fifths of a mile of new blood vessels to support it, so the cardiovascular system is overworked. The skeletal system (including back, feet and legs) is adversely affected and breaks down more quickly than a person with normal weight over the years. The metabolic system is unable to keep up with the excess demands put on it and diabetes and thyroid, liver and digestive disorders result. All these overload problems then lead to early disease, early aging and shortened life span.

Blood pressure — Elevated blood pressure, from whatever cause, increases each pumping effort of the heart. This leads to heart enlargement and arterial damage. The damage of the arteries in the brain leads to strokes; in the eyes, loss of vision and in the kidneys, loss of function and failure.

Cholesterol — High cholesterol levels in the blood lead to increased deposits of fats and lipids in arteries. This fat plus calcium when they unite in the walls of these blood vessels causes hardening to occur just as water with lots of calcium clogs water pipes. Hardened blood vessels lose their normal elasticity and are more apt to develop thrombosis, hemorrhages and other vascular problems.

Heart murmur — A heart murmur occurs when the heart valve is defective in some way. The turbulence of the moving blood then makes the sound associated with the murmur. Common causes are rheumatic fever, hypertension, heart enlargement and birth defects. Sometimes "innocent" murmurs, having no serious implications, are present. The medical worry is related to the leakage and poor function that results in the pumping action of the heart when murmurs are present.

Pneumonia/Asthma — Persons who have had pneumonia more than three times or much coughing associated with asthma have a lot of

134

scarring in the sensitive lung tissues. They may also have allergies, inadequate drainage, poor resistance to bacteria in respiratory tree and so are likely to have a high incidence of infection with additional damage to the lungs, lessened oxygen use and poor health in general. No one should smoke and especially those with these kinds of respiratory diseases. The irritation of tobacco smoke complicates the limited reserves of the lungs and increases the chances of other complications such as bronchitis, emphysema, tuberculosis and cancer.

Rectal polyps — Polyps are toadstool-like tumors that grow out of the wall of the rectum and lower colon. Most are benign. In patients over 40, however, there is a tendency for some to undergo malignant changes and early detection and removal is advised. Polyps seldom cause symptoms, so patients don't know they are there until the doctor sees one while doing a proctoscopic exam.

Diabetes — This common disease has well-defined presenting symptoms of weight change, frequent urination, increased thirst and frequent infections. There is a familial trend for development of the disease. Early control of diabetes can prevent many of its serious complications on vision, heart and kidneys.

Depression — The classic and dramatic hazard associated with severe and frequent depressions is suicide. It can, however, also produce a variety of psychosomatic complaints such as fatigue, gastrointestinal disturbances, insomnia, headache and weight loss. These symptoms can mask physical complaints associated with more serious illness making early diagnosis of other illness difficult.

Part II. Life-style and Family or Social History

Life-style — The various components that make up your life-style are complex. Self-induced illnesses that result from use of tobacco, abuse of alcohol and drugs, overeating, insufficient exercise and injuries from a variety of accidents are well recognized as adversely affecting your health. Why some people learn these bad habits and practice them all of their lives and others discard them after a trial (or never try them at all) involves poorly understood behavior patterns. Modern research methods over the next decade that involve behavior modication, biofeedback, hypnosis and other psychological methods such as transcendental meditation (T.M.) will do a lot to unravel the mysteries and suggest ways of prevention and treatment.

Family social history — If you could choose your own ancestors and pick ones that lived into healthy, active old age, then you would probably live long too — if you avoided accidental death. If you added to this formula a happy marriage, with all its associated benefits, and a home in the country, away from the stress of the city, you would have fewer medical problems and exceed the insurance company's expectancy tables by a decade or more.

Part III. For Women Only

Family history of breast cancer in mother or sisters — Breast cancer is more common in some families than others, although the reasons are not clear. Therefore, if your mother or sister has had a breast malignancy, extra vigilance is suggested. Your doctor will suggest a program of detection.

Examines breasts monthly — Every adult female should maintain awareness of cancer of the breast. Self-examination each month, after the menstrual period, is important for you in order to learn the normal texture of your breasts so that abnormalities may be detected early. Breast cancer is curable if detected early.

Yearly breast exam by physician — Breast examination should be performed each time a Pap smear is done.

Pap smear yearly — The Pap test should be done every two years between the ages of 20 and 30 (or at the time of the refill of oral contraceptive prescription) and every year thereafter. Cancer of the cervix is found with greater frequency in females who have had multiple pregnancies and start having their babies at an early age. Cancer of the cervix is usually slow growing and can be cured if detected early by the Pap test.

15 THAT ANNUAL CHECKUP — NECESSITY OR NUISANCE

ONE OF THE first things I noticed when I set up practice as a Nebraska country doctor in 1954 was the extraordinary number of Golden Wedding Anniversary celebrations reported in the *York Daily News-Times*. One summer I counted 20. Then, when the 1960 census turned up 15 people in York, Seward and adjacent counties who were 100 years of age or older, I understood why Ponce de Leon had failed to find the Fountain of Youth in Florida. He should have been looking in Nebraska.

One of my senior partners, Dr. Bob Karrer, usually took care of the woman reputed to be our oldest patient. One day, on his afternoon off, I was asked to call at Mrs. Clark's home. Her back was acting up.

"Well now, Mrs. Clark," I asked, "just when did this backache of yours begin?"

"About the time we moved in off the farm. That was shortly after the war."

Well, I knew it wasn't the Korean War, and I doubted it was World War II, so I confidently continued, "Oh, then it was about 1919 when your back first started giving you trouble?"

"No," she smiled, "1897. It was after the Spanish-American War."

Startled, I asked, "Just how old are you, Mrs. Clark?"

Her eyes twinkled. "If you weren't a doctor, I wouldn't tell you. But if you promise not to breathe a word to anyone — I'm 106." She paused to let that number sink in. And it did — I was really impressed! Then she went on briskly, "Doctor, I've had this backache now for 60 years, and it's time I got to the bottom of it. I want you to give me a complete head-to-toe checkup!"

Mrs. Clark, who had probably never had an annual checkup in her life, and lived more than 100 hale and reasonably hearty years, had surrendered at last to such pleas as the American Cancer Society's, "Fight cancer with a check and a checkup."

It's surprising she held out so long. Medical writers and doctors warn you from glossy magazine pages that you wouldn't run your car for

50,000 miles without a tune-up. Your daily newspaper reports on the V.I.P. who's checked into the Mayo Clinic or Walter Reed. Government H.E.W. spokesmen extol the virtues of H.M.O.s, in part because they offer periodic health checks as part of their prepaid insurance package.

Ah, but what happens when, dutifully following this advice, you pick up your phone and call the doctor's office for an appointment?

"Yes, I'd like a complete physical."

"Oh, you only want a checkup," says the voice impatiently. "Well, the doctor is only seeing emergencies this week, but I can work you in at ten o'clock six weeks from tomorrow. Is that okay?"

(You had a feeling you might be wasting the doctor's time. The voice seems to confirm it.)

"Yes, that's fine. Any special instructions?" (You want the voice to say, "Yes, I'll send you an interval history questionnaire for completion. You should come in fasting for blood chemistries one hour ahead of time. Please bring in your first morning urine for the lab, etc., etc.")

"No, goodbye."

As you put down the phone, you're angry. You have dutifully responded to the plea from TV: "Have a checkup. It can save your life!" But the voice at the doctor's office coldly put you down.

What happened? Was this just a grouchy secretary? Is that all Dr. Bowdon really thinks of annual checkups? Am I wasting my money?

The problem is a complex one. The Medical Establishment is a bit schizophrenic about regular preventive checkups. Dr. Jekyll says, "Yes, I believe in the value of a thorough annual examination. I can give you many examples of troubles I have spotted early enough to help a lot." Dr. Hyde retorts, "It's a waste of time and money. Wait till there are early symptoms and then move in."

What causes this split personality? What do the experts say?

Dr. Harry S. Lipscomb, formerly with the Xerox Center for Health Care Research, Baylor College of Medicine, Houston, says, "The level of disease detection in well populations usually has been too low to justify the high costs of health screening systems."

Katherine R. Boucot, M.D. MPH and William Weiss, M.D. of Philadelphia's Pulmonary Neoplasm Research Project report, "Five-year survival rates in our study were so poor that one may assume that semi-annual (x-ray) screening contributes little toward solving the lung cancer problem."

Editors of Lancet had this to say about the Pap smear, the most highly touted screening test of all, "Cervical cytology is, perhaps more than any other screening method, bedevilled by the fact that those most at risk for cervical cancer are those least likely to come forward for testing (e.g., most of the invasive cancers occurring in older women over 60 years)."

Robert Ray McGee, an internist from Clarksdale, Miss., writing in *Medical Economics* said "where a patient has normal weight and blood pressure and no excess glucose in the urine, I doubt whether all the ECGs, chest x-rays and blood lipid studies you give him will detect something like asymptomatic coronary disease, for instance."

The founder of the Medical Passport Foundation, Dr. Claude Forkner said, in personal communication with me, that most of the current health screening methods are much less effective in finding trouble than a well-developed medical history, with a chance for followup questions, costing much less. He's saying a person gets more for his money from a thorough questionnaire plus 40 minutes followup questioning time with the doctor than from that same amount of time and possibly greater cost in lab tests.

Dr. Joseph Trautlein of the Milton S. Hershey Medical Center concurs with Dr. Forkner. In *Patient Care* he emphasized "Of all the components of this data base, the history is far and away the most cost-effective."

On the other side of the fence, we find regular health screening has its strong supporters.

A *Parade* article by my collaborator Howard Eisenberg and his wife Arlene pointed out that "stress test" electrocardiograms done with treadmills — the patient's heart is monitored by a cardiologist while he exercises vigorously — can reveal significant abnormalities in patients who have shown no symptoms at all on traditional prone ECGs. They quoted Dr. Samuel M. Fox III, past president of the American College of Cardiology as saying "the evidence is very strong that exercise stress testing is a powerful predictor of future coronary disease. Very well substantiated data indicate that coronary events are from 6 to 20 times more frequent in people with abnormal responses to stress testing."

A particularly dramatic example of that is cited by Dr. Albert A. Kattus, Chairman of the American Heart Association's Committee on Exercise. When 310 supposedly perfectly healthy insurance underwriters took stress tests, thirty were found to have ECG abnormalities. Less than three years later, ten of those thirty underwriters had already suffered coronaries. Not a single one of the 280 who passed their stress tests had yet had one. That's a pretty good reason for choosing a clinic that includes a stress ECG as part of your physical.

Dr. Morris Collen from Kaiser-Permanente in Oakland, Calif. has reported detailed studies of 5,000 men and women between the ages of

35 to 55 showing that regular preventive health exams produced lower rates of disability, less income lost and fewer days off for illness, when compared to groups that did not have regular checkups over a period of seven years. And the famous Strang Clinic in New York City — where the Pap test was born and where "Preventive Medicine Institute" is as much a part of the Clinic's name as it is of its philosophy — reports even more striking results. The Institute has examined a quarter-million adults since 1963. Its examinations are believed to have saved 1,000 lives and prevented disease in another 10,000.

The Kaiser and Strang results emphasize the key issues: regularity, systematic methods, five to seven-year followup plans at one center. It's no good to go to Mayo Clinic one year, Lahey the next, Scott-White the third. Clinic shopping does not pay off. What you need is regular screening to discover what is normal for you. It's a matter of establishing baseline data on your blood pressure, hematocrit, cholesterol, electrocardiogram and chest x-ray. Then, if something goes awry, it shows up.

But, remember, it may take three years of consecutive testing to get your baselines. Statisticians emphasize the importance of getting an average of at least three tests before you can establish your baseline level to compare it with.

Example: A chest x-ray deals with a very subtle little blip that could be called "within normal limits." But if you saw three consecutive annual x-rays showing nothing on the first, a little spot that could be nothing but an artifact on the second, and something more visible on the third, you'd know you were tracking something.

Where, then, should you stand in this crossfire — should you duck out, leave the scene and not worry about a checkup at all? Remember the disagreements are not *against* the checkup, it's just that the "state of the art" is primitive. Improvements are arriving on the scene at a rapid rate.

Well, the advice I give depends on your age and health. Here is a plan that will be disputed by some as too skimpy — but endorsed by others:

(1) If you are well, not on regular medication (this includes the Pill), have no specific complaints or symptoms and have established your baseline tests, follow this schedule:

50–60, every two years

40–50, every three years

30–40, every five years

Under 30, every five years (This group begins at pre-school level exams when childhood immunizations are reviewed and boosters given, and continues at established points such as camp physicals at 10, sports exams at 15 and college, military and job checks at 20 years. But those physicals shouldn't be the perfunctory kind of school exam where the doctor, in effect, pulls a chicken through the pot of water and calls it soup.)

(2) If you have known medical problems, examinations should be on at least a yearly basis, or more often as your doctor directs.

If you opt for a mini checkup, what is the minimum you can expect for a "once over?" If you prefer to spend more, what is a maximum? The VW version should include the following.

Sed rate — The erythrocyte sedimentation rate, if normal rules out infectious disease, most cancers, blood disorders, liver trouble and collagen diseases like arthritis and its cousins. It can also tell your doctor other things about your blood and serum.

CBC (complete blood count) and hematocrit — This provides information on infections, allergies and anemias.

Cholesterol and blood lipids — This tells whether you may be a candidate for changes in your dietary habits and might give insight into likelihood of early heart problems.

Urinalysis — When this test is negative it rules out diabetes, urinary tract infections and some other systemic diseases that affect the kidneys.

Height-weight measurement — A stable, normal weight is a fair indicator of good health. Sudden changes up or down need further evaluation.

Blood pressure determination — This test is an essential in all exams.

Pap test — All female patients require this regularly if not annually. It is especially important for those on the Pill and women in their 50's and 60's.

Medical history — A thorough questionnaire (it may be manual or automated) plus a followup series of questions by your doctor on "positive" points.

Physical exam — Last, but not least, the doctor's exam should be aimed at positive points in the history or laboratory tests and other areas that he finds medically significant.

If your wish is a Cadillac version, it can be obtained at some clinics in your locale or from your personal physician. However, some medical centers across the country have developed high quality comprehensive packages that may be of interest to you.

You may of course, want to jump in between the compact and the luxury model and try a good Pontiac. This can be arranged with the help of your doctor. You might be able to have him add certain tests based on your age, sex and race because these do have a most important role in your specific health hazards. (Check the following simplified — top ten — version of the Geller-Gesner tables put out by the Methodist Hospital of Indiana for cause-of-death probabilities for persons in your particular group.)

When your health has been measured, when the doctor has given you your report — then you have your job to do. Correcting trouble spotted, and preventing future problems, as your own best doctor all the time.

CAUSE OF DEATH PROBABILITY TABLE

Rank	Age	White male	White female	Black male	Black female
	5–9				
1		Motor vehicle accidents	Motor vehicle accidents	Motor vehicle accidents	Motor vehicle accidents
2		Accidental drowning	Leukemia	Accidental drowning	Fire-related accidents
3		Leukemia	Pneumonia	Homicide	Pneumonia
4		Firearm-related accidents	Cancerous brain tumors	Fire-related accidents	Accidental drowning
5		Machine-related accidents	Circulatory birth defects	Pneumonia	Cancerous brain tumor
6		Circulatory birth defects	Accidental drowning	Firearm-related accidents	Circulatory birth defects
7		Pneumonia	Fire-related accidents	Leukemia	Leukemia
8		Cancerous brain tumors	Cystic fibrosis	Circulatory birth defects	Homicide
9		Fire-related accidents	Strokes, blood vessel disorders	Anemia	Anemia
10		Strokes, blood vessel disorders	Congenital hydrocephalus	Machine-related accidents	Rheumatic heart disease
	10–14				
1		Motor vehicle accidents	Motor vehicle accidents	Motor vehicle accidents	Motor vehicle accidents
2		Accidental drowning	Pneumonia	Homicide	Homicide
3		Suicide	Leukemia	Accidental drowning	Pneumonia
4		Firearm-related accidents	Suicide	Firearm-related accidents	Accidental drowning
5		Machine-related accidents	Strokes, blood vessel disorders	Pneumonia	Fire-related accidents
6		Homicide	Homicide	Fire-related accidents	Strokes, blood vessel disorders

143

Rank	Age	White male	White female	Black male	Black female
7		Leukemia	Circulatory birth defects	Machine-related accidents	Leukemia
8		Pneumonia	Accidental drowning	Leukemia	Anemia
9		Accidental falls	Cancerous brain tumors	Suicide	Cancerous brain tumors
10		Circulatory birth defects	Fire-related accidents	Kidney disease	Kidney disease
	15–19				
1		Motor vehicle accidents	Motor vehicle accidents	Homicide	Homicide
2		Suicide	Suicide	Motor vehicle accidents	Motor vehicle accidents
3		Homicide	Homicide	Accidental drowning	Strokes, blood vessel disorders
4		Accidental drowning	Pneumonia	Firearm-related accidents	Pneumonia
5		Machine-related accidents	Leukemia	Suicide	Suicide
6		Firearm-related accidents	Strokes, blood vessel disorders	Pneumonia	Abortions with sepsis[1]
7		Leukemia	Hodgkins disease	Machine-related accidents	Kidney disease
8		Pneumonia	Complications of childbirth	Strokes, blood vessel disorders	Firearm-related accidents
9		Air and space accidents	Cancerous brain tumors	Fire-related accidents	Leukemia
10		Accidental falls	Accidental drowning	Kidney disease	Rheumatic heart disease
	20–24				
1		Motor vehicle accidents	Motor vehicle accidents	Homicide	Homicide
2		Suicide	Suicide	Motor vehicle accidents	Motor vehicle accidents
3		Homicide	Homicide	Suicide	Strokes, blood vessel disorders
4		Machine-related accidents	Strokes, blood vessel disorders	Accidental drowning	Pneumonia

[1]This hazard now less because of legalized abortion.

5	Accidental drowning	Pneumonia	Pneumonia	Cirrhosis
6	Air and space accidents	Leukemia	Cirrhosis	Suicide
7	Pneumonia	Hodgkins disease	Strokes, blood vessel disorders	Rheumatic heart disease
8	Strokes, blood vessel disorders	Complications of childbirth	Arteriosclerotic heart disease	Anemia
9	Leukemia	Diabetes mellitus	Firearm-related accidents	Diabetes mellitus
10	Hodgkins disease	Rheumatic heart disease	Machine-related accidents	Hypertensive heart disease
25–29				
1	Motor vehicle accidents	Motor vehicle accidents	Homicide	Homicide
2	Suicide	Suicide	Motor vehicle accidents	Motor vehicle accidents
3	Homicide	Breast cancer	Arteriosclerotic heart disease	Strokes, blood vessel disorders
4	Arteriosclerotic heart disease	Strokes, blood vessel disorders	Cirrhosis	Cirrhosis
5	Machine-related accidents	Homicide	Pneumonia	Arteriosclerotic heart disease
6	Air and space accidents	Arteriosclerotic heart disease	Strokes, blood vessel disorders	Pneumonia
7	Strokes, blood vessel disorders	Diabetes mellitus	Suicide	Rheumatic heart disease
8	Cirrhosis	Cervical cancer	Accidental drowning	Cervical cancer
9	Pneumonia	Cirrhosis	Machine-related accidents	Breast cancer
10	Accidental falls	Rheumatic heart disease	Alcoholism	Diabetes mellitus
30–34				
1	Motor vehicle accidents	Motor vehicle accidents	Homicide	Arteriosclerotic heart disease

Rank	Age	White male	White female	Black male	Black female
2		Arteriosclerotic heart disease	Breast cancer	Arteriosclerotic heart disease	Strokes, blood vessel disorders
3		Suicide	Suicide	Motor vehicle accidents	Homicide
4		Homicide	Strokes, blood vessel disorders	Cirrhosis	Cirrhosis
5		Cirrhosis	Arteriosclerotic heart disease	Strokes, blood vessel disorders	Pneumonia
6		Machine-related accidents	Cirrhosis	Pneumonia	Motor vehicle accidents
7		Strokes, blood vessel disorders	Cervical cancer	Hypertensive heart disease	Breast cancer
8		Lung cancer	Pneumonia	Alcoholism	Cervical cancer
9		Pneumonia	Rheumatic heart disease	Suicide	Hypertensive heart disease
10		Air and space accidents	Homicide	Machine-related accidents	Kidney disease
1	35–39	Arteriosclerotic heart disease	Breast cancer	Arteriosclerotic heart disease	Arteriosclerotic heart disease
2		Motor vehicle accidents	Arteriosclerotic heart disease	Homicide	Strokes, blood vessel disorders
3		Suicide	Motor vehicle accidents	Motor vehicle accidents	Cirrhosis
4		Cirrhosis	Strokes, blood vessel disorders	Strokes, blood vessel disorders	Homicide
5		Lung cancer	Suicide	Cirrhosis	Breast cancer
6		Strokes, blood vessel disorders	Cirrhosis	Pneumonia	Hypertensive heart disease
7		Homicide	Cervical cancer	Hypertensive heart disease	Pneumonia
8		Machine-related accidents	Ovarian cancer	Lung cancer	Cervical cancer

9	Pneumonia	Rheumatic heart disease	Alcoholism	Motor vehicle accidents
10	Rheumatic heart disease	Lung cancer	Tuberculosis	Kidney disease
40–44				
1	Arteriosclerotic heart disease	Arteriosclerotic heart disease	Arteriosclerotic heart disease	Arteriosclerotic heart disease
2	Motor vehicle accidents	Breast cancer	Homicide	Strokes, blood vessel disorders
3	Cirrhosis	Strokes, blood vessel disorders	Strokes, blood vessel disorders	Cirrhosis
4	Lung cancer	Cirrhosis	Cirrhosis	Breast cancer
5	Suicide	Motor vehicle accidents	Motor vehicle accidents	Hypertensive heart disease
6	Strokes, blood vessel disorders	Suicide	Lung cancer	Cervical cancer
7	Pneumonia	Ovarian cancer	Pneumonia	Pneumonia
8	Intestinal and rectal cancer	Lung cancer	Hypertensive heart disease	Homicide
9	Homicide	Intestinal and rectal cancer	Alcoholism	Motor vehicle accidents
10	Rheumatic heart disease	Cervical cancer	Tuberculosis	Kidney disease
45–49				
1	Arteriosclerotic heart disease	Arteriosclerotic heart disease	Arteriosclerotic heart disease	Arteriosclerotic heart disease
2	Lung cancer	Breast cancer	Strokes, blood vessel disorders	Strokes, blood vessel disorders
3	Cirrhosis	Strokes, blood vessel disorders	Lung cancer	Breast cancer
4	Strokes, blood vessel disorders	Cirrhosis	Homicide	Cirrhosis

Rank	Age	White male	White female	Black male	Black female
5		Motor vehicle accidents	Intestinal and rectal cancer	Cirrhosis	Hypertensive heart disease
6		Suicide	Lung cancer	Pneumonia	Cervical cancer
7		Pneumonia	Ovarian cancer	Motor vehicle accidents	Pneumonia
8		Intestinal and rectal cancer	Motor vehicle accidents	Hypertensive heart disease	Intestinal and rectal cancer
9		Rheumatic heart disease	Suicide	Alcoholism	Lung cancer
10		Bronchitis and emphysema	Rheumatic heart disease	Tuberculosis	Kidney disease
	50—54				
1		Arteriosclerotic heart disease	Arteriosclerotic heart disease	Arteriosclerotic heart disease	Arteriosclerotic heart disease
2		Lung cancer	Breast cancer	Strokes, blood vessel disorders	Strokes, blood vessel disorders
3		Strokes, blood vessel disorders	Strokes, blood vessel disorders	Lung cancer	Breast cancer
4		Cirrhosis	Intestinal and rectal cancer	Pneumonia	Hypertensive heart disease
5		Motor vehicle accidents	Cirrhosis	Cirrhosis	Cervical cancer
6		Suicide	Lung cancer	Homicide	Pneumonia
7		Bronchitis and emphysema	Rheumatic heart disease	Motor vehicle accidents	Cirrhosis
8		Intestinal and rectal cancer	Ovarian cancer	Hypertensive heart disease	Intestinal and rectal cancer
9		Pneumonia	Motor vehicle accidents	Stomach cancer	Lung cancer
10		Rheumatic heart disease	Pneumonia	Tuberculosis	Kidney disease
	55—59				
1		Arteriosclerotic heart disease	Arteriosclerotic heart disease	Arteriosclerotic heart disease	Arteriosclerotic heart disease

#				
2	Lung cancer	Strokes, blood vessel disorders	Strokes, blood vessel disorders	Strokes, blood vessel disorders
3	Strokes, blood vessel disorders	Breast cancer	Lung cancer	Breast cancer
4	Bronchitis and emphysema	Intestinal and rectal cancer	Pneumonia	Hypertensive heart disease
5	Cirrhosis	Lung cancer	Hypertensive heart disease	Pneumonia
6	Intestinal and rectal cancer	Cirrhosis	Cancer of the prostate	Intestinal and rectal cancer
7	Pneumonia	Rheumatic heart disease	Cirrhosis	Cervical cancer
8	Motor vehicle accidents	Ovarian cancer	Stomach cancer	Lung cancer
9	Suicide	Pneumonia	Intestinal and rectal cancer	Cancer of the uterus
10	Arterial disease	Motor vehicle accidents	Motor vehicle accidents	Cirrhosis
60–64				
1	Arteriosclerotic heart disease	Arteriosclerotic heart disease	Arteriosclerotic heart disease	Arteriosclerotic heart disease
2	Strokes, blood vessel disorders	Strokes, blood vessel disorders	Strokes, blood vessel disorders	Strokes, blood vessel disorders
3	Lung cancer	Breast cancer	Lung cancer	Hypertensive heart disease
4	Bronchitis and emphysema	Intestinal and rectal cancer	Pneumonia	Pneumonia
5	Intestinal and rectal cancer	Lung cancer	Cancer of the prostate	Intestinal and rectal cancer
6	Pneumonia	Pneumonia	Hypertensive heart disease	Breast cancer
7	Cirrhosis	Rheumatic heart disease	Intestinal and rectal cancer	Cervical cancer
8	Arterial disease	Ovarian cancer	Stomach cancer	Arterial disease
9	Motor vehicle accidents	Cirrhosis	Arterial disease	Cancer of the uterus
10	Suicide	Motor vehicle accidents	Bronchitis and emphysema	Lung cancer

Rank	Age	White male	White female	Black male	Black female
	65–69				
1		Arteriosclerotic heart disease	Arteriosclerotic heart disease	Arteriosclerotic heart disease	Arteriosclerotic heart disease
2		Strokes, blood vessel disorders	Strokes, blood vessel disorders	Strokes, blood vessel disorders	Strokes, blood vessel disorders
3		Lung cancer	Breast cancer	Lung cancer	Hypertensive heart disease
4		Bronchitis and emphysema	Intestinal and rectal cancer	Cancer of the prostate	Pneumonia
5		Pneumonia	Pneumonia	Pneumonia	Intestinal and rectal cancer
6		Intestinal and rectal cancer	Arterial disease	Hypertensive heart disease	Breast cancer
7		Arterial disease	Hypertensive heart disease	Intestinal and rectal cancer	Arterial disease
8		Cancer of the prostate	Lung cancer	Stomach cancer	Cervical cancer
9		Cirrhosis	Ovarian cancer	Arterial disease	Cancer of the uterus
10		Hypertensive heart disease	Rheumatic heart disease	Bronchitis and emphysema	Stomach cancer
	70–74				
1		Arteriosclerotic heart disease	Arteriosclerotic heart disease	Arteriosclerotic heart disease	Arteriosclerotic heart disease
2		Strokes, blood vessel disorders	Strokes, blood vessel disorders	Strokes, blood vessel disorders	Strokes, blood vessel disorders
3		Bronchitis and emphysema	Intestinal and rectal cancer	Cancer of the prostate	Hypertensive heart disease
4		Lung cancer	Pneumonia	Pneumonia	Pneumonia
5		Pneumonia	Breast cancer	Lung cancer	Arterial disease
6		Arterial disease	Arterial disease	Hypertensive heart disease	Intestinal and rectal cancer

7	Intestinal and rectal cancer	Hypertensive heart disease	Arterial disease	Breast cancer
8	Cancer of the prostate	Accidental falls	Intestinal and rectal cancer	Stomach cancer
9	Hypertensive heart disease	Stomach cancer	Stomach cancer	Cancer of the uterus
10	Diabetes mellitus	Ovarian cancer	Bronchitis and emphysema	Cervical cancer

16 WHAT'S YOUR PROBLEM?

HERE ARE MANY of the health problems and questions that have been raised and asked during Courses for the Activated Patient. When a two-hour session is held, the doctors, nurses and other health professionals who teach the course are asked to present a one-hour lecture on a topic and then use the second hour for demonstration, patient involvement and questions from the class. It is from sessions such as those and my years of experience at desk- and bedside that I have selected the problems for this chapter. They are presented according to age and type of person most likely to have the problem, so that you can more quickly locate answers to problems that most concern you.

BABIES AND CHILDREN

Q— My daughter was out playing in the yard last summer when a small insect flew into her ear. We eventually got it out with warm oil but it was a big mess. What should I do if it happens again?

A — As you know from looking at the swarm of flying things around a light at night, insects are attracted to light. Therefore, use this same instinct to remove the bug. If you are outdoors, aim the affected ear at the sun and then gently pull the ear backward to straighten the ear canal. Most of the time the insect will take the hint and fly out — unless it is so covered with ear wax that it can't move.

If the sun is not bright enough to attract the bug, go indoors and turn on a bright light and follow the same maneuver: Aim the ear toward the light and straighten the canal.

The thing to remember is do the maneuver *first* and *immediately*. Don't poke your finger in your ear or fuss with cotton-tip applicators. You then limit the chances the insect can fly out on his own. If these simple measures fail, call your doctor.

Q — What signs should I look for in my 12-month-old baby if he swallows a button, stone, coin or similar small object?

A — It is quite common for infants less than 15 months of age to swallow such things. Most of them pass through the gastrointestinal tract without getting stuck or causing any symptoms.

Experts recommend that the object should be followed frequently with x-ray films. If it continues to move down, there is no treatment needed.

If a foreign body is going to get stuck, it will be either at the level where the food pipe (esophagus) narrows behind the voice box (larynx), or where the small intestine narrows. Should it get caught at the first spot, symptoms of coughing, gagging, choking and breathing distress will occur *when the child eats*. The child may also vomit at these times.

If the object reaches and becomes lodged at the second spot, there is usually no pain for a day or two. Then pain and vomiting develop. Should a tear (perforation) result in the intestine wall, it may cause tenderness, rigidity, pain and nausea.

A few words of caution: Avoid abnormal diets or unusual amounts of liquids. Trying to cover the foreign body with rubbish does no good and may result in diarrhea. This in turn may lead to a perforation and require prompt surgical care!

Q — My neighbor's baby had the croup last week. What should I know about it so that I can get medical help if needed?

A — Croup is dangerous because it involves the opening into the lungs at the site of the larynx. If the larynx gets too swollen, it causes breathing distress and can even result in suffocation if not handled properly.

Breathing distress can be spotted by listening and looking. If you hear croupy sounds and cries and the child isn't better after using a cool mist vaporizer for an hour or two in a homemade tent, help is indicated. One serious sign of trouble is sucking in (retraction) between the baby's ribs while breathing in. This should trigger your call to the doctor.

Q — Just what is diaper rash, anyway? Give some treatment tips. My baby keeps getting it over and over.

A — Diaper rash is an ammonia burn. Ammonia is created by the breakdown of urea — a waste product in the urine — by bacteria on the skin in the diaper area.

Treatment is aimed at

(1) Limiting the amount of meat and protein in the diet. Meat is a prominent source of urea.

(2) Changing diapers frequently to keep the skin dry. This prevents the chemical, urea, from breaking down.

(3) Covering diaper area skin with protective layer of petroleum jelly when the skin looks red and irritated.

(4) Avoiding soap on the diaper area when the skin is red as this removes the natural protective oil in the skin.

Q — What is the best treatment for diarrhea in babies? One pediatrician I know says weak tea and ice chips only for 24 hours; another one gives mashed bananas or scraped apples. I'm confused.

A — Most diarrhea is self-limiting and probably of viral origin, although good studies to prove this are not available. The vast majority of infants have a mild form of diarrhea and are helped by these general rules:

First 24 hours: No solid foods. Give diluted formula (one part of evaporated milk to two parts of water and white corn syrup) *or* GI drink (salt, one-half level teaspoon; white corn syrup, 2 oz.; orange juice, 8 oz. and add water to make 1 qt.). *Warm* and give the solutions in large and *infrequent* feedings (six-6 oz. every five to six hours). (*Note:* It is important to emphasize that frequent small feedings may increase the fluid loss in diarrhea. If the baby normally eats every four hours, decrease the frequency to every five–six hours. Warm the formula and solutions. Cold feedings may cause more diarrhea.)

Second day: If diarrhea has subsided, continue liquids as above and add mashed ripe bananas or scraped apple to each feeding and gradually work back from schedule of feeding every five –six hours to normal three-four hours.

Third day and thereafter: As recovery progresses increase concentrations of formula and add solid foods as hunger and strength returns.

Progress: Give a report of progress each day to your physician during the entire illness for babies under six months of age.

Q — I have a son who is always getting hiccups. I've tried all the old remedies like blowing up a paper bag and holding the breath, but they don't do much good. Is there anything new?

A — Yes, there is a remedy that I tell my patients to try. If the maneuver is done *promptly*, the hiccups usually stop within a few minutes.

Here is the maneuver for a young child.

(1) Put the child on your lap face up.

(2) Instruct him to bend backward as far as possible. Hold onto his arms.

(3) Have the child hold his breath as long as possible while in this upside-down position.

(*Note:* An older child or adult can obtain the same effect by leaning back over the edge of a bed or couch while legs and hips are on the bed.)

I don't know why this remedy works, but since hiccups are caused by periodic spasms of the diaphragm between the chest and abdomen perhaps this maneuver "stretches" the diaphragm and stops the spasm as you might stop spasms in the calf of your leg by stretching the muscle.

Q — I'm confused about the booster shots my baby is supposed to have, what are the latest recommendations?

A — Despite all the success of the 1950s with polio and the 1960s regarding measles immunizations, today we find much apathy and confusion on the part of parents. Recent estimates indicate one in three preschool children aren't immunized. That means that more than five million children one to four years old are now unprotected against either polio, rubella (German measles), measles, whooping cough, diphtheria or tetanus.

These illnesses are not just harmless childhood diseases. All can cripple or kill — but all are preventable.

Your child needs the protection outlined as follows.

(1) Combination diphtheria-pertusis-tetanus (DPT) at two, four, six and eighteen months and a booster when he starts school.

(2) Polio (oral vaccine) at same intervals as DPT.

(3) Measles, mumps, rubella combination shot at one year.

(4) Tetanus-diphtheria booster in junior high.

(5) TB skin test at age one and in junior high when tetanus-diphtheria booster given.

A reminder table for immunizations can be obtained by writing American Academy of Pediatrics, Dept. P., Box 1034, Evanston, Ill. 60204.

(*Note:* If you don't have a family doctor to give the shots, call your local health department. It usually has supplies of free or low cost vaccine.)

Q — Why do most young babies spit-up?

A — Some spitting up occurs in most babies when the baby is feed too much. There is no room left in the stomach. The spitting is an overflow. As the baby gets older, the spitting disappears.

Q — My kids are always eating junk food. What can I do about it?

A — Children — and indeed Americans of all ages — are on such a sweetness binge that Harvard's Dr. Jean Mayer has urged Congress to ban TV ads aimed at shoving sugary foods down young throats. He said, "Many children's food advertisements are nothing short of a national disaster."

You should forbid all chewy, sugary food as snacks. If tots want something to chew, provide sugarless gum. Encourage your kids to eat fruit and drink juices when they come home from school. Apples, oranges and other fresh or dried fruits offer quick energy with much greater nutritional benefits. Also, don't overlook that childhood favorite peanut butter. On crackers or whole wheat bread it's a nourishing, satisfying snack.

Q — Danny, my 4-year-old, hates tongue blades so much he won't open his mouth when he goes to the doctor. If he has a sore throat, we really have a wrestling match at the office. Any advice?

A — Next time you take him for a throat exam ask him to open his mouth wide, stick out his tongue and "breathe like a dog when he's hot." This should elevate the palate enough so that the doctor can see your son's throat without using a tongue blade! Along the same lines, since you are learning to become an Activated Patient, is to get your child in on the act. Gather family members together for a throat examination session with each person, including Danny, taking a turn "panting" and examining other throats. It will be good training for all.

Q — My two-year-old girl is bigger than her brother was at that age. I'm worried about her getting too fat. How can I tell if she's too heavy?

A — Your doctor has charts to determine this. One popular growth chart, prepared by Ross Laboratories of Columbus, Ohio, is given to physicians as a professional service. (We are including one such growth chart in the Family Health Record section at the back of this book.) Ask the doctor to show you how to graph the height and weight and then see if your child is above the average. If she is overweight, there is good reason to be worried. Fat babies become fat adults and more and more experts believe that obesity can be spotted as early as 12 months of age.

At that age fat cells in the body are still being formed. With *overfeeding* as much as *30% extra fat cells* can be formed. Once these cells get formed, they are with the person all the rest of their days and a life-long problem of obesity results!

Chubby babies are no longer considered the picture of health they once were. "Lean and healthy" is a better goal for your baby.

Q — I'm spending hundreds of dollars a year on allergy injections. Can I give them at home?

A — With the cooperation of your doctor — maybe. For many years, I have taught patients to give shots at home with these constraints: (1) Patient is stabilized; (2) family lives close to my office (no more than 15 minutes away); (3) injections are given during my office hours so staff can be called if needed.

TEENS/YOUNG ADULTS

Q — My son wants to go out for football. Just how dangerous is it?

A — The National Federation of State High School Associations reports that 1974 was an all time low for high school football deaths, one per 200,000 participants (1.2 million players). However, there is a high rate of injuries with one out of five needing some sort of medical care and one out of 13 having a serious injury.

There are some other general observations: the most injury-prone position is the fullback, the quarterback is next; the taller the player, the more likely he will be injured. Most injuries occur in first three weeks of practice and could probably be prevented with more pre-conditioning and certified trainers for the teams.

Q — My nephew is saving money for some "wheels" to take him to work. He doesn't know whether to buy an older car or a new motorcycle. Which is safest?

A — Statistics here in Washington, D.C. in 1974 show that motorcycle deaths for young adults are going up while the car fatalities are going down. Seven were killed on motorcycles — and all were wearing crash helmets when killed. Elsewhere in the U.S. cycle deaths are nearly four times that by auto accidents. It is predicted that by 1980, bikes and motorcycles will outnumber autos, therefore programs on cycle safety are urgently needed!

Q — With all the sex education going on, how come all these teenaged girls are pregnant?

A — A report by the Planned Parenthood Federation of America said in 1973 that despite the supposed sophistication of today's teenager, less than one in ten used a contraceptive. The reasons listed were: limited access to contraceptives, fear of the chemistry of the Pill and general ignorance of methods available.

Q — My daughter is on the swim team and gets earaches from being in the water so much. Is there anything I can do to control "swimmer's ear"?

A — Yes, I can give you a tip that will help control this problem. Have her take a box of Kleenex to the pool and put it in her locker. Whenever she finishes the workout, have her take a tissue, twist each of four corners into a tip. Then, with her head tipped to that side, she should gently place the tissue tips into the left ear canal. Each of the four should be held in place for the count of 10. For the right ear, the drying procedure should be repeated with a second tissue. This routine will help get the ears dry and minimize the chances of swimmer's ear (otitis externa).

Q — My son won't go to school parties with girls in his grade because they are all too tall for him. He's 13. When will he start to grow?

A — Well, boys don't have to wait as long as they used to to catch up with the growth of girls. The National Center for Health Statistics says, after a study from 1966 to 1970, that boys now reach puberty 1½ years later than girls instead of a two-year lag.

The study showed that at the age of 12 years, the average boy is 60 in. tall and at 17 is 69 in. tall. The girls are 61 in. at 12 and 64 in. at 17. The boys averaged 67½ in. at 15. As for bulk, the 12-year-old boy weighs 95 pounds and at 17 tips in at 150; the girls are 103 and 127 at those ages.

So if your son says, "I'm too short" (or too fat or too skinny), these new growth statistics might help allay his concerns.

Q — My 16-year-old daughter insists on getting her ears pierced. Is there any danger?

A — A recent report from Seattle to the American Medical Association says that seven girls there contracted hepatitis after their jeweler pierced their ears at his store. He said he used "cold sterilization" by soaking the instrument in alcohol. The A.M.A. emphasized that alcohol won't kill the hepatitis virus and that autoclaving or 20-minute boiling is required. I would therefore recommend that piercing be done by a doctor or nurse familiar with sterilizing procedures.

Q — Just how common is smoking pot, anyway?

A — Let me answer with some good news and then the bad news. The good news is that the pot-smoking fad is losing momentum among American youths. A recent study reported in the "Archives of Psychiatry" of medical students two years ago showed a substantial decline between their use as freshmen and sophomores when compared to their use as upperclassmen.

The bad news is that in a recent HEW report there is still a lot of pot smoking (especially in high schools). The study showed marijuana does these things.

    (1) Adversely affected driving ability and thinking skills.

    (2) Interferes with body's ability to resist disease.

    (3) Alters hormone levels that could interfere with normal adolescent development.

Other bad news is that although pot smoking is on the decrease, teenage drinking is on the rise. Unfortunately, too many parents don't see the danger of teens "sneaking a little nip now and then" until they are confronted by a son or daughter in an alcoholic stupor, acting erratically, or picked up by the police because of drinking. Fortunately, there is an organization that has had great success in helping adults and now, youngsters, and that's A.A.

Q — Recently, there were newspaper reports of a teenager in Falls Church who killed another student with a handgun after he was kidded by some schoolmates. There is one "peculiar" 15-year-old boy who lives near us. My kids tease him. Should I worry about it?

A — Experts at the University of Michigan have recently described the typical teen-age murderer and believe they can be spotted before they kill. There are three types.

    (1) One type of potential murderer dehumanizes others as "gooks," "honkies" or "niggers" — the actual murdered

159

person is considered "inconsequential." A killing is likely to occur if this teenager's wants are frustrated.

(2) In the second type, the murderer slaughters others because they represent an unacceptable part of himself. When they describe a fantasy of destruction, sexual excitement is shown. In a word, they get their "kicks" from fantasies of violence.

(3) In the third variety, the teenager is able to kill with the permission of his peer group who, in his mind, approve the action. The fantasy justifies the killing as seen in "gang murder."

There are some common traits in all three kinds that include these: the "enemy" is not viewed as human; all had either a violent father and a helpless mother or a violent mother and an absent father; all had been subjected to violence and dehumanization in their own families; were show-offs (exhibitionists) and had a willingness to display their aggressive fantasies to listeners who seemed interested. Seldom do the violent acts "just happen." They have usually occurred many times in flghts of fantasy and in the final grim act, the teenage murderer "acts out" the fantasy.

Q — I have a daughter who at 17 is 30 pounds overweight. Any good advice?

A — Reports from many experts agree that you should not nag or ridicule obese teens. Weight loss for some is impossible and nagging may only bring anger and alienation from the parents. Seek professional guidance. It's a complex problem.

Q — Is there anything new I can say to my son to discourage his interest in smoking?

A — Nothing new, but you might try the same thing my high school football coach told me when I was a student in Ellendale, N. Dak.: "Bank the cost of a pack of cigarettes each day; compound it at 5¼% monthly and save $30,000 over the next 40 years!"

Q — My son the basketball player is always getting ingrown toenails on his big toe. What is the treatment and prevention?

A — The usual treatment, if it is severely ingrown, is to have the doctor cut a V-shaped wedge out of the nail away from the inflamed area of the toe. This allows the nail to grow centrally and relieves the pain along the edge while healing occurs.

If it is not bad enough for the surgical wedge, the doctor may recommend pieces of cotton tucked in along the edge of the nail to push away the overlapping skin from the nail.

Prevention is aimed at making sure your son's shoes, both sports and school are wide enough and that his sox are smooth, dry and properly fitted.

WOMEN

Q — Since all the publicity about Mrs. Ford and Mrs. Rockefeller, I've read so many articles that I'm confused. I have two questions for you: First, please repeat the self-exam steps and second, give me a list of the new breast checkup centers.

A — First, the self-exam:

(1) Lie down with the right hand under your head. Examine your right breast with your left hand. Push down gently with your fingers flat until you can feel the chest muscle underneath.

(2) In your mind's eye, divide the breast into four areas like a clock: 12:00; 3:00; 6:00 and 9:00. Starting at 12 (at the nipple), move your fingers clockwise from 12 to 3 and on around in a little circle. Then, move your hand up 2" and make another circle in the same way; then up another 2" etc. until entire breast is covered. (If you notice a lump at, for example, 4 o'clock, you have a point of reference for yourself and your doctor.) Repeat this procedure with your left breast and right hand.

Then, follow these rules:

- Do this examination each month after your menstrual period so that you can be familiar with your breasts in their normal state.
- After menopause, check breasts each month on the *first day* of a new month.
- See your doctor without delay if any unusual lumps or dimples are noted.

Now, the second part of your question. In early 1975, the American Cancer Society and the National Cancer Institute established 27 breast screening centers around the United States. By making an appointment, women over 35, without symptoms of

BREAST SELF-EXAMINATION

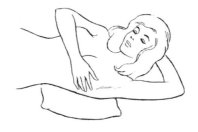

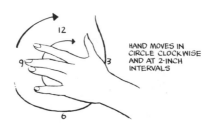

HAND MOVES IN
CIRCLE CLOCKWISE
AND AT 2-INCH
INTERVALS

breast disease, can have a free examination. It will include breast examination (palpation), x-ray (mammography) and heat graph (thermography).

The centers are listed below:

East

Rhode Island Hospital
Rhode Island Dept. of Health
Eddy St.
Providence, R.I. 02908
401-831-6970

Guttman Institute
200 Madison Ave.
New York, N.Y. 10016
212-689-9797

College of Medicine and
Dentistry of N.J.
15 S. 9th St.
Newark, N.J. 07107
201-484-9221

University of Pittsburgh
School of Medicine/
The Falk Clinic
3601 Fifth Ave.
Pittsburgh, Pa. 15213
412-624-3336

Temple University-Albert
Einstein Medical Center
York & Taber Rds.
Philadelphia, Pa. 19141
215-567-0559

Wilmington General Hospital
Chestnut & Broom Sts.
Wilmington, Del. 19899
302-428-4815

South

University of Louisville
School of Medicine
601 S. Floyd St.
Louisville, Ky. 40402
502-583-2894

St. Vincent's Medical Center
Barrs St. & St. Johns Ave.
Jacksonville, Fla. 32204
904-389-7751, ext. 8491 or 8492

Vanderbilt University
School of Medicine
Nashville, Tenn. 37322
615-322-2501

Duke University
Medical Center
3040 Erwin Rd.
Durham, N.C. 27705
919-286-7943 or
919-383-1060

Emory University & Georgia
Baptist Hospital
Atlanta, Ga. 30322
404-355-4940

Georgetown University
Medical School
3800 Reservoir Rd., N.W.
Washington, D.C. 20007
202-625-2183

Midwest

University of Kansas
Medical Center
Rainbow Blvd. at 39th St.
Kansas City, Kans. 66103
913-342-1338

Medical College
of Wisconsin
8700 W. Wisconsin Ave.
Milwaukee, Wis. 53236
414-257-5200

University of Cincinnati
Medical Center
Eden & Bethesda Aves.
Cincinnati, Ohio 45229
513-872-5331

University of Michigan
Medical Center
396 W. Washington St.
Ann Arbor, Mich. 48103
313-763-0056

Iowa Lutheran Hospital
University at Penn
Des Moines, Iowa 50316
515-283-5678

Cancer Research Center
Business Loop
70th & Garth Ave.
Columbia, Mo. 65201
314-442-7833

West

Oklahoma Medical
Research Foundation
800 N.E. 8th St.
Oklahoma City, Okla. 73190
405-235-8331, ext. 241

Samuel Merritt Hospital
Breast Screening Center
384 34th St.
Oakland, Calif. 94609
415-658-8525

163

Mountain States
Tumor Institute
215 Ave. B
Boise, Idaho 83702
208-345-3590

Virginia Mason
Medical Center
911 Seneca St.
Seattle, Wash. 98101
206-624-1144

Pacific Health Research
Institute, Inc.
Alexander Young Bldg.
Suite 545
Hotel & Bishop Sts.
Honolulu, Hawaii 96813
808-524-4337

University of Arizona
Arizona Medical Center
Tucson, Ariz. 85724
602-882-7401 or 7402

Los Angeles County-
University of Southern
California Medical Center
Los Angeles, Calif. 90033
213-226-5019

Good Samaritan Hospital
& Medical Center
1015 N.W. 22nd Ave.
Portland, Oreg. 97210
503-228-8331

St. Joseph's Hospital
1919 LaBranch
Houston, Tex. 77002
713-225-3131, ext. 301

Q — What are the things one can look for if you suspect depression in your family? I think my mother is depressed.

A — It is often difficult to spot a depression. It often "hides" itself in many ways. Some experts, however, have noted some observable signs that seem to give clues. Look for these things in your mother:
  (1) Weight changes
      (a) weight loss, loss of appetite
      (b) compulsive overeating
  (2) Changes in personality
      (a) gives up too easily
      (b) little facial expression
      (c) withdrawn, unable to interact with others
  (3) Cries excessively ("for no reason")
  (4) Careless about clothing, attire, home
  (5) Changes in sleeping habits
      (a) can't get to sleep at night
      (b) can't stay asleep, awakens early and can't get back to sleep
  (6) Chronic fatigue

Q — What's the danger of crash diets?

A — The danger of crash diets is usually not life threatening or that they won't work. In fact, most of them work. Experts agree 'that virtually every diet on the market today will help the dieter lose weight. Some will do much better than others. The danger is that nearly all are not nutritious. A past president of the American Nutrition Association, Dr. Morton Glenn, once said, "A crash diet, by definition, is an overwhelmingly quick way to lose weight . . . Giving someone a crash diet is the equivalent of telling your daughter, 'If you're late for an appointment, don't bother looking at the traffic lights.' "

A sensible diet plan is a goal of losing about two pounds a week. If the diet you are considering promises more than that it is a crash diet.

Q — I've heard that there are now do-it-yourself Pap smear kits. Do you teach that in your courses?

A — No, we don't teach that. However, I am aware of the large scale use of Pap smear kits by patients in Brazil. In the city of Santos, 40,000 women did their own cervical smear at home with a method called Gynecocyte Auto-Test. It was done under the direction of Dr. V. R. Cabral.

A report by Dr. Cabral at a recent International Congress of Cytology said that they got 96% acceptance among women approached at a cost 70% cheaper than with conventional Pap screening methods.

Q — I can't tell by reading the package stuffer from the Food and Drug Administration that my doctor gave me who shouldn't take "the Pill." Please advise.

A — Women having any of the following *must not* take the Pill:
(1) Cancer of the breast or uterus
(2) Pregnancy
(3) Active liver disease
(4) Elevated blood fats (hyperlipidemia)
(5) Coronary artery disease
Also, it is *not recommended* if a woman has any of the health problems below:
(1) Depression
(2) Migraine headaches
(3) Fibroid tumors of uterus

(4) High blood pressure (hypertension)
(5) Epilepsy
(6) Irregular or very light menses

Q — Why is it bad for pregnant women to smoke?
A — There are now two specific bad effects reported:
(1) For years it has been known that infants born to mothers who smoke tend to be smaller in size. For some reason these babies apparently get less nutrition from their mothers.
(2) Now additional studies show that each year about 4,600 babies are stillborn to women who smoke.
These same studies do show, however, that if the mothers stop smoking by the fourth month of pregnancy, the risk to the baby seems to disappear. Apparently the danger to the baby is not the result of the mother's long-term smoking habits, but specific toxic effects on the infant while she is carrying it.

Q — Why does the doctor make me drink lots of cranberry juice whenever I get a flare-up of my kidney infection? I don't like it in the first place and he asks me to drink 16 oz. a day.
A — If the urine is acidified, the bacteria that cause infections are discouraged from growing. If you have recurrent urinary tract infections, an alternative to cranberry juice that is recommended by some experts is vitamin C (ascorbic acid) 500 mg 4 times daily. It's simple, effective and less expensive than cranberry juice. Talk to your doctor about how long you should take the vitamin C and your individual situation, however.

MEN

Q — I have to stay away from coffee because it makes me jittery but can drink tea. Why?
A — It's a matter of the dosage of caffeine in it. The average amount of caffeine in a cup of coffee is 83 mg while there is only 42 mg per cup of tea. A 12-oz. can of cola drink, including the "diet" brands has 52 mg.

Q — My son and I have a small sheet metal shop and I wonder if there is something in the air at the shop that is affecting me. Whenever I get a cold, it just won't quit. I used to get over it in about a week and now one hangs on for a month or more. What should I do?

A — We know that the environment plays a big role in the normal defenses of the nose, throat and lungs. Industrial dusts, pollutants and cigarette smoking are known to lower the resistance of workers. The normal respiratory tracts cleaning methods are altered and the foreign particles, if they aren't removed, lead to infections, drying of the mucous membranes and other troubles. I would make a careful check of your shop and make sure the air conditioners, filters and so on are cleaned regularly. I'd wear a mask when you work with dust and put up "No Smoking" signs at the shop. If this doesn't help, see your doctor.

Q — It's easy for you doctors to say "cut down on cholesterol" but hard for us patients to do it. How about some easy tips.

A — The easiest tip I can give you is to become more and more like a vegetarian. Now by this I don't advocate giving up meat and dairy products completely, but rather a 20% to 30% shift away from them toward the low-cholesterol vegetables, fruits, breads, cereals and fish. As a baseline starter, the next time you go to the supermarket, keep track of the total food bill for things from the dairy products and meat departments (include milk, cheese, eggs, meat, butter, margarine, etc.) and the total from the produce department (plus items such as cereals, breads, bakery products, flour, nuts, beans, rice, macaroni, spaghetti, etc.). Compare the tape totals. (Please exclude all the *household extras* for this one-time study.) Calculate what percentage of the food budget goes to each sector, then plan a Family Food Policy that will allow an increased percentage of the budget toward the vegetarian side. Check the totals once a month and note changes.

Another easy tip, which might make the first tip even easier, is getting your hands on a recent publication, *The Whole Family Low Cholesterol Cookbook* by Helen Page, who runs a cooking school, and John Speer Schroeder, a cardiologist at Stanford University School of Medicine. The book includes over 400 recipes marked with a signpost guide that makes day-to-day low-cholesterol eating as easy as Pineapple Cheese Pie (one of the tasty recipes in the book). Also, you can write for the *New Metropolitan Cook Book,* Metropolitan Life Insurance Co., One Madison Ave., New York, N.Y. 10010, or ask the American Heart Association, 44 East 23rd St., New York, N.Y. 10010 for their low-cholesterol diet booklets.

Q — My brother just had a bad heart attack and his doctor talked to him about coronary risk factors. What are they? Should I worry?

A — There are seven principal factors that were established in the famous epidemiology studies done over a period of 16 years at Framingham, Mass. These are: age, sex, cholesterol level, cigarette smoking, hypertension, abnormal electrocardiogram, diabetes.

As to whether you should worry or not about how these affect you, there are some risks you can't affect, but some you can control. The three that can be controlled by you are cholesterol, blood pressure and cigarette smoking. When you add to this eating less salt and getting more exercise, your life style can greatly affect your risks of coronary artery disease.

Q — Shakespeare said a long time ago that alcohol increases the desire and decreases the ability. Anything new there?

A — Yes, Dr. Jack Mendelson, a Harvard psychiatrist and alcoholism expert, has recently shown that during heavy alcohol intake, there is a very significant fall in levels of male hormone (testosterone). He feels it is directly related to poor sexual performance.

Q — Is there anything new for jock itch? I've had it for so long and treated it with so many medicines that I've lost track. It still comes back every summer!

A — Your story is a familiar one. When you have had as much trouble as you tell me, I would insist on careful laboratory tests that would include a trip to a skin specialist who would do microscopic exam of skin scrapings, Wood's light examination and perhaps cultures. Cure is sure if the diagnosis is accurate — but it may require medication for a long term even when you have none of the bothersome symptoms. Also, keep in mind that if humid hot weather causes flare-ups, avoid tight pants and shorts that might cause sweating and use care in keeping the skin dry. Too, if you have athlete's foot, there may be some spread from the feet to your crotch, so treat it at the same time.

Q — I've heard that there is a male contraceptive pill now. Is it safe?

A — The "pill" you speak of is still being tested on animals. Dr. Charles Terner of Boston University says that results with rats have been encouraging. The results show prevention of sperm without impaired sexual drive. He uses a combination of male and female hormones.

Q — I hear a lot about the dangers of stress and heart attack, stomach ulcers and so on but the only person who doesn't have stress is the one who sits under a tree all day and doesn't do anything to or for anyone. What is one to do?

A — The best advice comes from the world's greatest expert, Dr. Hans Selye of Canada. In his book *Stress Without Distress* he says, "Stress is the response to any demand made upon the body. Distress is damaging or unpleasant stress. One can react to stress by running away, fighting it — or using the alternative of peaceful coexistence." So before getting into a fight ask yourself, "Is it worth fighting for?"

Q — Is there any simple method to help me stop smoking?

A — Well, a lot of new methods seem to be helpful if you really have decided to kick the habit. Two I've studied recently are those put out by the American Cancer Society: "I.Q. (I Quit) Club" and the one by Boehringer Ingelheim (a drug company) "37 Ways to Stop Wasting Your Breath." It was developed by the Max Planck Institute in Germany. If you want more details, contact your local Cancer Society or have your doctor write Boehringer at Elmsford, N.Y. 10523.

Q — I do a lot of camping and hiking and frequently have wood ticks digging into me. What's the best way to get them out?

A — A tick fastens itself to you not only with its teeth but reinforces the attachment by a cement-like secretion. It can voluntarily detach itself quickly but forcible removal usually leaves the mouth parts imbedded in your hide. The tick is a small crab-like creature that needs air to survive. Therefore, one of the best ways to get him to detach "voluntarily" is to coat him and the nearby skin with fingernail polish. Because this seals off the air, the tick will usually try to back out of the hole it has "dug" and can then be removed with tweezers or fingers.

17 TOWARD A HEALTH PARTNERSHIP

IN THE 1960s, Bob Dylan wrote words and music for a ballad that quickly became a classic American folk song because, though originally written to protest the Vietnam war, it spoke a timeless message — of change, "blowin' in the wind."

Today, similar winds are blowing in the field of health — winds of change that I confidently predict will waft you and your family toward a health partnership with your doctor.

I wouldn't have been quite as confident about that back in 1936, when I was a 10-year-old getting my medical care in Ellendale, North Dakota from Roy Lynde, M.D., in an office over his brother's Chrysler-Plymouth agency. In those days, medical knowledge was the exclusive province and property of the physician. I remember my mother's stern reprimand one day as we waited for Doc Lynde to return from a house call, when I sneaked a peek at his *Journal of the American Medical Association.*

Talk about change. Now the doctor who presents a paper at a medical convention may be on the *Today* show the next morning explaining his views or his "breakthrough" to millions of patients simultaneously. Little news about health is now "for doctors only." We doctors may not always like it. One physician, complaining about the new news-aware patient, wryly suggested that the best strategy was to hold off returning phone calls to such patients. "Most likely another 'startling fact' will appear in the newspaper tomorrow to refute the 'startling fact' that the patient read today."

It is a bit embarrassing to walk into your office and have to admit to a patient that you haven't heard of this drug or that treatment — often experimental, inconclusive, or sensationalized in the media. But there's not much we can do about it. And there's no denying the fact that the patient's stake — his or her own health — is much greater than our own. In many ways, the patient already is the doctor's partner. I say, let's make it official.

I guess it was Ralph Nader who started it all. He took on the auto industry first, then chemicals, and pharmaceuticals and plastics. It was inevitable that gusts from his winds of consumerism would eventually sweep into that area of so much concern to us all — health care.

Herbert S. Denenberg, the former Pennsylvania insurance commissioner, followed Nader's lead with his series of bluntly informative
pamphlets, like his "Shoppers' Guide to Hospitals" and "Shoppers'
Guide to Surgery" (14 rules on how to avoid unnecessary surgery). The
peppery plainspoken ex-college professor was frequently pictured
under a large scholarly plaque in his office which read, "Populus
imamdudum defutatus est." If your Latin is as weak as mine, you'll
have to accept the commissioner's liberal translation: "The consumer
has been screwed long enough."

Health care's most persistent gadfly though is himself a physician.
His name comes up often in Washington. Anxious officials of the Food
and Drug Administration, A.M.A. staffers, and representatives of the
Pharmaceutical Manufacturers' Association have been known to
remark aloud to one another, "Hmm, I wonder what Sidney Wolfe is up
to now."

Why are they all afraid of Big Bad Doctor Wolfe? Because, as director
of the Nader-based Health Research Group, he's into everything in
health care. Everything from the economic problem of too many beds in
our hospitals to the medical problem of too much x-ray radiation in our
lives. When he breaks new ground, physician resistance is often
immediate — as when his group put together the now famous "A
Consumer's Directory of Prince George's County Doctors." But the
medical establishment often about-faces and joins him, however reluctantly. The A.M.A. did when they announced recently that it is "not
unethical" to cooperate with consumer groups in publishing doctor
directories.

The "flower children" of the late 1960s, too, left a number of sandal-
prints in our society, many of them self-help health and consumer-
oriented. Initially staffed by interns and medical residents — most, of
course, under 30, because what flower child would trust a doctor over
30? — their Free Clinic movement reached its apex in 1970. Although
anti-Establishment in philosophy, most of the clinics depended heavily
on the Establishment for medical supplies and financial support. It was
pretty hard for the regional manager of ABC Pharmaceutical Co. to turn
down a chance to be photographed in front of the M-Street Free Clinic
as he handed the amply bearded doctors a month's supply of free
penicillin. Not only did he get his picture in the *Village Voice*
newspaper, but it went over well at the National Retail Druggists'
Association meetings, and back at the home office in Chicago.

But the shabby "Free Clinic" store fronts did more than dispense
penicillin. They went out of their way to educate the street people
about health. Mainly, the education concentrated on the big issues of

the 1960s — drug abuse, contraception, VD, mental illness, yoga, natural foods, megavitamins — but it included the basics of exercise, nutrition, maternal health and the like, too. At their peak, there were several hundred Free Clinics flourishing or struggling across the country. Washington, D.C. alone had about ten. But as this book goes to press in 1975, I'm hard-pressed to find a couple here still in operation. The counterculture may be dead, but it has left its mark on the medical establishment — a whole new interest in patient education.

Probably the best-known published product of the Free Clinic movement is the book *Our Bodies Ourselves*, put out by the Boston Women's Health Book Collective with a distribution assist from a large New York publisher. Along with generous servings of women's lib philosophy, the book offers a wide range of valuable information ranging from self-defense to breast self-examination. Out of the Headlands Clinic in Northern California came *The Well Body Book* by Samuels and Bennett, another important contribution to the emerging science of self-help medicine, and this one — again a clue that something important is happening — picked up for distribution by another major publisher.

With the positive contributions to self-help medicine, however, one must also report the negative. And that's unfortunately the only way I can describe the mother-daughter team of colorful women's activists recently touring the United States and lecturing on self-help gynecology. The daring duo tell their women's club audiences how to do Pap smears and show slides of the cervix. So far so good. But they also describe do-it-yourself extraction methods for self-abortion and recommend large doses of Vitamin C to abort the embryo in the first month of pregnancy — the former potentially dangerous, the latter distinctly dubious. They claim that pregnancy can be detected three to five days after conception because the cervix turns a distinctive bluish color. Personally, I wouldn't feel secure about color change clues until at least six weeks of pregnancy, and I don't know any OBG men or women who'd want to stake their hard-earned reputations on so uncertain a piece of clinical evidence.

At the "climax" of their lecture, both mother and daughter lower their pantyhose, get up on a doctor's examination table and invite the entire audience to pass by and examine their exposed cervixes! The Cervical Circus, as some reporters have called it, may make good copy, but it's doubtful patient education.

There is plenty of good patient education around though — more of it with every passing day. I've personally been involved in setting up a program for the National 4-H Foundation that is aimed at more than 7 million rural Americans. And at the Center for Continuing Health Education recently set up at Georgetown University with the help of an H.E.W. grant, I'm getting reports in as director from all over the country on promising patient ed programs.

In North Carolina, Dr. John Nowlin of Duke University has created a 12-session course called "Sickness Demystified" that includes practical self-evaluation and self-treatment methods for common ailments, such as skin rash, minor joint sprains and sore throats. Dr. Roland J. Weisser, Jr. of West Virginia University's School of Medicine dispatched a questionnaire to family practice patients, and developed a self-help course to fit their interests in first aid, reducing cost of medical care, early cancer warnings and much more.

The only way you can join Santa Rosa, California's 2,500-member Common Health Club is by participating in a mandatory introductory session on preventive medicine and undergoing multiphase testing that is intended to be even more educational than it is diagnostic. After results are in, an appraisal session is held, and periodic health education classes are an important part of club activities. They must be doing something right. Membership's been growing at the rate of 150 members a month.

And so it goes — with reports coming in from Boise Idaho (where TV is a component and where such clues as pharmacists noting the rising sales of syrup of ipecac indicate people are learning and doing); the New Jersey College of Medicine and Dentistry (parceling out more than $400,000 in grants to community hospitals to establish consumer health education classes and medical screening programs); Denver Clinic (where an RN health educator supervises a newly opened patient education center with three learning carrels for audiovisual equipment); and the Yarmouth Project in Maine, where multimedia methods were so successful with fifth graders that the program has been widened to include six more Maine school systems.

It's all part of a slow but steady movement toward what I visualize as a Health Partnership that will begin in grade school with students taking courses from texts that might be called *The Share-Care Course for Good Health*. Share-Care and self-help medicine will be taught by doctors, nurses and health educators to show individuals how they can become more responsible for their own health care. New programs of education will center on self-interest. School children will keep their own medical records and, when they're given immunizations or weighed and measured, they'll enter the information themselves — as children are already doing in a pilot program I've been able to start at two schools in Washington, D.C. Share-Care will emphasize that health information is shared by patient and doctor or nurse.

Students will be taught that symptoms are really the body talking to them in a special language — a kind of Body English they can learn much as they learn French or Spanish. They'll learn practical self-help medicine for their common ills and injuries. They'll learn how to use their doctor and hospital as a community resource, and when it's appropriate to use these professional services. They'll learn why this resource must be conserved.

As the elementary student progresses into high school, his knowledge of self-help medicine will be increased in depth and technique. No more will health be taught by a poorly trained instructor who is really a full-time coach or home economics teacher. Tomorrow's health educators will have available the kind of resources that were showered upon science teachers after Sputnik shook up the American education scene in the 1950s.

As students join the work force, they'll be encouraged to join self-help groups interested in nutrition, alcohol abuse, auto safety, environment, marital problems, child health and so on. As they and their families go to their doctors' offices and clinics, they'll find — in addition to the usual clinical departments of physical therapy, x-ray and lab — a new department of patient education. Departments started in 1974 with the help of such organizations as the American Group Practice Association and Core Communications in Health, Inc. will be commonplace.

They'll find, too, that their community hospital has an active department of health education that provides a variety of seminars, books, movies and closed circuit TV for that "teachable moment," when serious disease or accident in the family brings them to the hospital — not just to sit listlessly leafing through magazines in the waiting room, but learning at a time when they can really appreciate how important that good health we all take for granted really is.

Some will pay a registration fee and enroll in a Course for the Activated Patient being taught by their family doctor for his new patients, and to update his old ones. There they'll learn self-help methods applicable to their area. Health information about frostbite is appropriate for Farmington, Maine, but what to do about sunstroke is more compelling in Tucson, Arizona.

They'll find the doctor now devotes Wednesdays to teaching the course, instead of seeing patients or teaching at the medical school. He's found that the medical center is quite a long drive, and with the fuel shortage, he's stopped going there. He's found that teaching patients is more fun than teaching medical students anyway, and pays off in some direct ways: He has fewer telephone calls at the office, fewer night calls, and he enjoys a much richer relationship with his patients after they have become "in partners." The biggest pay-off of all is the peace of mind that comes with the discovery that malpractice suits decrease as a direct result of increased patient trust and understanding.

In the coming Health Partnership, others will find such pleasant bonuses as discounts on their share of the premium when they enroll in their employer's prepaid health insurance plan, if they take the course and successfully pass an exam on common injuries, illnesses and emergencies. Health Maintenance Organizations (HMOs), too, will offer preferential rates, just as some insurance companies do to nondrinking, nonsmoking, or safe-driving customers.

Will this Health Partnership come about because of more money for patient education? Through a directive from the Department of Health, Education and Welfare? Because of an A.M.A. resolution at the next annual business meeting? Not at all. It will probably come about because consumers will have beaten on the doors of the medical establishment long and loud enough so that it was no longer possible to ignore the message.

An example of what I mean took place in New Mexico when a group of patients, doctors, nurses and educators convened to discuss "The Role of the Consumer in Assuring Quality Health Care." Many issues were discussed — from access to health care to its quality, from doctor–patient communications to continuity of care, from outcome to cultural patterns and problems.

An arm-long list of demands for a changed relationship emerged. Some leaned on doctors. ("Consumers should receive education in the management of common illnesses, injuries and emergencies" and "The consumer must have the opportunity to work out treatment with the provider.") Others pressed responsibility upon the patient. ("The consumer must be willing to tell the health professional he does not understand what is being said about diagnosis, medication and treatment" and "Consumers should advocate provision of continuing health education programs from elementary school throughout the education system.")

The end result was a kind of Constitutional Convention. And, although held without Thomas Jefferson or Benjamin Franklin, it had its health equivalents and produced a notable document, embodying words consciously akin to those used by our nation's founders 200 years ago. Read these words drafted at the Albuquerque Conference:

175

"The consumer has a right to access to health care regardless of race, creed, religion, sex or ability to pay. The health care system must exist for the benefit of consumers . . . Both consumer and provider (must) recognize, allow and accept the input of one another. All consumers have expertise about themselves and their environment which is not recognized and utilized by health care providers."

The convention even had its own Patrick Henry — Dr. Walter B. Clancy of the University of Arkansas Graduate School of Social Work, whose keynote address stirred the delegates with these words: "This sleeping giant of a patient must bestir himself and become involved in issues concerning his own health care, if he is truly interested in the future quality of health care!"

Your health is your concern as a patient. It's your doctor's concern as a physician. When all is said and done, it is to build and strengthen that health partnership of mutual interest and concern that this book is dedicated. Now, with the book-within-a-book *Self-Help Medical Guide* on the blue pages that follow, your junior partnership officially begins.

A NOTE TO THE READER

The 128-paged blue section which follows — entitled *The Self-Help Medical Guide* — corresponds to pages 179–306 of this book. Regular paging is picked up following the book-within-a-book.

THE SELF-HELP
MEDICAL GUIDE

The book within the book
HOW TO BE YOUR OWN DOCTOR— SOMETIMES

by Keith W. Sehnert, M.D.
with Howard Eisenberg

Grosset & Dunlap
Publishers   New York

HOW TO BE YOUR OWN DOCTOR — SOMETIMES
Copyright © 1975 by Keith W. Sehnert, M.D. and Howard Eisenberg

CONTENTS

CONTENTS

CONTENTS

INTRODUCTION

This "book within a book" is the portion of HOW TO BE YOUR OWN DOCTOR — SOMETIMES that you and your family will find yourselves referring to most often. Medical experience shows that each year the average person in the United States has four illnesses, injuries or emergencies serious enough to prompt visits to a doctor. It has long been recognized that the reasons for the visits are usually not the complicated and unusual conditions depicted on television medical shows, but common, real-life health problems that plague normal people year in and year out. Until recently, however, the specific health problems that prompted most of the visits remained unverified and uncounted.

The dilemma facing authors of doctor books such as home medical encyclopedias, emergency care guides and various family first aid texts in the past was: "What to choose from the infinity of medical knowledge." One author might decide to put in EVERYTHING — including interesting but unlikely diseases such as hemophilia — but the result was a huge book or collection of books which was often unmanageable. Or an author could choose to make the book smaller by speaking in GENERALITIES. But this did not provide the specific details that people needed to deal with particular health problems.

The thirty-six illnesses, injuries and emergencies covered in this self-help guide have been found, through recent computer analysis of medical practice, to represent over 70 percent of the reasons you might go to a family doctor, pediatrician, internist or obstetrician/gynecologist this coming year. By following the simple step-by-step procedures given for handling these common health problems, another by-product of modern computer technology, you should be able to eliminate unnecessary trips, cut down on frantic dashes to the doctor's office and make each visit a purposeful one.

G7

The medical protocols, plus the general advice, treatment and concepts provided, are designed to help you enter a satisfactory HEALTH PARTNERSHIP with your physician. By learning to make some clinical observations by yourself and following the medical procedures outlined here (which clearly indicate when it's important to call the doctor), you will cut medical costs, use your doctor more appropriately and generally save your time and his for the more complex medical situations that do turn up.

The concept on which this Self-Help Medical Guide is based is new — some say even revolutionary. The working guide, therefore, is still in the developmental stage, and should be used as such. But constant field testing is planned and future editions will incorporate improvements that will shape the guide into a bible of paramedical care in the home.

THE SELF-HELP
MEDICAL GUIDE

14 MOST COMMON ILLNESSES

ARTHRITIS
Osteoarthritis, Degenerative Arthritis

Description Most people over the age of 50 have osteoarthritis to some extent but very few (about 5 percent) have serious or disabling symptoms. The joints that get the most use (knees, back, hips, neck and fingers) are the ones usually affected by this common type of arthritis.

There are several other kinds of arthritis: nonarticular rheumatism called bursitis or fibrositis, gout and connective tissue diseases — including rheumatoid arthritis and arthritis due to infection. These other arthritic conditions usually cause more crippling and disability than osteoarthritis.

The usual symptoms are stiffness and pain. Redness and heat are almost never present. There is seldom any fever.

Practical Pointers 1. Pain in a joint may result from overuse, but frequently it is caused by nothing more than changes in the weather or a drop in barometric pressure.

2. Pain from stiffness is common in the morning, before and just after getting out of bed. It is relieved by movement and local heat application. It usually lasts about 10 minutes and seldom longer than 30 minutes.

3. Pain will usually travel from one joint to another.

4. Bumps (Heberden's nodes) are commonly seen in the knuckles of women after menopause. These are knobby, thickened lumps over the joints of the fingers. The main complaint is cosmetic rather than pain, and the nodes should not be taken as an indication of a serious or crippling form of arthritis.

5. Laboratory studies, when you see the doctor, are almost always within the normal range. Commonly reported normal

G11

are the sed rate (erythrocyte sedimentation rate), and the complete blood count. The sed rate involves putting blood in a special tube (Westergren) and checking it after an hour to ascertain the rate at which the red blood cells settle to the bottom of the tube.

Treatment Tips 1.   Take aspirin if needed. It is still the medication that gives you the most help for the least cost. (See Drug Index, p. G78.)
2.   Use heat applications as needed. (See Treatment Index, p. G94.)
3.   Apply elastic bandage in a figure 8 across a painful knee. It provides support and eases the pain.
4.   Wear knitted wool cylinders (8 in. long) over arthritic knees in the winter. The extra warmth is helpful. Windproof nylon or synthetic fiber gloves for the hands are also beneficial and should be worn under mittens or woolen gloves.
5.   Massaging the muscles surrounding the joint may be helpful, but rubbing the joint itself is of little value.
6.   Lose weight if indicated. Less weight decreases the wear and tear on the joints.
7.   Be as active as possible. If the joints are painful, rest in bed or an easy chair for 30 minutes every 4 hours. If you are free of pain, you may have as much activity as comfortable; it helps psychologically and physically. Muscles should be kept stretched as well as strong. (See Treatment Index, p. G89–G94.)

When to Call the Doctor 1.   If aspirin makes you dizzy, causes ringing in the ears, indigestion, heartburn or constipation.
2.   Pain seems limited to one joint and there is history of gout in the family.
3.   If you are taking medicines such as liver extract or a thiazide diuretic for high blood pressure that may cause elevation of uric acid in the blood (hyperuricemia).
4.   There is increasing fatigue and general weakness.

ASTHMA
Bronchial Asthma

Description   Asthma is a distressing and, at times, frightening lung disease associated with allergies. An attack may be caused by dust, pollen; infection, smoke, food, medication, exertion, cold damp weather, emotional upsets or fatigue. The severity and duration of an attack depends on your general health, age and attitude as well as the early treatment offered. Surroundings offered by your family and home are also important.

Bronchial asthma occurs when the bronchial tubes go into spasm and the mucous membrane on their inner lining gets inflamed, swollen and choked with sticky mucus. When this occurs it becomes difficult for you to move air in and out of the lungs. This causes labored breathing (wheezing) and produces shortness of wind (dyspnea).

Acute attacks usually require treatment in your doctor's office or a hospital.

Associated symptoms may include runny/stuffy nose, coughing, sinus problems, fever and muscle pains in the neck and chest.

Practical Pointers

1. Whenever you have an attack, it is a good time to review the probable cause and think of the many things you can do to reduce the frequency and severity of future attacks. Was the attack caused by irritating smoke from cigars, cigarettes, fires, car fumes, some food or an emotional stress?

2. Asthma frequently leads to emphysema, so the number of attacks must be kept to a minimum.

3. Prevention of wheezing is possible by rigidly following certain rules.

(a) Create an allergy-free bedroom and install electronic precipitator. (See Treatment Index, p. G81–G82.)
(b) Don't lie on any carpet unless separated from it by a clean blanket, plastic sheet, linoleum or masonite panel.
(c) If certain events always cause an asthma attack (playing or running hard, the excitement of holidays or birthdays, anger) take asthma medicine BEFORE the event.
(d) Treat all colds, sore throats and infections promptly. Ask your doctor to give you these prescriptions to have on hand: an antihistamine or decongestant for the nose, an asthma medicine for the wheeze and an antibiotic for the infection.

4. Maintain a good level of physical fitness and include daily exercise as a part of your everyday life.

5. Drink lots of liquids. This reduces the thickness of the bronchial secretions and keeps them watery. A good goal is one glass of water every hour.

6. Stop smoking, and avoid situations in which smoking does occur.
7. Keep windows closed in cars and at home and use air conditioning as much as possible.
8. Consider allergy shots (skin testing followed by regular desensitization injections). Discuss it with your doctor.

Treatment Tips
1. Get away from and stay away from whatever makes you wheeze.
2. Retire to an allergy-free room as soon as wheezing starts.
3. Start medicine as soon as possible and continue it until squeaking or wheezing has stopped for at least 24 hours.
4. Drink one glass of warm liquid (tea, soup, lemonade or liquid gelatin) every hour. (NOTE: If you are unable to keep or get solid foods down, YOU MUST HAVE LIQUIDS.)
5. Don't let anyone smoke in your home or car during recovery.
6. It is better if you can relax, lie flat and sleep.

Tips about Children
1. Children sometimes get bellyaches by swallowing large amounts of sticky, irritating mucus. They may feel better if they can vomit and rid themselves of this mucus.
2. Don't allow children to use asthma medicine that is given by spray. It may make the asthma worse.

When to Call the Doctor
1. When you can't talk, eat or lie flat in bed and sleep.
2. When it HURTS to breathe. Wheezing can make the chest ache dully, but pain caused by breathing is a bad sign.
3. If vomiting occurs more than twice in several hours — particularly if the patient is a child.
4. If sputum changes in color from clear white to yellow, green, gray or if it becomes bloody.
5. If fever is present several times daily. (See Testing Index, p. G126–G127.)

BLADDER INFECTION
Cystitis

Description Bladder infections are usually caused by bacteria but sometimes a virus is at fault. The most common bacteria is *E. coli*, an organism normally found in bowel movements.
　　Cystitis is more frequently experienced by women, especially young married women, than men. The mild trauma

of sexual intercourse is a common cause. The exact cause of other bladder infections is uncertain but the shorter urinary tube (urethra) of women and the frequent presence of bacteria on the skin in that part of the body make this a likely cause of infections. Women may also experience cystitis after having a vaginal infection.

Other urinary tract causes of infection may be an enlarged prostate, a narrowing of the urethra from past infections or an obstruction in the ureter (the tube from the kidney to the bladder).

Symptoms of cystitis may be a burning on urination, chills and fever, increased frequency of urination, a feeling of urgency to empty the bladder, pain over pubis, backache, blood in the urine and occasionally a urethral or vaginal discharge.

Practical Pointers
1. Properly treated, cystitis is usually a self-limiting illness that runs its course in about three days.
2. Cystitis is quite often associated with an infection ascending to the kidneys. This causes the lower back to become tender. A gentle kidney punch will elicit pain on one or both sides. (See Testing Index, p. G125.)
3. The temperature should be checked three times daily. (See Testing Index, p. G126–G127.)
4. Shaking chills with actual chattering of the teeth may indicate a severe infection with involvement not only of the bladder and kidneys but some spread to the system (septicemia).
5. Sometimes there is a discharge of infected urine or pus that may make a male think he has the venereal disease gonorrhea, commonly called the clap.

Treatment Tips
1. Rest in bed when there is fever. This saves your healing energy and shortens the illness.
2. Increase liquid intake (8 oz. every hour). This helps wash out the urinary tract. It is probably also an important PREVENTIVE measure. Women who have frequent cystitis are often found to be habitually low on liquid intake. (Along this line, since it is known that sexual intercourse often is a factor in cystitis, European doctors have for years recommended the "French Flush" to these women, i.e., drink two large glasses of water or liquid after intercourse. It is a helpful tip to remember.)

G15

3. Take aspirin. It has an analgesic effect on the pain of cystitis and may be used particularly before bedtime. (See Drug Index, p. G78.)

4. Take sitz baths. Use them during the stage of the illness in which there is lots of burning. (See Treatment Index, p. G95.)

5. Avoid alcohol, tea and coffee during this illness as they are urinary tract irritants.

When to Call the Doctor

1. You have a personal history of kidney disease (such as chronic pyelonephritis, kidney stones or glomerulonephritis).

2. You are a diabetic.

3. There is a possibility of pregnancy.

4. Shaking spells or vomiting have occurred within the last 12 hours (this may indicate septicemia).

5. Cystitis is associated with an irritating vaginal discharge.

6. Red blood in the urine (hematuria) persisting for one or two days, or if you have had abdominal or back trauma within the two weeks prior to the symptoms that might have injured your kidneys.

7. Symptoms and fever increase after 48 hours of above treatment.

8. You have high blood pressure.

BRONCHITIS

Description Bronchitis may be caused by bacterial or viral infections of the lower windpipe (bronchi). It can be occasional, or repeat and become chronic. Frequently, it is the end result of a common cold or upper respiratory infection that is not completely cured. Bronchitis is much more common among smokers and people who work in polluted air or have respiratory allergies.

As the cells in the mucous lining of the bronchi are damaged by the virus particles or bacteria they secrete a sticky mucus. The normal "clean-up crew" of the bronchi, the cilia cells, find this sticky mucus difficult to move out. The cells normally work like a group of volleyball players who pass the ball along and over the net. But in the case of bronchitis, the ball is so sticky the players aren't able to pick it up off the floor. The bacteria then grow causing the infection to spread rapidly. The cough associated with bronchitis is the body's way of helping the cilia cells clean out the sticky mucus. (See Symptom/Concept Index, p. G114–G115.)

Chronic bronchitis can lead to chronic obstructive lung disease (C.O.L.D.), the cause of death of 45,000 people each year in the United States.

In addition to the cough, bronchitis symptoms are tiredness, muscle ache, fever, runny nose and sore throat. Untreated, it spreads and can lead to pneumonia.

Practical Pointers

1. Bronchitis is usually associated with clear yellow or white sputum. But if the sputum is colored green or brown, the problem is most likely a bacterial infection and antibiotics will be required for a cure. Morning sputum is often concentrated and hard to judge. Sputum coughed up throughout the day is more reliable regarding the color.

2. Sticky mucus causes changes in the breath sounds — called wheezing.

3. Chest pain with bronchitis is common in adults, but seldom seen in children. The pain, caused by coughing, is occasional and is located on the midline under the breast bone (sternum).

4. Chest pain that is STEADY can mean heart attack (myocardial infarction), ballooning out of an artery wall (dissecting aneurysm), blood clot to lung (pulmonary embolism) or other serious problems.

5. Other types of chest pain can be chest wall syndrome (a pain associated with muscle tenderness at certain points between the ribs) or pleurisy. This pain occurs with coughing or deep breathing and is not midline as in bronchitis.

6. Fever is a good indicator of general condition. (See Symptom/Concept Index, p. G115–G116.) Check and record your temperature three times a day.

7. Bronchitis is a contagious disease and precautions should be taken to isolate the patient from the rest of the family.

Treatment Tips

1. Avoid breathing in irritating substances and tobacco smoke until all symptoms are gone.

2. Go to bed. Depending on the degree of illness you should either stay in bed or greatly limit your activity. It takes a lot of healing energy to cure your infection and the less you do the more rest your lungs will get.

3. Drink lots of liquids — a good goal is a gallon a day! This extra fluid will help make the mucus in the lungs less sticky, closer to its normal water-like consistency, and the "clean-up crew" will have an easier job.

G17

4. Take your temperature three times daily. (See Testing Index, p. G126–G127.)

5. Use steam inhalation. It is most helpful. The microscopic water vapor loosens the sticky mucus. (See Treatment Index, p. G100.)

6. Use postural drainage twice daily. (See Treatment Index, p. G100.)

7. Take cough medication as needed — especially at night. (See Drug Index, p. G79.)

8. Massage the chest and back muscles. Products such as Vicks VapoRub and similar over-the-counter preparations help some people. The massaging will bring increased blood flow to the chest muscles and help you relax.

When to Call the Doctor

1. You have frequent bronchitis or C.O.L.D.

2. You are short of breath when not coughing or when you are resting.

3. You suffer from increasing chest pain and are over 30 years old.

4. Bloody mucus is coughed up frequently.

5. Your fever is often over 101°.

6. If mucus continues to thicken despite efforts as directed. (If this occurs, collect the mucus in a clean covered jar and take it to the doctor for examination and culture.)

7. You are wheezing (this means another person in the room can hear you when you breathe with your mouth open).

8. You are older than 60 years.

9. If cough persists for more than 10 days.

10. You have diabetes.

11. If you smoke one pack or more of cigarettes per day.

12. If pulse rate is greater than 100 beats per minute or less than 50 beats per minute. (See Testing Index, p. G124–G125.)

COMMON COLD
Viral Upper Respiratory Infection

Description The common cold is a virus-caused inflammation of the membranes of the nose and throat. It also frequently involves the chest and ears.

Viruses are very tiny particles, much smaller than a red blood cell, that cause disease when they invade susceptible cells. Viruses need living tissue in order to grow and reproduce. Scores of different viruses have been found in patients with colds. Probably 45 percent of the infections in the common cold are caused by one virus called rhinovirus.

According to the 1973 National Health Survey, respiratory diseases such as pharyngitis, laryngitis, rhinitis, common cold, bronchitis and sinusitis cause at least half of all acute minor illnesses seen in the doctor's office. They may occur any time of the year but are most common in late winter and early spring and often follow an epidemic pattern.

Symptoms associated with viral upper respiratory infection (URI) include watery nasal congestion, sneezing, sore throat, sinus pain, cough and fever.

Practical Pointers

1. Serious complications rarely occur although viral pneumonia may occur under certain conditions.
2. Antibiotics such as penicillin and tetracycline are of no value and may make things worse by creating antibiotic-resistant strains of bacteria, upsetting the digestive tract's normal, helpful bacteria and causing diarrhea.
3. Colds last from three to seven days with a gradual one or two day onset. Low-grade fever usually occurs on the third day with full-blown symptoms for about three days. After the third day, symptoms should gradually subside.
4. Yellow or white exudate in the throat may be seen with viral infections but usually indicate bacterial infection. (See Testing Index, p. G127–G128.)
5. The common cold is spread primarily by viral particles on the hands and face. Personal cleanliness during the illness, with generous use of soap and water, will help limit its spread to other members of the household.

Treatment Tips

1. Avoid excessively cold temperatures and overfatigue.
2. Go to bed if you have a fever. If not, get extra rest.
3. Increase your liquid intake. Set a goal of 8 oz. of juice or water every 2 hours.
4. Stop smoking (and don't resume it afterward).
5. Gargle with hot salt solution. (See Treatment Index, p. G97.)
6. Use throat lozenges if helpful.
7. Use nose drops. (See Drug Index, p. G79.)
8. Use oral nasal decongestant if needed for relief of symptoms. (See Drug Index, p. G78–G79.)
9. Take aspirin if needed. (See Drug Index, p. G78.)
10. Check temperature three times daily and record. (See Testing Index, p. G126–G127.)

When to Call
the Doctor

1. Temperature over 101° several times each day.
2. Increase in throat pain.
3. White or yellow spots on tonsils or throat.
4. Shaking chills and chattering teeth.
5. Chest pain.
6. Shortness of breath.
7. Earache.
8. Pain in sinuses.
9. Coughing produces green or gray sputum during the day.
10. No improvement by fifth day.

EARACHE
Otitis Media

Description Otitis media, inflammation of the middle ear, is most common in children and adolescents but may occur in people of all ages.

Earache is usually caused by a bacterial infection, but it can also be caused by viruses or allergies. These infections extend up into the middle ear following nose, tonsil, throat and adenoid conditions.

The bacterial infections require penicillin, tetracycline or erythromycin — all types of antibiotics. In patients less than 3 years old, ampicillin is preferred by many physicians because it is effective against a bacteria called *Hemophilus influenzae* frequently seen in children.

Serous otitis media is a painless, more chronic form of middle ear inflammation. It usually resolves itself without the use of an antibiotic.

Symptoms associated with earaches include pain (often severe), dizziness, fullness of ear, hearing loss, ringing in the ears, fever, headache and runny or stuffy nose.

Practical 1. Serous otitis media is usually not painful. You may
Pointers complain mainly of hearing loss and fullness in the ear.

2. Ear infections can, on rare occasions, be associated with meningitis. If the patient can touch his chin to his chest without pain, this serious complication is probably not present.

3. A probable cause for ear infections is the careless, hard blowing of the nose or excessive sniffing that drives infected mucus up into the middle ear. (See Symptom/Concept Index, p. G111.)

4. The symptoms of otitis media may be similar to other disorders around the ear and may require direct visualization of the drum and external canal with an otoscope (See Testing Index, p. G122–G123). In regular otitis media, the drum is bright red while in serous it is dull and bluish.

5. In young children (3 years old or less), if otitis media is not treated with an antibiotic a high percentage will suffer hearing loss.

6. In children, especially those under three years, there may be no pain of the usual kind, but the youngster may tug or pull at the affected ear.

7. The reason otitis media is so common in children is that they have narrow tubes from the middle ear to the throat (eustachian tubes) that can fail to drain properly.

Treatment Tips   1. It is important to rest, either in bed or sitting in a chair, if there is fever or pain.

2. Apply heat to the ear. In children or adults having intense pain (as might be caused by a rapid change of altitude in airplane landing or auto descent from mountain), heat may be applied by the juice glass method. (See Treatment Index, p. G94–G95.)

3. Use nose drops four times daily. (See Drug Index, p. G79.)

4. Take oral nasal decongestants. They come in the liquid, capsule or tablet form. They may be used in addition to the nose drops. (See Drug Index, p. G78–G79.)

5. Make sure the external ear canal is free of wax. (See Treatment Index, p. G88.) It will allow your doctor to better examine the canal and eardrum and, if indicated during the illness, perform a surgical puncture of the drum (myringotomy) to relieve pressure.

6. Do not give aspirin for earache. Pain is a valuable signal regarding the ear condition and it should not be masked.

When to Call   1. Increasing pain in ear or headache despite treatment.
the Doctor   2. If the ear drum ruptures. A telltale sign is reddish fluid draining from the ear.

3. Temperature over 102°.

4. Convulsive twitching of face muscles.

5. Dizziness.

6. Patient is 3 years old or less.

EMPHYSEMA
Chronic Obstructive Lung Disease (C.O.L.D.)

Description Emphysema is a chronic lung condition brought on by repeated infections, allergies and irritants such as tobacco smoke, dusts and chemical fumes. Over the years, the elastic fibers in the air sacs of the lungs and the bronchioles and bronchi of the air tracts lose their normal elasticity and are unable to spring back to their normal state after the person has inhaled air. Because breathing requires this elastic effect to help during exhaling, there is a loss of useful lung volume, a decreased ability to oxygenate the blood and a tendency toward frequent attacks of bronchitis. A decreased ability to transfer oxygen (perfusion) and carbon dioxide across the membrane of the air sac causes oxygen shortages.

Emphysema is now the primary cause of death for 45,000 people each year in the United States and the secondary cause for 100,000 more.

Associated symptoms are shortness of breath on exertion, frequent respiratory infections and bronchitis, wheezing and chronic cough.

Practical Pointers 1. It is difficult for modern patients — geared as they are to an instant cure for everything — to accept the fact that there is no cure for emphysema. There are, however, many ways to cope with the problem and help the patient live a fairly normal life.

2. All experts agree that emphysema sufferers who smoke MUST STOP SMOKING. It not only worsens the illness but cuts down the chances of success with other therapy.

3. If you work where the air is polluted, do everything you can to decrease the pollution. Install filters, improve the air conditioning, control the source of dusts and irritants and — if all else fails — change jobs.

4. Treat concurrent allergic conditions with desensitizing injections prepared by an allergy specialist.

5. Lose weight if you are overweight.

6. Maintain a physical fitness program of daily exercise and work to improve your general strength and stamina. The psychological benefits of a person being able to make his own bed, go to the store and do other self-care activities are substantial.

7. Do daily breathing exercises. (See Treatment Index, p. G91.)

8. Do postural drainage routine. (See Treatment Index, p. G100.)

9. Maintain high fluid intake with goal of 8 oz. of fluid six times daily (for example, on all the even hours from 10 A.M. to 6 P.M.). This helps keep your bronchial secretions thinner, less harmful, easier to cough up and less likely to cause infection.

10. Avoid sudden changes in temperature, humidity, exertion and loud talking or shouting. These may trigger a coughing episode.

11. Sleep with 5 in. blocks under foot of bed. This will help drain the secretions during the night and in the early morning.

12. Avoid stressful situations as much as possible. The bronchial tree seems to be as sensitive as the gastrointestinal (GI) tract and responds to stress by going into spasm and triggering wheezing.

13. Have at least one air conditioner with a good filter available for bedroom use.

Treatment Tips 1. Use steam inhalation. This helps many patients. (See Treatment Index, p. G100.)

2. Eat small meals taken 4 or 5 times a day.

3. Use the medications as prescribed by your doctor such as:

(a) antibiotic

(b) anti-cough preparation

(c) bronchodilator

(d) aerosol bronchodilator

(e) throat lozenge

(f) oral nasal decongestant

(g) sedative for bedtime use

(h) steroid

4. Take temperature 3 times a day and record it. (See Testing Index, p. G126–G127.)

When to Call 1. Temperature over 101°.
the Doctor 2. Blood in the sputum.

3. Increasing chest pain.

4. Shortness of breath without coughing or when at rest.

5. Thickening of sputum despite treatment (plan to take sputum sample to doctor for culturing and ask him for collection procedure).

6. Vomiting.

HIGH BLOOD PRESSURE
Hypertension

Description Recognized as the most common serious health problem in America, hypertension is an elevation of blood pressure above normal levels. Untreated it causes strokes, kidney damage, visual problems and many heart and blood vessel disorders. An estimate of the number of hypertensives in the United States is 5 to 6 percent of the total population (that translates into 20 to 25 million people!).

What is blood pressure? It is the force exerted against the walls of the arteries as the blood is carried from the heart to all parts of the body. The force is created by the pumping action of the heart.

There are two phases of the heart's pumping action, systole and diastole. The peak action is called systolic pressure. When the heart relaxes between beats, the lower level diastolic pressure results. An example of a "normal" reading would be 120/80. These numbers refer to the millimeters of mercury (in the glass tube part of a sphygmomanometer) pushed by the blood pressure.

Until the early 1960s, the diastolic was considered more important than the systolic pressure, but now most experts regard both pressures as having equal significance.

Normal blood pressure varies with age. Most insurance companies now say that if you are under 40 years of age, it should be 130/80 or less. If over 40, the upper limit of normal is 140/80. Increased insurance ratings begin at 150/90 and most doctors start medical treatment at that level.

There is no such illness as "low blood pressure" except in certain rare conditions. A reading under 120/80 rarely causes trouble and is usually an asset since less strain is placed on the circulation system in its daily work.

Eighty-five percent of the patients with high blood pressure have ESSENTIAL HYPERTENSION. "Essential" doesn't mean "necessary" here but that no apparent cause has been discovered that explains the abnormal pressure. SECONDARY HYPERTENSION, on the other hand, is usually caused by specific organic conditions such as kidney disease, adrenal tumors and certain other hormonal disorders.

Called by some the "silent disease," hypertension may exist for many years without symptoms. When symptoms do

G24

occur, the most frequent are dizziness, fatigue, headaches, weakness, nervousness and insomnia. More serious symptoms include small strokes, speech or visual difficulties, and heart failure.

Practical Pointers

1. Hypertension is more common among urbanites, especially blacks. One survey showed an incidence of 21.1 percent in blacks compared to 13.5 percent in white city dwellers. The stress of inner city life is a major factor because rural whites and blacks have an incidence of only 5 or 6 percent, the average rate of hypertension.

2. Blood pressure like body temperature varies during the day and may be elevated by the stress of going to your doctor's office or clinic. Have someone check your blood pressure at home at various times to determine your normal average (see Testing Index, p. G119–G122). If it is elevated, you should have your blood pressure verified by your doctor or his nurse (on at least four visits at different times of the day over a four-week period) before antihypertensive medication is begun.

3. Check your weight. If you are 20 percent overweight for your age and height you will be asked by your doctor to take off those extra pounds. Frequently, the mere loss of this extra baggage will bring your blood pressure down to normal range.

Treatment Tips

1. Lose weight. Estimates show that each pound of fat requires about ¾ mile of blood vessels to support it. Thus, if you are 30 pounds overweight, there are about 23 miles of extra "pipeline" that the heart (as a motor and pump) must push the blood through. This extra effort, required 60 times each minute, is frequently the cause of high blood pressure (see Symptom/Concept Index, p. G110–G111).

2. Avoid coffee, tea and cola drinks including "diet" colas as all contain caffeine. Caffeine is a stimulant that increases the heart rate and blood pressure. You may drink decaffeinated coffees, such as Sanka, or weak tea and still get most of the pleasures of an "after dinner cup" without blood pressure problems.

3. Stop smoking. Tobacco causes spasms of the blood vessels and increases blood pressure. It must be avoided.

4. Stay away from stressful personal and environmental settings that can raise the blood pressure. Encourage hobbies

and situations that are known to be relaxing and pleasant.

5.   Drink moderately. Alcohol is not harmful to hypertension if used in moderation (e.g., 2 oz. of whiskey per day or 2 cans beer per day), and if there is no other reason to abstain.

6.   Maintain physical fitness. Emphasize regular daily exercise such as hiking, walking, biking, swimming, etc.

7.   Take regular vacations and use weekends wisely for extra rest and recreation.

8.   Maintain a well-rounded diet. Try to avoid salty and high fat foods. Most Americans need only about 1 gram of salt per day but many take in 10 to 15 grams!

9.   Take medication as prescribed by your doctor. Arrange for and make follow-up visits to his office as directed.

When to Call the Doctor   1.   Possible reaction to medication such as weakness, sleepiness, dizziness, depression, fatigue, blurred vision, constipation, light-headedness when standing upright or other symptoms your doctor may warn you about. (Please ask him, if he hasn't mentioned any.)

2.   Unusual weight changes, either gain or loss.

3.   Palpitations, skipped heartbeats or shortness of breath with usual exertions.

4.   Unexplained numbness of face, arms or legs.

5.   Changes in vision such as blurring, blind spots or loss of vision.

PERSISTENT STUFFY NOSE
Allergic Rhinitis, Hay Fever

Description   Nasal allergies are the usual cause of the persistent stuffy nose. If it is a common cold, the nasal stuffiness lasts a week. If it lasts longer you must suspect allergic rhinitis. The word rhinitis means inflammation (-itis) of the nose (rhinos) — think of the rhino at the zoo with his big nose.

"Hay fever" is not necessarily caused by hay and very seldom produces a fever. About 10 percent of the entire population has some kind of nasal allergy at some time during the year, so you have many members in the club.

Eyes are also frequently affected by allergies, so that both watery eyes and runny/stuffy nose may be present.

Nose and eye allergies result when your mucous tissues react to pollen, dusts, animal dander, smoke, bacteria, viruses, food, drugs, chemicals, light, changes in temperature, emotional stress and many other possible irritants and factors.

Associated complaints may include sinus problems, sneezing, coughing, wheezing, muscle aches and fever.

Practical 1. The nasal mucosa has a typical pale, boggy
Pointers appearance with a clear watery discharge. Have an assistant look at your nasal passages. (See Testing Index, p. G125–126.)
2. Keep away from whatever makes your allergy worse. Wear a mask if the allergies are bad that time of year or if you are cleaning a dusty place or cutting grass. Ask the pharmacist at the drugstore for a cold weather mask.
3. Avoid sweeping with a broom — use a vacuum cleaner if possible. If a broom is used, cover it with a damp cloth to reduce irritating dust.
4. Make sure your room is allergy free. (See Treatment Index, p. G81–G82.) If symptoms flare up, check filters in furnace air ducts, air conditioners and room air cleaning devices. (See Treatment Index, p. G82.)
5. Wear big curved sunglasses to keep tree, grass and weed pollen from blowing into your eyes during your allergy season.

Tips about Children may rub, pick or wiggle their itchy noses (the
Children allergic "salute"). They tend to sneeze a lot in the morning and are "mouth breathers" at night — they may snore. Allergic children may have dark circles under their eyes.

Treatment Tips 1. Take oral nasal decongestant or antihistamine 3 times a day to relieve symptoms. (See Drug Index, p. G78–G79.)
2. Get extra rest in allergy-free room when symptoms are present. Stay inside on windy days.
3. Wash the hands and face often during the allergy season or on bad days. Use warm water.
4. Keep an antihistamine at work, at school and in the car.
5. Use nose drops for supplemental relief at bedtime. (See Drug Index, p. G79.) LIMIT USE TO 3 TIMES A DAY FOR NO MORE THAN 3 DAYS. Overuse of nose drops may lead to loss of sense of smell and other complications.
6. Stop smoking (an irritant) and avoid alcohol. Antihistamines combined with alcohol produce extreme drowsiness.

7. Increase fluid intake. Much body fluid is lost in sneezing, coughing and nasal discharge.

When to Call 1. Thick green or yellow mucus in nose.
the Doctor 2. If you work around dangerous machines, in high places, or must drive and antihistamines make you sleepy.
3. If symptoms cause increasing problems over the years and are not helped much by general preventive measures. Ask about desensitizing allergy shots.

PINK EYE
Conjunctivitis

Description Inflammation of the outside mucus covering of the eye is called conjunctivitis. It is often characterized by pink or beefy red streaks over the surface of the eye, hence the name pink eye.

Conjunctivitis is usually caused by viral or bacterial infections but can also be related to irritation from smoke, wind or dust, or exposure to intensely bright light such as produced by electric arc welding, a sunlamp and strong sunlight reflecting from snow or beaches. It may also occur with the common cold and childhood diseases such as measles.

Occasionally, eye conditions such as acute iritis, herpes simplex, acute narrow angle glaucoma and foreign bodies in the cornea may present symptoms similar to conjunctivitis.

Pink eye is associated with a mucoid or yellow discharge which may cause the eyelids to be stuck shut in the morning. Sufferers may complain of a sandy feeling under the lids. Eyes are extrasensitive when exposed to light, and there may be some blurring of vision.

Practical 1. It is important to determine if there is real PAIN in the
Pointers eye or merely DISCOMFORT. If it is a sandy, scratchy, itching discomfort, it is probably conjunctivitis.
2. The common acute form of pink eye has a STICKY discharge, while the chronic forms do not have this type of discharge.
3. If you complain of a transient blurring of vision with the discharge, it is usually simple conjunctivitis. If there is real pain in the eye plus persistent difficulty in seeing, you do not have conjunctivitis alone.

G28

4.   A common cause of pink eye occurs when a tiny (size of tip of small needle) sliver of foreign matter hits and lodges in your eye while you are using a grinding wheel or chipping paint. The injury may occur 6 to 8 hours before symptoms start.

5.   Frequently the first evidence of eye strain is pink eye. You unconsciously rub your eyes, bacteria on your hands is tranferred to the eyes.

Treatment Tips   1.   Conjunctivitis is usually contagious, so take precautions to prevent its spread. Use your own towel. Wash hands carefully and frequently.

2.   DO NOT USE EYE DROPS CONTAINING CORTISONE. Prescription eye drops commonly include cortisone or cortisone-like medicines for their potent anti-inflammation characteristics. But if you have herpes simplex, instead of conjunctivitis, such drops will worsen the condition, slowing the normal healing action of the eye, and cause an ulcer and bad scarring.

3.   Apply warm, wet compresses to the eye 4 times daily. (See Treatment Index, p. G95.)

4.   Avoid constant wiping of the eye and lid as this frequently causes chapping.

5.   Use aspirin to ease distress. (See Drug Index, p. G78.)

6.   Leave the affected eye unbandaged. Do not use an eye patch.

7.   Wear protective sunglasses.

8.   After getting your doctor's approval for use of prior prescription or new prescription for antibiotic eye ointment or drops, apply as directed. (See Treatment Index, p. G82–G83.)

When to Call the Doctor   1.   No improvement in eye after 24 hours of above treatment.

2.   Distinct pain in eye itself, or pain radiating into the temple.

3.   Change in usual ability to see.

4.   Difference in size of pupils. (See Testing Index, p. G123.) A constricted or small pupil may indicate iritis in that eye.

5.   If you experience visual changes after putting in eyedrops for refraction before a glasses prescription or when you return to a well-lighted area after prolonged exposure to darkness (particularly if this is accompanied by severe pain in the eye or head).

G29

SINUS INFECTION
Sinusitis

Description When the nasal sinuses are inflamed and infected, sinusitis results. Everyone who watches TV ads knows that there are eight sinus cavities. The ones most commonly involved are the two frontal sinuses in the forehead and the two maxillary sinuses in the cheek bones. Sinus infections are seldom seen in children because the sinuses do not develop fully until late adolescence.

The most common reasons for sinusitis are viral or bacterial infections and allergies. Over 50 percent of acute infections are bacterial and due to *D. pneumonia* or *Hemophilus influenzae.* In children it may be *Staphylococcus aureus.* Acute infections are by definition those that last less than three weeks and chronic types last longer. Growths in the mucous membrane (polyps) and tumors can also interfere with proper drainage of the sinus cavities and cause infections.

Strenuous blowing of the nose (hard like blowing a bugle) is a probable cause of many sinus infections. (See Symptom/Concept Index, p. G111.)

Deep swimming or diving and jumping into deep water may carry infected mucus into the sinus areas — as will pressure change from rapid descent in an airplane.

Associated symptoms may be runny/stuffy nose, sneezing, bad breath, muscle aches, fever and some swelling of facial area.

Practical Pointers 1. Maxillary sinusitis is the commonest of all sinus infections, and headache or tenderness in the cheek bones on one side is the most common symptom.
2. Headache is worse when stooping over.
3. If the nasal discharge is thick and yellow, the cause is bacterial. Sometimes the mucus is bloodstained.
4. A common problem associated with sinusitis is postnasal drip. This in turn leads to sore throat and hoarseness.
5. If the problem is ethmoid sinusitis, a rare condition, pain will be felt along the area between the nose and inner portion of the eyelid. Before the present era of antibiotics, this was a very grim complication that often led to meningitis and death.

Treatment Tips 1. At the first sign of sinus distress, use alternating hot and cold compresses (see Treatment Index, p. G95) to stimulate flow of mucus from sinuses followed in sequence by nose drops (see Drug Index, p. G79) and then hot gargles (see Treatment Index, p. G97). Repeat every 3 to 4 hours.

2. Check temperature three times daily and record. (See Testing Index, p. G126–G127.)

3. Take oral nasal decongestant 3 times daily. (See Drug Index, p. G78–G79.)

4. Take aspirin as needed for pain. (See Drug Index, p. G78.)

5. Increase fluid intake. Set a goal of one glass of liquid every two hours.

6. Rest until fever, pain and acute symptoms have subsided.

7. Stop smoking.

When to Call the Doctor

1. Temperature elevation over 101°.

2. Bleeding from the nose.

3. Severe headache that does not go away after you have taken aspirin.

4. Increased swelling over the face (forehead, eyes, side of nose, cheek).

5. Changes or blurring in vision.

6. Increased thick nasal discharge.

SORE THROAT
Pharyngitis

Description Most (about 80 percent) sore throats are caused by viral infections or irritations from smoking, shouting, coughing and postnasal drainage. Some pharyngitis, however, is caused by bacteria. If this bacterial infection is of the "strep" type (Group A, beta hemolytic streptococcus), it frequently will require penicillin or erythromycin for proper treatment.

In addition to the local pain on swallowing, a sore throat may be associated with a runny or stuffy nose, sinus symptoms, fever, headache, enlarged and tender lymph nodes at the angle of the jaw and generalized aching.

Practical Pointers

1. The diagnosis of strep throat is made after a throat culture has been obtained by your doctor. He may do the culture in his office or send you to a laboratory. It takes 48 hours to grow the bacteria on a culture plate. Only then will it be known whether it is a "positive" or "negative" culture. If it is "positive," certain changes will be noted on the plate and

an antibiotic will usually be prescribed by your doctor. And when he gives it to you, take the full amount for seven to ten days. DO NOT STOP when you feel better after three days!

2.   Studies have shown that about 5 percent of the people in a community are strep carriers; that is, they may not be sick from the bacteria, but they carry it in their throats and may give it to others.

3.   Recent or simultaneous acute viral respiratory illnesses increase the chances of strep infections.

4.   Three factors should make you suspect strep pharyngitis: exudate (yellow or white mucus that may give a cobblestone appearance to the throat), lymph node enlargement (swollen nodes at the angle of the jaw and along the front of the neck) and fever (greater than 101°). (See Symptom/Concept Index, p. G115–G116.)

5.   Exudate may also be present with viral infections, but it is more common with strep infections.

6.   The neck nodes in bacterial infections are enlarged, quite tender and may make you wince when they are touched. The node enlargement is caused by increased blood flow to the lymph tissue to fight the bacteria. It may help to think of the area as a battleground.

7.   If the throat has been sore for more than two weeks, it is called chronic (long lasting) pharyngitis and is usually due to smoking or nasal allergies. Other causes that must be considered and evaluated by your doctor include chronic infections of tonsils or sinuses, mono (infectious mononucleosis) or a possible malignancy or blood disorder.

Treatment Tips   1.   Gargle every 2 hours. (See Treatment Index, p. G97.) This relieves local pain and cleans off the sticky mucus.

2.   Take frequent sips of hot liquids. Lemonade or weak tea and increased amounts of all juices and liquids with the goal of six 8 oz. glasses per day is suggested. This replaces water lost by sweating, nasal discharges, sneezing, etc.

3.   Check temperature three times daily and record. (See Testing Index, p. G126–G127.)

4.   Take aspirin if pain or fever is a problem. (See Drug Index, p. G78.)

5.   Use lozenges if they are helpful.

6.   Rest in bed. This conserves your healing energies.

G32

7. Stop smoking.
8. Rest your voice.

When to Call 1. Chronic sore throat has persisted for two weeks.
the Doctor 2. Associated with severe headache. You can't touch chin to chest without pain. (Sore throat can also be the presenting complaint of meningitis.)
3. You have a history of rheumatic fever, kidney disease or problems with frequent strep infections.
4. Throat is not better after three days of home treatment as above.
5. If fever is over 101° several times daily.
6. Pain in throat seems to be increasing.
7. Earache develops.
8. Shortness of breath, coughing, chest pain.
9. Persistent thick mucus from nose.
10. Skin rash.

STOMACH FLU
Gastroenteritis

___

Description The symptoms of nausea/vomiting/diarrhea are commonly known as the "stomach flu" or some say "the bug going around."

Nausea is a sickness in the stomach area with an inclination to vomit. "Throwing up" is vomiting. Diarrhea means loose, liquid, frequent bowel movements.

Virus is the cause of 90 percent of the gastroenteritis cases, but it can also be due to food poisoning by staphylococcus, *E.coli* or salmonella bacteria. Other parasites are *Giardia lamblia* and *Endamoeba histolytica* which cause amoebic dysentery.

Overindulgence in alcohol, certain types of food or medicines and emotional states may cause similar distressful symptoms.

Occasionally, these common symptoms may herald more serious problems such as appendicitis, gall bladder infection (cholecystitis), pancreas inflammation (pancreatitis), infectious hepatitis, diverticulitis or other digestive disorders.

Associated symptoms for gastroenteritis include abdominal pain, back pain, muscle aches and fever.

G33

Practical 1. Review food intake. It will often reveal the cause of
Pointers the gastroenteritis and give your doctor a chance to give
better advice. Think about these questions:

(a) Is anyone else sick who ate the same meal — the same
individual foods? Have you eaten meals away from home
within the last 24 hours?

(b) Have you just returned from a trip? Such upsets as
"Montezuma's revenge" from Mexico or "New Delhi belly"
from India may be an unexpected postlude to an otherwise
pleasant vacation or business trip.

(c) Is there a similar outbreak of illness among people you
have been in contact with? Illness among classmates,
relatives and clusters of people probably indicate a viral
origin.

2. If you are pregnant, nausea and vomiting may be
associated with it in the first three months.

3. Diarrhea may be PROTECTIVE as Mother Nature speeds the
offending viral particles or bacteria through your body before
they can penetrate the mucosal cells. Don't take antidiarrheal
medication too early, i.e., the first 6 to 8 hours.

4. Viral gastroenteritis runs its course in 24 to 48 hours. There
is acute onset with crampy pain, relief of pain with bowel
movement and lack of fever.

5. Appendicitis is usually distinguished by pain that
intensifies gradually and shifts to the right lower quadrant of
the abdomen. (See Testing Index, p. G119.)

6. The pain associated with cholecystitis and pancreatitis
may radiate to the back or up under the right shoulder blade
(cholecystitis) or left upper quadrant (pancreatitis). (See
Testing Index, p. G119.)

7. A common feature of diverticulitis is a small amount of
pasty stool. Diverticulitis is a colon condition in which pockets
develop in the wall and become irritated (inflamed). When
inflammation is NOT present it's called diverticulosis.

8. Infectious hepatitis may be accompanied by low fever,
joint pains and jaundice.

9. Clues to a diarrhea of emotional state are the following:
pain is relieved by heat; symptoms related to situational stress
or life style changes (new job, divorce, bereavement); pain
that moves from one location to another; morning diarrhea
only (nervous diarrhea rarely occurs at night); vomiting

immediately on ingestion of food and history of irritability, insomnia and various other symptoms associated with "nervousness."

Treatment Tips 1. Rest in bed until nausea, vomiting, diarrhea and fever are gone. An upright position increases the amount of fluids lost in diarrhea and saps more of your energy.

2. Watch foods carefully:

(a) ICE CHIPS ONLY until vomiting stops during the first day.

(b) Clear liquids on second day — sweetened tea, ginger ale, Coke, broth or "special drink" — when diarrhea and vomiting have stopped. (See Treatment Index, p. G97–G98.)

(c) Soft diet on third day — such as custard, pudding, Jello, cooked cereal, baked potato — when symptoms have disappeared.

(d) Avoid fruits, alcohol and highly seasoned foods during recovery for five days.

3. Treatment of uncomplicated diarrhea may at times require medication. (See Drug Index, p. G77.)

Tips about Children Infants (newborn to two years) should be treated by stopping all juices, fruits and formula. Give only sugar water until you call the doctor. (See Treatment Index, p. G98.)

When to Call the Doctor 1. Nausea/vomiting/diarrhea is usually risky for infants, young children, the elderly, the debilitated and diabetics. Also a person with heart, kidney or other chronic disease might get into trouble in a hurry.

2. Black or bloody stools or vomit are noted.

3. History of head trauma within last 48 hours (head injury may result in increased pressure on the brain which can also cause nausea and vomiting).

4. If symptoms have lasted more than four days.

5. If unable to retain liquid intake after 36 hours, or no improvement after 24 hours of above treatment.

6. If temperature is over 101° several times.

7. More than eight stools per day.

8. Convulsion (infants or children).

9. Worms in bowel movement (pinworms or round worms may cause diarrhea).

10. Persistent pain in abdomen or rectum.

11. You are taking special medication that may cause diarrhea.

G35

VAGINAL DISCHARGE
Vaginitis

Description Vaginitis is an inflammation of the mucous surface of the vagina, its lips (labia) and the glands and tissue surrounding it.

The most common causes are a fungus (*Monilia albicans*), a parasite (*Trichomonas vaginalis*) and several bacteria such as strep (streptococci), staph (staphylococci), coliform (*E. coli*) and *Hemophilus vaginalis*.

The most frequent cause is trichomonas, an organism slightly larger than a red blood cell. It survives best in the vagina although it may also gain access to the bladder and cause symptoms there. It is also found in the male and may cause cross infection if both husband and wife are not treated at the same time.

The next most frequent offender is monilia. Such infections are more likely to occur during pregnancy and in diabetic patients. They also occur after antibiotics have been taken or when panty hose are worn too often. The inadequate ventilation of panty hose sets the stage for infection.

Your final unwelcome visitors are the bacteria. Sometimes your doctor may call this infection, nonspecific vaginitis.

All the infections cause discharge, itching, burning and sometimes pain. The "trich" discharge may be associated with an unpleasant odor.

Practical Pointers 1.   Infections in the vagina may result from a generally lowered resistance secondary to other illness, lack of sleep, poor diet and insufficient liquid intake.

2.   Monilial vaginitis has a characteristic cottage cheese-like discharge. It is also at times accompanied by fungus infections in other parts of the body besides the vagina such as the groin, skin around the rectum and in the armpits, and under toenails and fingernails.

3.   The discharge associated with trichomonal vaginitis is thin and foamy and is yellowish-green or gray in color.

4.   Vaginitis in children is usually of the bacterial type, from germ-ridden dirt trapped in tight pants or clothing in close proximity to the vaginal opening, but it can also be caused by pinworms, or from foreign objects such as a peanut, small bead, pebble, etc. inserted into the vagina by the child.

5. "The pill" (any oral contraceptive) is a frequent reason for monilial vaginitis because it alters the normal pH of the vaginal mucosa.

6. Nylon underwear and panty hose retain moisture and heat which help the infecting organisms grow.

7. Eat yogurt (1 cup three times daily) while taking an antibiotic. It may help prevent monilial vaginitis — particularly if you've had trouble with this in the past.

8. Clean the bathtub carefully after bathing to prevent the infection from spreading to others.

Treatment Tips 1. Take vinegar douches. They are helpful in trich and fungal infections. (See Treatment Index, p. G98.)

2. Vaginal infections usually require a doctor's prescription. While undergoing treatment from your physician, you should:

(a) Avoid scratching, it will irritate the tissue and spread the infection.

(b) Don't wear pants or body suits that are tight in the crotch and thighs.

(c) Don't stop the medication as soon as symptoms disappear. Continue it until the prescription is all gone.

(d) Abstain from sexual intercourse until the medication prescribed by your doctor is completed and you are free of symptoms.

When to Call the Doctor 1. If you have a vaginal discharge or itching, you can usually wait several days before seeing the doctor without any serious problems resulting.

2. Call and make your appointment if discharge continues (constant or intermittent) after three or four days of douche treatment.

13 MOST COMMON INJURIES

BLEEDING NOSE
Epistaxis

Description Bleeding from the nose may be caused by injury, the common cold, dry weather, allergies, infection, blood disorders, blowing the nose, foreign bodies, exposure to high altitude, medication, high blood pressure and other factors.

The most common causes are injury, nasal congestion associated with a viral upper respiratory infection or nasal allergies. The common fear that nose bleeding is caused by hypertension is overrated and in reality quite a rare cause.

Associated complaints may include runny nose, sinus problems, allergy/hay fever, muscle aches.

Practical Pointers 1. Epistaxis involves bleeding from the front of the nose. Coughing or spitting up blood from mouth or lung bleeding (hemorrhage) indicates a totally different problem.
2. Nosebleeds are generally more annoying than serious and self-limited if properly handled.
3. Improper treatment by disturbing clots may cause an increase or resumption in bleeding. Common IMPROPER TREATMENTS — stuffing cotton, gauze or tissue into the nose; applying cold cloths to the back of the neck; inserting a paper towel under the upper lip and other nostrums — delay and disrupt the normal healing process!
4. As in the case of any external bleeding, direct pressure on the site is the only action necessary to control nosebleeds.

Treatment Tips 1. Apply direct pressure to the site by clasping the nose firmly between your thumb and index finger — as though you smelled a skunk. (See Treatment Index, p. G86.)
2. Squeeze hard enough to stop the bleeding — but not enough to cause pain.

3. Breathe slowly and easily through your open mouth.

4. Continue applying pressure for a full 5 minutes, without letting go. If bleeding should resume, immediately apply pressure one or two more times. If properly done, bleeding stops with one application of pressure in about 90 percent of the cases.

5. After bleeding has stopped, keep quiet in a sitting position leaning forward. If this is not possible, try a reclining position with head and shoulders on three or four pillows.

6. After bleeding has stopped, do not blow the nose, talk or laugh. It might disturb the clot. These precautions should be observed for three or four hours.

7. Gentle direct pressure may be applied to the nose, even if the bones higher up in the nose (nasal septum) are broken.

When to Call the Doctor
1. If bleeding is not controlled after three attempts.
2. Fracture of the nose has occurred during the injury. This is usually apparent by deformity of the contour of the nose.
3. Injury to nose is causing difficulty in breathing.
4. Lacerations to skin on outside of nose.
5. History of blood and bleeding disorders.
6. Severe or moderate hypertension.

BROKEN WRIST
Fractured Wrist or Forearm

Description The wrist is broken more often than any other part of the body. The fracture can affect any one or more of the bones which join at the wrist: radius and ulna (the two bones of the lower arm) and eight carpal bones. Fractures occur with falls or when the wrist is bent backward beyond the range of motion.

"Sprained wrist" is a common layman's diagnosis that is usually wrong. A true sprained wrist is uncommon and symptoms after a fall are frequently caused by a fracture, dislocation or perhaps arthritis. Persistent pain may be due to fracture of the scaphoid bone at the base of the thumb or one of the other carpals. Unfortunately, these small bones (arranged in two rows of four each) have irregular shapes and surfaces are difficult to visualize in X-ray films. Even with careful X-ray technique, fractures can be overlooked, especially on wet film readings.

G39

Fractures of the radius and ulna are quite easily seen by your doctor on both direct exam and X-ray films. Frequently they are both broken. Another common fracture is that of the lower end of the radius (a Colles fracture).

Associated complaints are pain, swelling, discoloration and loss of function.

Practical Pointers
1. Fractures of the wrist, especially the Colles or radius/ulna fractures, are extremely painful and, like all major fractures, may precipitate shock. Therefore, lie down if you feel faint.
2. Since it is difficult to determine by the amount of swelling or pain whether a wrist is indeed fractured, MEDICAL OR ORTHOPEDIC EVALUATION IS ESSENTIAL.

Treatment Tips
1. Lie down flat on your back in a comfortable position with the forearm on a pillow or blanket. Loosen collar and sleeves.
2. Apply ice packs or cold wet compresses to minimize swelling for at least 30 minutes before splinting. (See Treatment Index, p. G87.)
3. Splint the arm and wrist and support forearm in sling with elevation of wrist. (See Treatment Index, p. G85.)
4. Check finger tips repeatedly to note swelling or bluish discoloration. If this occurs loosen the ties of the splint, straighten the arm and elevate the arm and wrist above the heart.
5. Aspirin may be given to ease the pain, but the pain in many cases will be too intense for much relief. (See Drug Index, p. G78.)

When to Call the Doctor
1. As soon as the traditional first aid steps outlined above have been carried out, medical help and X-rays should be obtained as soon as possible.

BURN WITH BLISTERS
Second-Degree Burn on Hand/Foot
___

Description Burns are injuries that result from heat, chemicals or radiation. Milder burns, called first degree, cause redness, mild swelling and pain. The second-degree burn, a deeper injury to the skin, produces redness plus blisters, with more swelling and pain. The blistering occurs when blood plasma bubbles through the damaged layers of the skin. The more severe burn, third degree, causes charring and much more destruction of the skin.

The most common causes are deep sunburn, contact with hot liquids such as boiling coffee or cooking grease or flash burns from gasoline or kerosene.

Second-degree burns seldom cause death but adults with as little as 15 percent and children with 9 percent of the body surface burned must be hospitalized because of fluid balance problems, pain and the danger of infection. (See Symptom/Concept Index, p. G112–G113.)

Prevention is paramount in this type of injury, especially in children under 14, because such a large percentage of the 8,000 deaths each year occur in this age group — all too often involving small children left unattended at home.

Related complaints are fever, loss of appetite, nausea, sweating and tingling sensations in the hand or foot.

Practical Pointers   1.   The skin is broken in second-degree burns so you must take care to avoid infection. When the skin is broken, the bacteria that are on normal skin, grow quickly in the plasma that has leaked from the blood vessels.

2.   The more aged you are (or if the burn victim is a young child) the greater are the complications and problems associated with burns.

Treatment Tips   1.   Apply cold water to cut the pain and minimize the swelling of the skin tissues. Keep these applications on the burned area for at least one hour. (See Treatment Index, p. G87.)

2.   Wash the skin gently with mild soap and water.

3.   Apply medicated ointment or sterile petroleum jelly, if available, to SMALL BURNS ONLY. Larger burns may need to be seen by a doctor to assess the extent of the burned area and should not be covered with oil-based substances.

4.   Cover with gauze dressing or strips of clean cloth. Tape to keep the coatings in place. Keep the dressings on the burned area for one week unless they become soaked with plasma or develop an unpleasant odor. If removal of the dressing seems necessary, rinse the part with large amounts of water to free the dressing from the sticky burn surface.

5.   Elevate the burned part. Keep it at rest to help healing. Bed rest is essential if legs or feet are involved. Even if burns are small, weight bearing greatly delays healing.

G41

6.   Aspirin may be taken to control pain. (See Drug Index, p. G78.)

When to Call the Doctor   1.   If you are younger than 14 or older than 64 and burn covers about 10 percent of body surface. (See Symptom/Concept Index, p. G.112–G113.)
2.   Areas of third-degree burn present (skin burned black or brown).
3.   Persistent pain not relieved by aspirin.

CUTS/WOUNDS
Lacerations of Face, Hand, Scalp

Description   A wound is a break in the skin. It can be an ABRASION (the outer layer of skin is rubbed or scraped away); CUT (a wound made by a sharp object such as a knife or glass); LACERATION (a torn or irregular edged wound which may have some crushed tissue) or PUNCTURE (the penetration of a nail, needle, or other sharp and pointed object).

All types of wounds have certain treatment in common: they require control of bleeding; cleansing; closing of the skin; dressing for protection and immobilization to hasten healing and prevent or minimize infection. Many also need specific protection, as against lockjaw infections (tetanus). Immobilization must be emphasized for all wounds.

Prompt and proper care of wounds minimizes scar tissue, disability and complications.

Associated symptoms include the sensation of heat, throbbing, tenderness and pain.

Practical Pointers   1.   If the wound is a minor one, you can usually tell whether or not it will need stitches by the length and depth. (If it is OVER 1 IN. LONG AND GAPES OPEN, deeper layers of skin have been cut and surgical repair is indicated.) Lacerations can easily be treated at home but many people, not knowing the guidelines, become frightened at the bleeding and make unnecessary trips to their doctors.
2.   Over 80 percent of the bleeding associated with common injuries can easily be stopped with direct pressure on the site using a clean handkerchief or gauze pad. The use of tourniquets and pressure points in stemming blood flow generally went out of style at the end of World War II. Except for rare, serious injuries like the near severing of an arm or foot, they are seldom used today.

G42

3. The heart is a pump and the more excited you get the faster it pumps and the more blood escapes from a wound. Keep a cool head. Sit or lie down.

NOTE: Although the greatest frequency of wounds involve the face, hands and scalp, the information and treatment given can usually be applied to wounds elsewhere on the body. Because the scalp is usually covered with hair, however, scalp wounds are treated in a different manner when it comes to dressing. After the bleeding is controlled and the wound is cleansed, few need to have a dressing applied. Unsightly scar formation is less of a concern because the area is covered with hair. Also, because of the great vascularity of the skin in the scalp, the frequency of infections is much less than other wounds.

Treatment Tips 1. Apply direct pressure with any clean cloth available (handkerchief, gauze, towel) to control bleeding. Keep the pressure on for three minutes before you examine it again. (See Treatment Index, p. G86.)

2. If bleeding is not a problem, apply ice or cold water to minimize swelling. Ice in a plastic bag or ice cold soaks should be applied for 10 minutes. (See Treatment Index, p. G87.)

3. Wash the wound if it is dirty. Use clean water and some mild soap. Make sure that particles of dirt, sand, glass, etc. have been flushed out by running water on it for about five minutes. While cleansing, don't worry about a small amount of bleeding, as this helps to irrigate the wound and brings healing cells to the area. (See Symptom/Concept Index, p. G112–G113.)

4. If the wound is not gaping but the skin is not evenly closed, use butterfly closures and immobilize the area. (See Treatment Index, p. G84.)

5. Apply anti-bacterial ointment and dress the wound. (See Drug Index, p. G80.) Apply gentle pressure with roller gauze. Change dressing in 24 hours. (See Treatment Index, p. G84.)

6. To immobilize a cut finger or toe, tape it to an adjacent digit or use sufficient tape or a splint to keep the injured part from moving. (See Treatment Index, p. G104.)

Follow-up and Rehabilitation 1. Wounds should be kept dry, dressed, protected and immobilized for one week.

2. Dressings may be changed daily for both cosmetic and medical reasons.

When to Call the Doctor

1. Persistent bleeding and blood soaking through dressing.
2. Gaping wound. (Usually, if it is greater than 1 in. in length, deep tissues have been cut and sutures are needed.)
3. Temperature over 100°.
4. Numbness at a point below the wound.
5. Red streaks (lymphatic streaking associated with infection) radiating away from the wound.
6. Persistent and increasing pain at the site of the cut.
7. Inability to move a joint below the wound (this may indicate a cut or injured tendon).
8. Swollen nodes (lymph glands) in the leg, groin, armpit or neck.
9. If laceration is caused by a human or animal bite.
10. Wound is a puncture and lockjaw (tetanus) is a possibility (as in "dirty" outdoor wound, farm accident, etc.).

FINGER NAIL/TIP INJURY
Subungual Hematoma

Description A common injury that results when the tip of a finger gets slammed in a door is called the subungual hematoma. In nonmedical words, the fingernail gets black and blue and you have an intense throbbing pain in the finger tip.

The crushing causes bleeding under the nail and because both the nail and finger bone under it are hard, there is no soft tissue to absorb the pressure. The blood tumor (hematoma) that forms tries to push the nail away from the bone and an intense, throbbing pain results that can keep you awake all night. The blood usually forces its way back toward the body (proximal) end of the nail near the half moon (lunula).

Although the injury described above is the end result of slamming the finger (digit) in a door, other joint injuries and tendon injuries can result. One such injury results in the "mallet" finger in which the finger is cocked up like a piano mallet. In this condition you cannot straighten the finger tip and it hangs down in a position like a mallet in a piano. The extensor tendon has been torn loose and will require surgical repair.

Practical Pointers 1. A pinching or crushing injury of the finger or any other part of the body goes through the entire inflammatory reaction. The tissue progresses from white to red to black and blue, etc.

2. The decision as to whether or not the nail needs drilling is based on the amount of pain and the degree of discoloration. If pain is gradually increasing over a period of three or four hours and if the nail is about half purple, then drilling is indicated. NOTE: Although many people these days are reluctant to drill a fingernail, carpenters frequently do this when they accidentally whack their fingers with their hammers.

Treatment Tips 1. Cool the finger as soon as possible with crushed ice or cold compresses. (See Treatment Index, p. G87.)
2. Drill nail if indicated. (See Treatment Index, p. G98.)
The drilling is a painless procedure. The fingernail has no feeling in it and the blood has pushed the nail away from the bone so it won't hurt if you drill slowly and carefully and the patient's finger is firmly held.
3. When the hole is through the nail, use a handkerchief or piece of gauze dressing to absorb the blood. Cloth will act as a wick and absorb the fluid quickly with extreme relief of pain.
4. Put a gauze type Band-Aid (not one covered with Telfa, the "ouchless" dressing) over the nail for protection and continued absorption. Keep the nail covered for several days.

When to Call the Doctor 1. Drilling the nail does not seem feasible (no assistance available, patient is uncooperative, eyesight is poor, etc.).
2. If there is bony deformity that indicates fracture or dislocation.
3. Unusual amount of pain.
4. Pain persists after hematoma has been relieved.
5. Mallet finger deformity indicates damage to extensor tendon on back of finger.
6. Laceration of finger in addition to fingernail injury.
7. Finger tip is so badly swollen that drilling is difficult.

FOREIGN BODY
Foreign Objects in Hand, Arm, Foot

Description Various kinds of foreign objects can penetrate the skin and become imbedded. Examples are fishhooks, wood splinters, metal chips, glass fragments, thorns, buckshot and pieces of pencil lead. The most common sites for such foreign bodies are the hand, forearm and foot, but the general methods for care presented here can be applied to other parts of the body.

Usually such splinters and fragments remain close to the surface and can frequently be removed without a trip to the doctor. They cause irritation but usually do not incapacitate you or cause serious infections. Some, however, can cause infections eventually so some attempt should be made to extract them. If your attempts and later those of the physician are unsuccessful, however, no harm results in leaving them in the site. They will usually work their way out — and if not, few cause problems. Tiny particles in an arm or hand should not cause great concern. (Some former soldiers have carried shrapnel bits for decades without ill effect.)

Practical Pointers
1. Before extraction is attempted, scrub the skin surface carefully and sterilize the tweezers and needle over a flame or in boiling water.
2. If you can't see and feel the object easily, leave it alone and go to the doctor.
3. If a foreign object is deeply imbedded and can't be easily removed (such as a broken sewing machine needle in a finger, an ice pick or wire in a foot) then the object should be left in place and the extremity splinted to prevent further injury during transportation to the doctor.

Treatment Tips
1. Cleanse the surface around the entry site with soap and water.
2. Examine the injury carefully and determine by feeling and visual inspection the direction of entry and the depth of the foreign body.
3. Make the area numb with the help of an ice cube, then with the tip of a large needle (No. 10), slightly enlarge the puncture. This makes extraction easier.
4. Flick out the splinter or particle with the needle or grab it with the tweezers.
5. If the foreign body is a fishhook, another technique is used. (See Treatment Index, p. G99.)
6. After the extraction, cleanse the area again with soap and water and dress the wound. (See Treatment Index, p. G94.)
7. Immobilize the wound by splinting for one or two days. (See Treatment Index, p. G104–G105.)

Follow-up and 1. Change dressings daily as needed.
Rehabilitation 2. Hot soaks for 30 minutes one to three times daily while dressings are removed. (See Treatment Index, p. G94.)
3. Continue protective dressing for seven days.

When to Call 1. If foreign body is too deep for easy extraction.
the Doctor 2. If booster shot for tetanus is needed. The current recommendations of the American College of Surgeons is "a booster of absorbed tetanus toxoid every 10 years after the third initial injection or 10 years after an intervening wound booster."
3. Swelling of the affected part.
4. Red streaks (lymphatic streaking) radiating away from the wound.
5. Temperature over 100°.
6. Persistent and increasing pain at the site of the foreign body.
7. Swollen nodes (lymph glands) in the leg, groin, armpit or areas near the foreign body.

FOREIGN BODY IN EYE

Description Foreign bodies that get in the eye include dust, chips of paint, rust or wood, sand, bark and a wide variety of other irritating objects. Few people have managed to avoid this unpleasant experience.

The eye is acutely sensitive and responds by immediately sending tears to wash off the offending foreign substance.

The presence of the foreign body also usually causes spasm of the eyelid, pain and sensitivity to light.

The human eye is covered with several layers of specialized skin that regenerate rapidly if there is infection. The center of the eye over and around the pupil (cornea) also heals remarkably well in one to three days.

Practical 1. You may need an assistant to see the foreign
Pointers object. If it isn't readily visible, a flashlight illuminating the eye from the side may be helpful. (See Testing Index, p. G124.)
2. Prevention plays its usual role with this type of injury. The eyes should be protected by glasses when you are in dusty or windy places. Goggles should be used when working around

machines that throw out particles of sawdust, plastic chips or metal shavings.

3. Don't rub the eye. Rubbing usually only drives the foreign body deeper into the eye tissue making removal more difficult.

4. Ask your assistant to carefully wash his hands before examining your eye.

Treatment Tips NOTE: An assistant is needed to help you.

1. Wash out the eye thoroughly with cold water, then lie down and face ceiling.

2. If the offending object can be located, it can often be removed easily by touching it with the corner of a clean handkerchief while the victim is looking in the opposite direction and the lid is fixed.

3. If the foreign body is lodged beneath the upper lid, have assistant grasp the lashes of the lid between the thumb and forefinger and, while the victim looks down, pull the upper lid down and over the lower lid.

4. If the above maneuver doesn't work, depress the upper lid with a matchstick and "flip" the lid. (See Treatment Index, p. G99.)

Follow-up and Rehabilitation
1. Reduce your visual activities for 24 hours.
2. Protect your eye from bright light or sunlight by wearing sunglasses.

When to Call the Doctor
1. If foreign object cannot be removed easily with two or three attempts.
2. You have only one good eye.
3. History of previous corneal injury and known scarring.
4. Foreign object was impelled with high-speed impact from grinding wheel or high-speed equipment.

FRACTURED ANKLE

Description Fractures of the ankle are similar to those affecting the wrist. They may involve the lower end of the two bones of the lower leg, the fibula and tibia, or one of the six heel tarsal bones.

The most common fractures involve the tibia and fibula. Powerful twisting forces frequently fracture the outer (lateral) malleolus of the tibia. The sports injuries that may cause this fracture include trampoline accidents (see Symptom/Concept Index, p. G108) and skiing mishaps when the boot is too low.

Other accidents may, of course, cause similar fractures by the ankle twisting, being run over or hit by a heavy object.

Practical Pointers 1. As noted previously, sprained ankles tend to be underdiagnosed and undertreated. For that reason, I give very cautious advice about things that can be done at home. It is generally urged that after the basic first aid instructions are carried out, medical advice and X-rays should be obtained.

2. Prevention is often apparent only after the injury has occurred but proper sports equipment, general construction safety procedures and an extra ounce of care are worth reviewing while the pain is present!

Treatment Tips 1. Remove shoes and stockings.
2. Lie down with the foot elevated on a pillow or blanket.
3. Apply ice or cold compresses to minimize swelling. (See Treatment Index, p. G87.)
4. Have an assistant splint the ankle with towel or pillow or immobilize the entire lower leg and foot with splints. (See Treatment Index, p. G104–G105.)

When to Call the Doctor 1. Because of the difficulty in evaluating ankle injuries, it is RECOMMENDED THAT ALL SUCH INJURIES BE SEEN BY THE DOCTOR for advice and X-ray evaluation. During the transfer of the patient to medical help, ice or cold compresses should continue to be applied.

INSECT BITES/STINGS

Description The most painful and common insect bites are those caused by the yellow jacket, honey bee, hornet and wasp. The arrival of spring with its lush foliage and flowers signals the return of these bothersome neighbors of the insect world.

In a few people (estimated at 4 per 1,000), these stings may cause severe systemic reactions which, if left untreated, can lead to shock and even death. The persons most likely to have these severe reactions are those who have a history of asthma, hay fever or a family history of allergies. There is also a correlation between these reactions and patients who have had adverse reactions to penicillin, sulfa, etc.

The normal reaction includes the sharp pin prick that lasts several minutes followed by a small red area at the site, a whitish zone and an outside ring with a red flare. A welt forms and subsides in three or four hours. This is followed by irritation, itching and heat. Most traces of the sting are gone in 24 hours.

If a generalized systemic reaction does occur, it can begin with these symptoms: dry hacking cough followed by sense of tightening in the throat or chest, swelling and itching of nose, eyes, lips, sneezing, wheezing, rapid pulse, pallor or bluish color of skin and a sense of uneasiness.

Once established, the reaction can produce constriction of throat, shortness of breath, asthma, more intense bluish color of the skin, nausea, vomiting, diarrhea, chills, generalized hives, shock and loss of consciousness.

Practical Pointers
1. Prevention plays a key role with this type of injury. Some points to remember are:

(a)   If a bee or stinging insect approaches you, avoid sudden movements. Move away in a slow, deliberate manner.

(b)   Beware of blossoms and fermenting fruit in orchards. They are havens for yellow jackets.

(c)   Approach picnic areas with caution. Food left behind attracts not only flies but bees.

(d)   Never go barefoot outside. Bees and yellow jackets love ground clover.

(e)   Avoid bright colors, flowered prints, hair spray and especially perfume if you are going to be outside a lot.

(f)   Cover your body as much as possible when gardening or hiking near bees and similar insects.

2.   Prevention also necessitates the knowledge that:

(a)   Yellow jackets burrow in ground for their home.

(b)   Honey bees nest in caves or hollows in trees.

(c)   Wasps live in open comb nests in any protected place.

(d)   Hornets live in large oval hives that hang in trees or are nested under leaves.

Treatment Tips
1.   Remove the stinger, if possible, by scraping with a fingernail or knife blade.

2.   When the stinger is removed, wash the sting area thoroughly with soap and water.

3.   Apply meat tenderizer generously on a 4 in. x 4 in. gauze square or handkerchief and apply it to the site for 20 to 30 minutes. (See Treatment Index, p. G95–G96.)

4. If tenderizer is not available apply ice or cold compresses. (See Treatment Index, p. G87.)
5. Rest the injured part. Activity will spread the insect venom.
6. If itching persists apply baking powder/ammonia paste. (See Treatment Index, p. G97.)
7. For the next two or three days do not exert yourself to the point of becoming hot.
8. Take aspirin for relief of pain or itching. (See Drug Index, p. G78.)

When to Call the Doctor
1. If evidence of generalized systemic reaction:
(a) Swelling and itching of eyes, lips.
(b) Abdominal cramps or nausea, vomiting, diarrhea.
(c) Pallor or bluish skin, "shocky" appearance.
(d) Shortness of breath, wheezing, hoarseness.
(e) Loss of consciousness.
NOTE: If these complaints are noticed, it is essential that the spread of the bee venom be slowed by continuous ice or cold compresses to site and application of a tourniquet above the sting to slow lymphatic spread during trip to doctor. (See Treatment Index, p. G87.)
2. Past experience with bad reactions to stings.
3. Allergic problems with history of asthma or hay fever.
4. History of drug allergies such as penicillin or sulfa.
5. Family history of unusual sensitivities to insect stings.

SCIATICA
Disc Syndrome

Description A common back disorder labeled with such diverse names as disc trouble, lumbago, slipped disc, ruptured disc and even "hexenschuss" (a German word meaning witches' brew), sciatica occurs when the disc irritates nerves leaving the spinal cord in the lower end of the spinal column. The pain that results may radiate down the leg. (See Symptom/Concept Index, p. G115.)

Located between the bony vertebrae are semi-cartilaginous "shock absorbers" called intervertebral discs. After 20 years of age, it is normal for these discs to age and start to degenerate. The degree and rate of degeneration is related to amount of injury and general wear and tear that the spine has received.

Normally the vertebra have a sliding movement in six directions — forward, backward, laterally to the right and left and rotate a bit clockwise or counterclockwise. In most adults the ligaments that attach the vertebra to each other become stiffened and shortened and lose their normal elasticity. Some people such as those who practice yoga-like exercises maintain their normal spinal flexibility.

Unfortunately, such vertebral health is uncommon in most of the Western world and disc degeneration and damage to the paravertebral ligaments may cause disc syndrome. (See Symptom/Concept Index, p. G109–G110.)

Poor physical fitness, improper seating, bad posture, careless lifting habits, lack of training regarding helpful exercises and positions as taught in yoga, lead to disc disease and its related disabilities.

Practical Pointers
1. A key example of "body talk" is that associated with the disc syndrome. The distress is always provoked by certain positions, chairs, car seats or types of lifting. If you can "listen" to your body and avoid the provocative positions, much of the pain and resulting disability could be avoided. Keep a diary and log in the history of your backache. It may help you discover the causes of pain.

2. Sitting habits associated with poor chair design (especially those in most of today's cars) are the cause of much back trouble. Good chair design should include:

(a) Seat height 16 in. from floor (typical kitchen chair).

(b) Seat length 16 in. long.

(c) Tilt to chair back to at least 105° (most tilt only 90°) for more curve to lower spine.

(d) Moderate cushioning (not really soft).

(e) Open space beneath seat to allow sitter to curve legs inward.

(f) A bulge in chair back to give support to lower lumbar region (like a typist's chair).

3. Once reinjury has occurred, a commitment for special back exercises should be established with daily plan starting as soon as pain has disappeared. (See Treatment Index, p. G89–G91.)

Treatment Tips
1. Lie on firm mattress or thick rug in a position of comfort. Move around until more or less free of pain. One good rule is to rest with the painful side down and knees flexed a bit.

2. Limit activity and rest as much as possible for 24 to 48 hours until pain has subsided.

3. Take aspirin. (See Drug Index, p. G78.)

4. Splint the lower back with tape. (See Treatment Index, p. G106.) It will give some support and should be tried on the second or third day. (NOTE: Massage to the lower back and heat WON'T be of much help with the disc syndrome, which is of bony and internal origin, even though this type of physical therapy helps lower back strain which has a muscular and external origin rather than the disc disorder.)

Follow-up and Rehabilitation
1. Great care should be observed in sitting habits during recovery phases. Sit only on a kitchen chair.

2. Do daily exercises to improve mobility of vertebrae and increase strength of abdominal and back muscles. (See Treatment Index, p. G89–G92.)

3. Establish plan of general physical fitness such as biking, hiking or swimming. It is best to plan on a sport that you can do yourself at YOUR own time and YOUR own speed.

4. Sleep on a firm mattress.

5. Do moderate activity but no heavy work.

6. Take great caution in sitting habits and maintain good posture.

7. Get extra rest at night and if possible take a 20 minute rest period at noon lying on a floor or firm couch.

When to Call the Doctor
1. If pain in leg persists despite above treatment.

2. Numbness in leg persists.

3. History of frequent repeated attacks of disc syndrome.

SHOULDER/ELBOW PAIN OR STIFFNESS
Bursitis

Description This disorder may affect the weekend athlete, the housewife painting the ceiling, the elderly patient who tackles a long distance automobile drive and others for various reasons. The cause is soft tissue injury of the shoulder or elbow. Although replete with many names such as bursitis, subdeltoid bursitis, tennis elbow, bartender's elbow, painter's shoulder or golfer's elbow, a common name could be "overuse syndrome."

Rather than focusing on the specific sport or action, it is more useful to think of the motion that is involved — jumping, throwing, serving, painting. Even if there is no underlying

G53

systemic disorder, several insistent forces may put the squeeze on you — the normal aging process, improper conditioning and warm-up, pre-existing defects and old injuries that can cause calcium deposits.

Frequently, in addition to the pain and limitation of motion that results, these disorders may cause an accumulation of fluid in the joint that can be removed by your doctor.

Associated complaints are arthritis, loss of sleep and loss of muscle strength.

Practical Pointers
1. The pain in both shoulder and elbow types of bursitis is characteristic in that even the slightest move will cause you intense distress.
2. The bursitis swelling can at times be large and visible.
3. Pain begins to taper off in five days.
4. Prevention from the next attack should start with the current attack. If a certain activity, motion or grip triggered the pain, it should be avoided or altered. (EXAMPLES: If the tennis overhead smash caused the trouble, stick to the less strenuous ground strokes; if the crawl causes pain, do the breaststroke; if a long drive in the car did it, try a higher car seat.)
5. Warm-up periods with stretching of muscles. Range of motion of joint are preventive for some.
6. A good motto to follow: "If it doesn't hurt, do it — but don't be a hero!"

Treatment Tips
1. Relax completely with the arm resting on a pillow or in a triangle sling until the pain becomes more bearable.
2. Apply cold compresses or ice the first day to minimize swelling. (See Treatment Index, p. G87.)
3. Take aspirin for pain. (See Drug Index, p. G78.)
4. On second day apply wet heat. (See Treatment Index, p. G94.)
5. Gentle massage is useful for limbering up the stiff muscles and the joint after an attack has subsided. Massage should always be done toward the heart and be stopped if it causes pain.

Follow-up and Rehabilitation
1. As soon as the acute episode is over, isometric exercises should be started for muscles around the involved joint. These exercises strengthen your muscles by setting them firmly and then relaxing them with little or no movement of joints.
2. After you resume normal sports activity, take a warm bath

or shower immediately after each active session. Don't let
your muscles stiffen by lolling around in the locker room.
3. Some practical exercises for the shoulder and elbow are
important. (See Treatment Index, p. G92–G94.)
4. Massage before exercise will help the tight-jointed aging
athlete. It should be used both before and after exercise.

When to Call 1. If pain isn't substantially less in two or three days.
the Doctor Bursitis usually subsides in five days and attacks that last
longer may be due to tendonitis.
2. If swelling of the joint is a problem. The doctor may have
to tap the joint and drain out the fluid.
3. History of previous and repeated attacks of bursitis.

SPRAINED ANKLE

Description Sprains occur when the tissues around the ankle joint are torn
or overstretched through stress during athletics, work,
recreation or other activity.

A sprain is damage to the ligament or joint capsule during
a twisting fall. In the most common (athletic) injury a person
running forward may find his foot caught or fixed in a position
with the toe pointing inward (inversion). Then, as he falls, the
body weight moves suddenly outward (laterally) putting great
stress on the joint and causing the ligaments to tear. (See
Symptom/Concept Index, p. G108.)

Associated symptoms include pain, swelling, redness and,
a day or so later, black-blue discoloration.

Practical 1. Sprained ankles tend to be UNDERDIAGNOSED and
Pointers UNDERTREATED. This can lead to a lifelong disability that
includes limping, unstable ankle ("I sprain my ankle every
time I turn around."), difficulty in walking on rough terrain,
foot pain and swollen ankles.
2. Prevention is the key to treatment. In athletic endeavors
(football, baseball, soccer, rugby, lacrosse) that have often
resulted in ankle injuries, a swivel shoe (the Swivler™
available from Wolverine World Wide, Inc. of Rockford, MI.)
has proved to be protective, reducing such injuries by
approximately half.
3. If you hear a "popping" sound or feel something give
way, it is usually a sign that a tear has occurred in the
ligament.

G55

Treatment Tips 1.   Ice the ankle or apply cold applications immediately. (See Treatment Index, p. G87.) This reduces the swelling and stops the bleeding in the joint. The icing should be continued for one hour.
2.   Next, immobilize the ankle by elevating it on two or three pillows for 24 hours with a cold wet towel wrapped around it.
3.   Use crutches when upright. DON'T PUT ANY WEIGHT ON THE ANKLE.
4.   There are two schools of medical thought governing the care of sprains. The treatment selected should be decided by your doctor following examination.
(a)   Early weight bearing: It is better to cast unnecessarily than to undertreat and risk chronic problems. A cast is applied or basket weave tape splint put on. The patient is put on crutches for three weeks with a program of exercises. When the cast or tape splint (see Treatment Index, p. G106) is removed, an elastic wrapping is used for another week or so.
(b)   Nonweight bearing: The patient stays off the foot completely for mild sprain (one week) or moderate sprain (two weeks) with ankle wrapped by elastic bandage. The bandage is rewound and tightened three times daily and worn night and day until the swelling is gone. On the third day, a program of exercises and physical therapy is started.

Follow-up and 1.   The rehabilitation routine will vary depending on the
Rehabilitation severity of the injury and the method of management.
2.   Hot soaks for 15 minutes twice daily and massage to the ankle will hasten recovery. (See Treatment Index, p. G94.)
3.   During recovery the patient should avoid wearing high heeled shoes.
4.   During hunting or hiking on rough ground ankle-supporting boots should be worn to minimize reinjury.

When to Call Because of the difficulty in evaluating ankle injuries
the Doctor (see comments above in "Practical Pointers"), it is RECOMMENDED THAT ALL SUCH INJURIES BE SEEN BY A DOCTOR. The severity of the sprain often bears no relation to the severity of the complications.

SPRAINED BACK
Backache

Description A sprained back causes pain along or beside the spinal

G56

column, but not down into the legs. The presence of leg pain points to sciatica (disc syndrome) covered earlier.

The patient usually reports the back injury as coming from a twisting or straining, without direct trauma such as being hit or tackled in football. At other times, there may be no recollection of a twisting effort and the pain is related as "the way I slept" or "it happened when I bent over to tie my shoe." You may also believe it occurred after sitting for a long time at a meeting.

Whatever the cause, the back — a very complicated structure with 140 muscles attached to 26 articulated bones separated by cartilage, discs and scores and scores of ligaments — is prone to give pain when mistreated. The bones (vertebrae) are like a radio or TV tower of building blocks held upright by guy wires. (See Symptom/Concept Index, p. G109–G110.) The muscles and ligaments become stretched, torn or shortened and pain begins.

Associated symptoms are pain, spasm, fatigue, muscle aches, tingling, tender spots and irritability and tension.

Practical Pointers
1. Backache is a prime example of "body talk" (see Symptom/Concept Index, p. G109–G110) because it results after months or years of back abuse — inadequate exercise, poor lifting habits, improper posture, faulty chairs or car seats, and so on. This disorder can be prevented 90 percent of the time by timely exercise — when the back feels GOOD, BEFORE the pain.

2. Although there are 28 million Americans with backache, it is unfortunate that almost all of the emphasis on exercise is aimed at competitive and recreational sports. Little time is spent on skills for backache prevention like yoga exercises (see Treatment Index, p. G89–G91), Dr. Kenneth M. Cooper's AEROBICS exercises, or the therapy methods of Dr. Arthur Michele in his book ORTHOTHERAPY.

3. Backache, occasionally confused with sprained back, may at times be caused by a urinary tract infection but there will usually be other symptoms such as abnormal frequency, pain on urination or blood in the urine.

Treatment Tips
1. Rest on a firm bed or on the floor (preferably with a thick rug) in a position that gives the greatest relief of pain and comfort. "Listen" to your back and move around until you are quite comfortable. (If props of pillows or blankets are helpful, please use them.) If you have a soft or sagging bed use a

bedboard (¾ in. plywood) under the mattress for extra
support. Stay in bed for 24 hours.
2.   Use aspirin as needed. (See Drug Index, p. G78.)
3.   Apply heat several times daily. This relaxes the muscles of
the neck and back. (See Treatment Index, p. G94.) After heat,
use gentle massage.
4.   After the first day, with the pain subsiding, splint the back
with tape. (See Treatment Index, p. G106.) Keep the tape on
three or four days (longer if possible). Keep the tape dry.
5.   After the first day, sit only on a straight KITCHEN CHAIR for
the rest of the week. All low, overstuffed easy chairs and most
car seats are to be avoided.

Follow-up and   1.   After seven days, normal activity may be resumed
Rehabilitation   — with caution.
2.   Gentle stretching exercises should be started — if they do
not produce too much pain. (See Treatment Index,
p. G89–G91.)
3.   Good posture should be practiced carefully.
4.   Avoid fatigue or heavy lifting for the next two weeks.
5.   Choose the type of chair you sit on with great care.

When to Call   1.   Substantial pain persists after two days of above
the Doctor   treatment.
2.   Pain radiates down leg or into shoulder or arm.
3.   Associated symptoms of urinary tract infection.
4.   Other symptoms such as associated with gynecologic (or
female) problems or abdominal pain.
5.   History of previous repeated back problems including
"disc trouble."
6.   Industrial or on the job injury covered by Workman's
Compensation Insurance.
7.   You are pregnant.
8.   Sports injury in which team doctor must offer special
examination and prepare a report.

9 MOST COMMON EMERGENCIES

This section of your Self-Help Medical Guide is aimed at what you can do to help OTHER persons when they are the victims of illness, injury or intoxication. In these common emergencies the emphasis is not on treatment but recognition of possible causes of the problem and appropriate actions to protect the victim while arranging for proper medical help.

ABDOMINAL PAIN

Description Abdominal pain, stomachache, bellyache — whatever you may call it — can be divided into one of three categories: (1) an acute abdomen, potentially an emergency that requires immediate action; (2) a chronic organic condition; or (3) nervous stomach (functional disorder).

Categorization would be much simpler if pain and tenderness were always felt over or at the anatomical site of the trouble, but such is not usually the case. Pain may start at the site but then shift (radiate) elsewhere through complex pain pathways making it difficult to unravel not only for the patient but also the physician.

The type of pain can be a helpful guide and probably gives more information than the location of the pain. The general burning pain of a perforated peptic ulcer contrasts with the sharp, breath-taking pain of gall bladder (biliary) colic. (Colic is a pain that comes for a while and then subsides in a regular pattern.) The gripping pain of intestinal obstruction differs from the tearing sensation of a ballooning of the wall of the abdominal aorta (aneurysm). The increasingly severe right lower abdominal ache of acute appendicitis can be differentiated from the constant ache of kidney infection (pyelonephritis).

The origin of abdominal pain is complex. In the walls and

linings of the stomach, intestines and various organs in the abdomen, there is no sensation of touch as in the skin. It is possible to crush, tear or cut intestine without the patient feeling pain — but if you stretch or balloon them up (distention), severe pain is produced.

Referred pain — pain that originates in one part of the abdomen but is felt in another more distant site — follows rather complicated patterns. It is helpful to understand the origin of the various organs (embryologic development) in order to explain the pathways involved. An example of referred pain is that associated with the gall bladder. Although the gall bladder is in the FRONT under the ribs on the right side of the abdomen, the pain may be felt in the back under the right shoulder blade. (See Symptom/Concept Index, p. G116–G117.)

In evaluating abdominal pain, the history and details of the pain are most important. Laboratory tests and X-rays can be most helpful, but the story you tell your doctor is usually the key to the decision as to whether the pain may require immediate hospitalization — perhaps surgery — or whether the body talk means it is another type of disorder.

These self-help instructions for abdominal pain will give you insight into the possible causes of pain so that appropriate medical consultation can be more effective.

Practical Pointers
1. Describing pain is difficult. Pain scares people and hurts enough to make it difficult to describe. If it has never happened before, there is no baseline to compare it with. Much also depends on your physical self-awareness, degree of articulateness and pain threshold. It may be difficult under the misery of the situation, but an exact description is often vital. Your goal should be better than that frequent complaint, "Oh, Doctor, it just hurts ALL OVER!"

2. There are four types of pain: cramps, constant ache, intermittent colicky pain and constant colicky pain. (See Symptom/Concept Index, p. G116–G117.)

Cramps are short-term, poorly localized and episodic. When mild they are probably insignificant. The most common cause is stomach flu (gastroenteritis). Cramps may be associated with nausea, vomiting, faintness, even mild panic which may be more upsetting than the pain itself.

Constant ache means pain that steadily rises in intensity. It is comparable to a toothache. An example is the pain caused by a swollen, inflamed gall bladder. It may also suggest a chronically swollen condition such as pancreatic disease.

Intermittent colicky pain increases to a maximum, then it suddenly relents. After an entirely PAIN FREE INTERVAL, that may be short or long, the cycle is repeated. This may be associated with mechanical obstruction of the intestine.

Constant colicky pain has a variable degree of intensity but there is ALWAYS SOME PAIN PRESENT. It comes in waves of pain and is typically observed in obstruction secondary to kidney or gall bladder stones.

3.   What makes the pain worse or causes it?

(a)   Eating: Probably the most significant feature of the pain associated with peptic ulcer is its tendency to occur one to four hours after meals. The pain can be present day after day for weeks and months.

Distress three to five hours after eating, once or twice monthly may be due to gall bladder disease.

Pain within minutes after eating may be caused by reduced size of the stomach. Diseases to be considered are cancer of the stomach, hernia of the stomach (hiatal hernia), inflammation of the stomach wall (gastritis) and similar problems.

(b)   Specific food problems: Fatty foods such as butter, salad dressings, rich pork, etc. can cause gall bladder tenderness and pain. Roughage from fresh vegetables or fruit can cause or aggravate lower abdominal pain in people with diverticulitis or irritable colon. Food allergies also may trigger gastrointestinal irritation.

(c)   Bowel movement or passage of gas: If lower abdominal pain is relieved by a bowel movement (defecation) a functional disorder such as nervous or irritable colon may be present. Some painful conditions may be started by excessive use of laxatives. One classic example is appendicitis.

(d)   Breathing: Pain that is aggravated by deep breathing suggests disease of the diaphragm muscles separating the chest from the abdomen. Examples of this are inflammation of the gall bladder (cholecystitis) or rupturing (perforating) stomach ulcer.

(e)   Physical effort: Definite positional relationship of pain exists with a sliding hiatal hernia. Pain occurs when you lie down at night and is relieved when you get up and walk around. Pain following a jolting ride in a car or after riding on a horse suggests a kidney or gallstone.

(f)   Nervousness: Intense pain is more frequently caused by serious organic disease while milder pain is commonly due to nervous (functional) disorders. Close relationship of pain to emotional distress is a good clue that the classification is functional. (NOTE: The final diagnosis of FUNCTIONAL gastrointestinal disease must be based on the exclusion of organic illness and requires careful evaluation by your doctor.)

Treatment Tips   1.   Limit all fluid intake to ice chips or small sips of water.
2.   Assume a position of comfort and rest quietly (in bed if possible).
3.   Do not take a laxative or enema.

When to Call the Doctor   1.   After a pattern of pain, intensity and history of possible causes have been observed and recorded.
2.   When temperature has been taken and recorded. (See Testing Index, p. G126–G127.)
3.   When blood pressure and pulse are noted. (See Testing Index, p. G119–G122.)

CONVULSION

Description   Convulsions or fits involve involuntary twitchings of muscle groups and usually unconsciousness. A shaking tremor may involve the whole body or only a part and last for a few seconds or minutes. The unconsciousness may range from moments of confusion to a deep sleep from which the person awakens in four or five minutes with little or no knowledge of what happened.

Convulsions are most frequently seen in children in association with high fever. Various forms of epilepsy such as GRAND MAL (big seizure) and PETIT MAL (little seizure) are also fairly common.

Convulsions, in themselves, rarely produce death. The principal hazards are associated with injuries to mouth or head during the seizure, especially if the person falls near a busy street or in a crowded subway. It is then possible for severe injury or death to result.

Practical 1. The most important priority is to prevent the patient
Pointers from being injured on surrounding objects.

2. Convulsions may occur in children, especially those under three years of age, if there is a high fever. In these youngsters the brain's heat regulating mechanism has not been completely developed. The children cannot sweat as easily as older children and adults in order to lose the heat generated from the infection. In addition, if these children are all bundled up in tight sleepers and covered with blankets, they can get such dangerously high fevers in a few hours that fever (febrile) convulsions occur. A practical preventive measure is to dress them in loose summer-weight pajamas when fever is detected.

If the fever persists or a convulsion is in progress or has been witnessed and is over, a cooling bath is urgently needed (see Treatment Index, p. G87–G88) and aspirin is indicated (see Drug Index, p. G78).

Convulsions may be self-limiting or indicate more serious problems.

3. Time the length of the convulsion if possible.

4. Examine the patient for medical card or ID tag to see if he is a known epileptic. Do this preferably in front of a witness so that you are legally covered and not accused of theft! Check victim's belongings for medication.

5. Look for evidence of injury.

Treatment Tips 1. The crucial first step is to assure that the victim has an adequate airway. An effective airway can often be maintained by rolling patient on side. (See Treatment Index, p. G101.) Clear mouth of vomitus.

2. If there is any evidence of injury or laceration, apply local treatment as indicated.

3. Make the victim as comfortable as possible.

4. Keep curiosity seekers away.

When to Call 1. As soon as an adequate airway has been
the Doctor established, AN EMERGENCY CALL SHOULD BE PLACED for the rescue squad.

2. If a doctor's name is known or can be identified from personal effects, the doctor should be called.

3. Any useful medical information that has been observed should be written down, if possible, and given to the rescue squad for use by doctors at the emergency room.

HEART ATTACK
Chest and Heart Pain

Description The first few hours are the most critical in dealing with a heart attack. The majority of patients who die from acute heart attacks, do so within the first hours (one to three) according to studies from the United States and Scotland.

Most heart experts agree that ignorance of symptoms and inappropriate self-treatment cause delays that are deadly. People are usually aware of the classic symptoms of heart attack: nausea, clammy skin, difficulty in breathing, pain in chest that radiates into the left arm and perhaps irregularity of heartbeat. Unfortunately, those classic signs are present in only 60 to 70 percent of the cases. At least 30 percent or more don't have those characteristic features.

To further complicate matters, a great many people with chest pain don't have heart attacks, but muscular chest pain, stomach ulcers, heart pain from angina, imaginary pains or problems such as biliary spasm, hiatal hernia or anxiety states.

In possible heart attacks, the need to get help within the early critical hours is uppermost. INAPPROPRIATE SELF-TREATMENT must be minimized. Valuable time is lost as people treat their "indigestion" with antacids and their "constipation" with laxatives instead of getting PROMPT CARE AT THE HOSPITAL. Getting to the hospital quickly and the prompt transfer to a coronary care unit whenever heart attack is suspected may save your life.

Practical Pointers 1. Prevention is the key to treatment, especially in coronary heart disease. Overwhelming evidence shows that before the heart attack, the scene was set with high cholesterol levels, high blood pressure, physical inactivity, excessive cigarette smoking, obesity and behavioral predisposition (the Type A personality). The "Type A" is described by experts as "continually under pressure for time" — one who converts life events, responsibilities and social situations into stress.

2. Several conditions that cause chest pain also give symptoms similar to a heart attack; they are the angina of coronary heart disease, gall bladder spasm, hiatal hernia and anxiety states. A table of symptoms has been prepared

to highlight the important differences. (See Symptom/Concept Index, p. G113–G114.)

3. If the above conditions seem to present a clear pattern, then appropriate medical advice is indicated. However, if there is still uncertainty, the following 13-Step Screening Quiz should be used:

13-Step Screening Quiz

Step 1 Place tip of index finger over center of chest discomfort and estimate distance (inches) from centerline of chest (draw an imaginary line from belly button to Adam's apple). If tip is 2 in. or less go to STEP 2.

Step 2 Is the discomfort BELOW or ABOVE the nipple?
If pain is above or even with nipple, go to STEP 3.
COMMENT: Pain BELOW nipple and to the LEFT is RARELY HEART pain.

Step 3 Is the discomfort between nipple and centerline?
If yes, go to STEP 4.
COMMENT: If pain is localized COMPLETELY to the LEFT, it is LESS LIKELY to be the heart.

Step 4 Do you feel discomfort on the right side of chest?
If yes, go to STEP 5.
COMMENT: Pain on BOTH SIDES of chest is MORE LIKELY to be from the HEART.

Step 5 Is discomfort "dull" pressure or a squeezing sensation "under the necktie"? If yes, go to STEP 6.
COMMENT: If pain is "sharp" you can usually be assured the pain is NOT that of a heart ATTACK.

Step 6 Is discomfort continuous? If yes, go to STEP 7.
COMMENT: If pain COMES and GOES it is probably NOT your HEART.

Step 7 How long does discomfort last? If it lasts 5 to 10 minutes, go to STEP 8.
COMMENT: If pain lasts only a FEW SECONDS, it is probably NOT heart. If pain lasts 1 to 5 minutes, it is probably ANGINA, NOT heart ATTACK.

Step 8 Does discomfort go up into neck or jaws? Is discomfort in arms? If yes to neck and jaws go to STEP 11. If yes to arms, go to STEP 9.

Step 9 Is discomfort on outside of arm? If yes, go to STEP 10. Distress on INSIDE of arm is HEART ATTACK SYMPTOM, go to STEP 11.
COMMENT: With pain in OUTSIDE of arm, it is NOT LIKELY from HEART.

Step 10 To further evaluate arm discomfort, raise it above your head. If painful, STOP.
COMMENT: This type of pain is MOST LIKELY that of BURSITIS or shoulder ARTHRITIS.

Step 11 Are you sweating with the discomfort? If yes, go to STEP 12.
COMMENT: Pain associated with SWEATING suggests a HEART ATTACK.

Step 12 Is your discomfort worse while lying down? If yes, go to STEP 13. If MORE COMFORTABLE lying down, LESS likely to be HEART.

Step 13 CALL DOCTOR
COMMENT: It is quite likely you NEED MEDICAL EVALUATION. You have ruled out most of the less serious problems that give chest pain.

When to Call
the Doctor
1. If the pain has persisted more than 15 minutes, ask someone to take you to the nearest hospital. If no one is there to help you, call the rescue squad. DO NOT DRIVE THE CAR YOURSELF. Lie down and rest.
2. Ask the emergency room nurse to call your doctor.
3. Tell the emergency room nurse that you may be having a heart attack. Insist on going to the CORONARY CARE UNIT (CCU) — even if you only SUSPECT a heart attack. This kind of insistence may be difficult in a busy emergency room where the staff can get "immune" to "emergencies," but do your best! Anxiety and anger on your part is dangerous, but so is lying there with heart rhythm abnormalities (see next section).

The above 13-Step Screening Quiz is a modification of a longer telephone screening quiz developed by Dr. Glenn O. Turner, a cardiologist from Springfield, MO. It has been used by him and his staff in Southwestern Missouri since 1971. In MEDICAL OFFICE STAFF (Nov.–Dec., 1974), Dr. Turner said, "Probably 95% of all phone complaints about non-ischemic, harmless chest discomfort can be conclusively identified as such."

Dr. Turner has pioneered in public education programs on the early warning signs of heart attack and his ideas have been adopted in a number of other states and communities.

HEART RHYTHM ABNORMALITY

Description An arryhthmia is an irregular heart rhythm. Instead of the regular, metronome-like beat that would sound like lub-dub, lub-dub, lub-dub, a heart with an arryhthmia might sound like lub-lub-dub, lub-dub, lub-lub-lub-dub.

The basic flaw is a conduction disturbance. The finely tuned electrical circuit in the heart develops a short circuit and sets up a chain of events that can lead all the way from mild inconvenience (palpitations) to sudden death (ventricular fibrillation).

There are a whole series of specific arryhthmias that have complex names, among them: premature atrial contractions, supraventricular tachycardias, A-V conduction impairment or heart block.

The specific details of these complex medical names are usually only known by heart specialists (cardiologists) after detailed studies that include electrocardiograms, careful histories and detailed physical exams. They may also require portable monitoring of the heart rhythm. This involves wearing a five-pound portable electrocardiograph (ECG) such as the Holter system (manufactured by Del Mar Engineering Labs of Los Angeles) for up to 24 hours. The typical cost to you for this service is about $90.00.

Practical Pointers
1. Typically, an arryhthmia will make you feel like your heart is "turning over" in your chest or "running away." However, it is known that about half of the patients with arryhthmia are without this type of classic symptom.
2. Dizzy spells or lightheadedness will occur, particularly when changing position from sitting or lying down to an upright posture.
3. Fainting spells or marked mental confusion for several minutes may indicate arryhthmia.
4. One type of arryhthmia, bradycardia (slow heart), is frequently observed if you have a very slow pulse — less than 60 beats per minute.

G67

5. Some heart medications such as digitalis and its various cousins can cause arryhthmias.

6. Conditions such as hyperactive thyroid (hyperthyroidism) or low blood potassium (from too much diuretic) and low grade infections can cause arryhthmias.

7. Adverse drug interaction may cause you to be extra sensitive to digitalis. This can happen with phenobarbital (a common sedative), Dilantin (taken for epilepsy), phenylbutazone (an arthritis medication) and antithyroid prescriptions.

8. After your doctor has determined the exact diagnosis and you have had the irregularity several times without serious problems, you will be less anxious when they occur — although you may need reassurance.

Treatment Tips Avoid cardiac stimulants such as caffeine (coffee, tea and cola drinks) and nicotine (all forms of tobacco). Ephedrine and its "cousins" (most types of cold tablets and syrups) must be avoided.

When to Call the Doctor 1. All patients with arryhthmias should be carefully evaluated by a doctor with the consulting advice of a specialist in cardiology or internal medicine.

2. If you are taking digitalis of some type and have nausea, loss of appetite, bizarre changes in your vision ("seeing through cracked glass") or mental confusion, consult with your doctor.

3. If you are anxious and need reassurance from him about the present episode.

POISONING

Description Poisoning can occur when solids, liquids or gases known to impair health or cause death are taken into the body or enter through the skin surface.

Children under the age of five are especially common poisoning victims because they are curious and tend to put into their mouths and taste, eat or drink nearly everything they pick up. Adults, however, are also subject to poisoning through accidental ingestion or injection, suicide attempts, industrial or occupational exposures and other causes.

The following are the most frequent causes of poisoning.

1. Overdoses of aspirin taken by children.

2. Medicines not properly controlled with safety caps or storage and left by careless parents to be ingested by young children or teenagers.

3. Use of poisons such as cleaning solvents, gasoline, kerosene or weed killers that were transferred from original containers and stored in soft drink bottles.

4. Improper use and mixing of volatile solvents and pesticides, insecticides and weed killers.

5. Combining of drugs and alcohol.

6. Ingestion of poisonous plants and nonedible mushrooms.

7. Careless taking of prescriptions from medicine chest with illegible instructions or confusing dose on labeling.

Poisoning can be prevented in nearly all situations by better supervision, informed handling, education of children regarding the hazards of various compounds and chemicals, careful storage (if you have young children in the house, regularly "childproof" the house for all substances that could cause trouble), and care in use of prescription drugs. (Don't keep medicines, including iron pills, on the kitchen table and NEVER take medicine in front of young children: they learn to copy your actions.)

The symptoms and signs vary according to the poison. They may range from an unconscious person, one in a stuporous or dazed condition to one that is irritable, jittery or even affected by violent convulsive movements.

There are a wide variety of contact poisons from plants (poison ivy, poison oak) and marine life (Portuguese man-of-war, jellyfish, scorpion fish and surgeon fish) that can cause serious trouble. These are not common, however, and are not discussed in this general section. Seek local medical advice.

Practical Pointers
1. History, related circumstances and significant objects near the victim are of vital importance. Such things as remnants of food, used drinking glasses, medicine bottles, cans and other containers may provide clues to the nature of the poison. Keep such objects in a safe place for the experts. Accident, suicide or even murder may be involved and legal questions may have to be answered.

2. The victim's breath may give a valuable clue. Such well-known odors as alcohol, kerosene, turpentine or acetone (as in fingernail polish remover) should be noted and recorded.

3. If the scene of the poisoning is a closed room, open the windows and doors as quickly and safely as possible.
4. Note lips and mouth for evidence of burns that could come from caustic poisons such as lye (found in drain cleaners).
5. Note the eyes for evidence of morphine or similar drugs that cause pinpoint size pupils.

Treatment Tips 1. Since the most common and serious poisoning results from toxic substances ingested by mouth, the first objective in treatment is to dilute or neutralize the poison as quickly as possible by diluting poison with water or milk. Check for SPECIFIC antidotes on the LABEL of poison container.
2. Next, it is important to induce vomiting — EXCEPT when caustic alkaline poisons such as drain cleaner are swallowed, the victim is unconscious or having convulsions, petroleum products such as gasoline or kerosene were used, or a strong acid such as toilet-bowl cleaner is involved. Vomiting can be induced by tickling the back of the victim's throat with your finger or giving nauseating fluid such as syrup of ipecac (see Drug Index p. G77)or universal antidote or a mixture of mustard and water. (NOTE: When poisoning victim vomits, position the person on side with mouth lower than chest so vomited material will not reenter airway and cause more trouble.) (See Treatment Index, p. G101.)
3. Maintain breathing and pulse while help is coming. Check and record breathing and pulse rates and give information to rescue squad or the health professional (see Treatment Index, p. G101–104.)
4. Call Poison Control Center, report problem and ask for advice and rescue squad.

When to Call the Doctor All patients who are poisoning victims should be carefully evaluated by a doctor. Arrange for transportation to the nearest hospital immediately.

PSYCHIATRIC PROBLEM

Description There are several common acute psychiatric emergencies. These are associated with alcohol, psychedelic drugs, schizophrenia, acute manic states and depression. The danger may be real, imaginary — or somewhere in between.
    The most common "emergency" is the difficult drunk. The

drunk is too agitated to sleep it off and lacks the judgment to keep quiet. Other frequent types of emergencies caused by alcohol include: D.T.'s (delirium tremons) which can cause death in 10 percent of uncomplicated cases to 25 percent in patients with medical or surgical complications; ALCOHOLIC HALLUCINATIONS where the patient hears voices or ALCOHOLIC PARANOIA when the person can have full-scale delusions and take such paranoid action that violence results.

Psychedelic or mind-changing drugs such as LSD, marijuana, amphetamines and narcotics can produce delirium, confusion and various other types of emergencies.

A confrontation with a paranoid schizophrenic can be a frightening experience. Ordinary rules of logic do not follow and behavior is completely irrational — the classic picture of a crazy person. Although they can be dangerous, this is fortunately the exception rather than the rule.

A patient afflicted with acute mania also exhibits a madness or deranged behavior. They usually speak grandiosely, of "big plans." They may seem sensible at times, but have a nervous restlessness about them.

Depression, probably the most common of all the psychiatric emergencies, except alcohol intoxication, is the easiest to miss. It may be readily apparent, as in the grief associated with the loss of a loved one, or hidden, such as the usual depression of middle age. The possibility of suicide in all these melancholic patients must not be overlooked.

Practical Pointers
1. If a person is a known alcoholic and is disoriented and seeing things (hallucinating) he is a likely candidate for delirium tremons.

2. A person with alcoholic hallucinosis may switch back and forth between normal behavior and states of visual and auditory hallucinations.

3. Victims of acute excitement (maniacs) have a characteristic rush of speech and a restless state that makes it hard for them to sit down for any length of time.

4. In addition to the brooding sadness frequently noted in depressives, there may also be a history of increasing insomnia (with reversal of sleep/wake patterns), loss of appetite, diminished sex drive and other physical complaints. Depressions, called the "common cold" of mental illness, are seen in all age groups. Suicide attempts are common emergencies connected with this state.

G71

Treatment Tips 1. A general rule is to remain calm and get the agitated person to a hospital as soon as possible.
2. A person on a marijuana high can frequently be brought back to a normal state of mind by a hot shower.
3. If a suicide attempt is encountered, "talking down" may be attempted while professional help is on the way. The method should involve nonthreatening, supportive talk. Establish empathy through some common bonds, if they can be established. Identify the problem, if possible, and encourage low key discussion about it.
4. If a person becomes berserk or violent, he may need to be restrained. A good rule of thumb for this is four men per patient. The more help available the less likely they are to resist.

When to Call the Doctor In most cases AID SHOULD BE REQUESTED as soon as possible. Because of the nature of most of these conditions, the special facilities of an emergency room or hospital are required. "Detox" (detoxification) Units are trained to handle the alcohol and drug problems mentioned and the Psychiatric Ward is needed for the mental patients.

SHOCK

Description Shock is a condition resulting in a depressed state of many vital body functions. It can be life threatening if it is not properly handled.

There are several types of shock: traumatic shock from injury, electrical shock, insulin shock, shock from types of infections and other forms of shock.

Causes include blood loss, loss of body fluids (after prolonged vomiting, diarrhea or burns), heart attack or stroke and poisoning by chemicals, gases, alcohol or drugs.

The degree of shock may be altered by body temperature, age, general resistance of the victim (that is, his ability to handle stress), pain, rough handling of the patient and delay in treatment.

Practical Pointers 1. In the early stages of shock, the skin is pale or bluish and cold to the touch. Victims with dark skin will show pallor of nail beds and the mucous membrane of the eyelids.
2. As the condition progresses, the skin becomes moist and clammy.

G72

3. The victim will report general weakness.

4. The pulse is rapid (over 100 beats per minute). If it is too weak to be felt at the wrist, the pulse may be felt on the artery at the angle of the jaw or heard at the apex of the heart with a stethoscope. (See Testing Index, p. G124–G125.)

5. The rate of breathing is usually increased (over 20 breaths per minute). (See Testing Index, p. G122.) It may also be irregular in rhythm with some deep sighing.

6. The victim may feel nauseated and vomit.

7. As the condition worsens, three serious signs appear.

(a) The skin becomes mottled and blanched.

(b) The pupils become enlarged (dilated).

(c) The victim becomes apathetic and at times unresponsive.

Treatment Tips
1. Check on airway. If there is mucus or vomitus, remove it. Lie patient on side to maintain safe position. (See Treatment Index, p. G101.)

2. Keep the patient lying down. This keeps blood flowing to the brain and other vital centers. Elevate legs 10 to 12 in. on folded blanket or other prop.

3. Cover the victim only enough to keep him from losing body heat. Cover him where he lies unless it is necessary to move him away from danger, protect him from further injury or provide other urgent first aid care.

4. If rescue squad or medical care is delayed for an hour or more, fluids may be given by mouth. The best drink is a salt-soda solution. (See Treatment Index, p. G97–G98.) Give one-half glass or 4 oz. every 15 minutes.

When to Call the Doctor
All patients with shock should be carefully evaluated by a doctor. Arrange for transportation to the nearest hospital as soon as preliminary first aid is completed.

STROKE

Description
A stroke is a spontaneous rupture of a blood vessel or formation of a clot that interferes with circulation.

It may vary all the way from a major stroke or cerebrovascular accident (CVA), with paralysis or weakness along one entire side of the body, to a transient ischemic attack (TIA). TIA occurs when too little blood flow reaches the brain yet complete shutdown, as in strokes, has not occurred.

Experts agree that TIA is the principal warning signal for a stroke. Some studies show it is experienced by about 10 percent of stroke victims prior to their attacks. Other research reports show it present in 70 to 75 percent of patients who eventually have a stroke. But, whatever the percentage, it constitutes an important figure and about one-third of those who experience TIA will have a stroke within five years!

The factors that lead to TIA, and eventually a stroke, are high blood cholesterol (and other fats in the blood), heart disease, diabetes and high blood pressure. Control of these specific factors, especially hypertension, slows down the tendency and decreases the likelihood of this sometimes lethal and always serious disorder.

Practical Pointers 1. The signs and symptoms of a major stroke are generally well known and include: paralysis or weakness on one side of the body, inability to speak (if the stroke causes paralysis of the right side), difficulty in breathing or swallowing and unconsciousness.

2. The minor stroke can cause headache, confusion, dizziness, and, a few days later, minor difficulties in speech, weakness in an arm or leg, and memory and personality changes.

3. The TIA is noted by its variety of symptoms. If properly recognized and treatment is begun promptly, these symptoms can LEAD TO PREVENTION of a major stroke. This recognition of TIA as a precursor to stroke is especially important in the age range of 55 to 65. Suspect symptoms might include:

(a) Numbness of the hand or foot (the same feeling that your gum has when a dentist injects novacaine into it for tooth repairs). The numbness stays in the extremity in one place and does not move up. It may be noticed in the right hand more often then the left one.

(b) Dizziness (vertigo) is the commonest single symptom. It must, however, be differentiated from lightheadedness. Dizziness means an actual change in the ability to walk. Staggering may take place. You will have to stop and hold on to something. Objects may seem to whirl about or you may feel like you are walking on the aisle of a moving train. Lightheadedness is less severe and involves being a little unsteady for two or three seconds when you change position quickly while getting up from a bed or jumping up from a chair.

G74

(c)   Double vision — in this symptom you will report two-for-one vision for several seconds at a time and then the image will return to its normal state.

4.   Check the blood pressure and pulse of the patient and record the results.

Treatment Tips   1.   If the stroke seems to be a major one follow these rules.

(a)   Maintain an open airway and place the patient on his side so that secretions will drain from his mouth. (See Treatment Index, p. G101.)

(b)   Give rescue breathing if necessary. (See Treatment Index, p. G102.)

(c)   Do not give victim fluids by mouth unless conscious and able to swallow normally.

(d)   Keep the victim at rest.

2.   If the stroke is a minor one, take the following steps.

(a)   Protect the victim against accident or physical exertion.

(b)   Keep the victim at rest.

When to Call the Doctor   All patients with strokes or TIA should be carefully evaluated by a doctor. Call and get medical advice as soon as possible.

UNCONSCIOUS PATIENT

Description   Coma or unconsciousness may be the result of intoxication, illness or injury. It is not a disease in itself. A baffling situation under the best of circumstances, unconsciousness requires prompt medical evaluation and treatment.

The most common cause of unconsciousness is intoxication from alcohol or sleeping pills (barbiturates). The second most frequent cause is head injury. Other leading causes are strokes, diabetic coma, insulin reactions, overdoses of prescription drugs and poisons such as carbon monoxide, industrial gases, heroin and other chemicals from our present-day drug scene. Some psychiatric conditions can even cause a coma-like state.

Practical Pointers   1.   When a person is unconscious, the usual medical sequence of history, examination and treatment is reversed. TREATMENT IS FIRST. Check the lips. Are they blue? Ensure an adequate airway and do emergency breathing if needed. (See Treatment Index, p. G102.)

G75

2.   Smell the victim's breath. The strong odor of alcohol may give you valuable information. If the cause is diabetic coma, the breath may have the odor of acetone (the principal ingredient of fingernail polish remover). Another clue to diabetic coma (blood sugar too high) is a flushed face — cherry red in color — and very dry skin. Breathing is erratic in this condition.

3.   Look at the head and scalp. Is there evidence of a cut or big bruise to indicate head injury? If there is skull or neck injury use great care in moving the patient.

4.   Check the skin of the arms. Are there scars or black and blue marks to suggest drug habits such as "main-lining" (taking heroin or narcotics by injection into the vein)?

5.   Examine the personal belongings of the person — preferably in front of a witness. Is there an ID bracelet that identifies an existing illness such as diabetes, hypertension, epilepsy, etc.? Is there a medical card or empty prescription bottle available that might help get in touch with the unconscious person's doctor or family? Is there evidence of crime or a suicide attempt?

6.   A clue for insulin reaction (blood sugar too low) is the ashen white face. The skin is moist and clammy and covered with cold sweat. There is NO ODOR OF ACETONE on the breath.

Treatment Tips   1.   The best treatment in some cases is no treatment. An old medical rule is: "First Do No Harm."

2.   Make the victim as comfortable as possible and loosen tight clothing.

3.   Keep curiosity seekers away. Their presence may only aggravate the condition.

4.   If the victim has vomited, clear the mouth of vomitus and mucus to prevent aspiration and other complications. Ensure a good airway. Place patient on side. (See Treatment Index, p. G101.)

When to Call   1.   As soon as an adequate airway has been
the Doctor   established, an EMERGENCY CALL SHOULD BE PLACED for the rescue squad.

2.   If a doctor's name is known or can be identified from the personal effects, the doctor should be called.

3.   Any useful medical information that has been observed should be written down, if possible pinned to the victim, and given to the rescue squad for use by the doctors at the emergency room.

G76

DRUG
INDEX

This Drug Index lists items that are available to you without a prescription. In the pharmaceutical industry, they are called over-the-counter (O.T.C.) products.

I DO NOT ENDORSE any particular products, but name those listed here in order to familiarize you with the general line of product. By looking at the ingredients listed on the various bottles or boxes in your drugstore, you will see that many products for a particular purpose are similar if not identical in makeup. Some, in fact, vary only in the "name," and the cost of the promotion that went into making it known to consumers. In making your selection among O.T.C. products for a specific disorder, you should consider cost, prior experience with the product or a product having the same ingredients and the recommendations of others — including your pharmacist. The reason I use specific trade names here is simply because that product is widely distributed and will usually be AVAILABLE in your drugstore, no matter where you happen to live.

ANTIDOTE
Syrup of Ipecac

Indications For treatment of poisoning to help induce vomiting

Directions For children 1 to 5 years of age, ½ oz. (or a little over 1 tbs.) with one cup of water. If no vomiting occurs after 20 minutes, this dose may be repeated ONE TIME only

ANTINAUSEANT
Emetrol

Indications For treatment of uncomplicated nausea and vomiting

Directions 1 or 2 tsp. every 1 or 2 hours as needed for vomiting

G77

ANTIPRURITIC
Caladryl Lotion

Indications For relief of itching due to mild poison ivy or oak, insect bites, or other minor skin irritations and soothing relief of mild sunburn

Directions Apply to skin 3 or 4 times daily. Cleanse skin with soap and water and dry area before each application

ASPIRIN AND ANALGESIC
Aspirin: Adult aspirin tablets are 5 grain; children's, 1¼ grain

Indications For relief of pain associated with simple headache, common colds and neuralgia

Directions ADULTS — 1 or 2 tablets every 3 to 4 hours as needed
CHILDREN — (3–12) ½ to 1 tablet every 3 to 4 hours as needed
(under 3) The general rule is 1 grain per year of age every 3 to 4 hours as needed

Caution If allergic to aspirin, or if taking anticoagulants or drugs for gout, use Tylenol

Tylenol

Indications As noted above in aspirin

Directions ADULTS — 1 or 2 tablets every 3 to 4 hours as needed
CHILDREN — (6–12) ½ to 1 tablet every 3 to 4 hours as needed
(3–6) 1.2 cc drops every 3 to 4 hours as needed
(1–3) 0.6 cc to 1.2 cc drops every 3 to 4 hours as needed
(under 1 yr) 0.6 cc every 3 to 4 hours as needed

COLD PREPARATION
Oral Nasal Decongestant
Dristan Tabs

Indications For relief of symptoms such as nasal congestion and postnasal drip associated with colds, nasal allergies, sinusitis and rhinitis

G78

Directions ADULTS — 2 tablets to start followed by 1 tablet every 4 hours not to exceed 4 tablets daily
CHILDREN — (6–12) One-half adult dosage
(under 6) Only as directed by physician

Triaminic Syrup

Indications As noted above

Directions ADULTS — 2 tsp. every 4 hours
CHILDREN — (6–12) 1 tsp. every 4 hours
(under 6) Only as directed by physician

Caution Do not exceed 4 doses in 24 hours

COUGH PREPARATION
Triaminicol

Indications Symptomatic relief of coughs especially when accompanied by stuffed and runny nose due to common cold

Directions ADULTS — 2 tsp. every 4 hours
CHILDREN — (6–12) 1 tsp. every 4 hours
(under 6) As directed by physician

Caution Unless directed by physician do not exceed 4 doses in 24 hours

NOSE DROPS
Neosynephrine

Available as ¼ or ⅛% solutions

Indications Temporary relief of nasal congestion

Directions ADULTS — Instill 2 or 3 drops (¼% solution) in each nostril every 3 to 4 hours as needed
CHILDREN — Instill 2 or 3 drops (⅛% solution) in each nostril every 3 to 4 hours as needed

Caution Do not use more than 3 times daily or for more than 3 days

SKIN OINTMENT
Neosporin Ointment

___

Indications To help prevent infection in minor cuts, burns and abrasions and as an aid to healing

Directions Apply directly to affected area and cover with sterile dressing if necessary; may be applied 2 to 5 times daily as needed

TREATMENT INDEX

This index has been prepared to give you practical help in treating the common health problems discussed under the illnesses, injuries and emergencies sections of your Self-Help Medical Guide.

ALLERGIES
Prepare an Allergy-Free Bedroom

Bed Wipe bed and springs. Cover box springs, pillows and mattress with plastic covers from the department store. If the plastic covers tear, patch them. No feather pillows! Bedspreads should be plain and easily washed (no chenille, corduroy or ruffles). No quilts or comforters. Blankets must be cotton, orlon or acrylic material that can be washed every 2 weeks.

Closet Clean carefully and use for current clothing. No storage.

Floor No carpets or rugs. If existing carpet is old, remove it. Tile, wood or new linoleum are fine.

Furniture Only wood or plastic chairs allowed. No stuffed chairs. No bookcase. Dresser for current clothing. No storage.

Walls Remove all old, torn wallpaper, repair plaster and paint with a water-based paint. No wall decorations or bulletin boards.

Windows Use a shade but never shutters or Venetian blinds. Curtains that can be washed every 2 weeks or plastic material that can be wiped off weekly are fine. Keep windows closed as much as possible.

In general, the above plan is proposed to avoid dust collectors and makers. A general rule is to strip the room of all clutter and junk. (The room should look like one that would make a Marine drill instructor happy!) Vacuum the floor daily. Keep the door shut. PETS are NOT allowed in the room. Only

G81

nonallergenic toys are permitted. Stuffed toys are not allowed on the bed.

Room Air Cleaning Machine

There are several of these electronic air purifiers on the market that do a good job of cleaning the air of the particles that float in the air and cause allergies. Room units can be purchased or rented from medical supply stores or larger department stores. Central units can be obtained from heating and air conditioning dealers or service companies.

APPLYING MEDICATIONS

Eye Drops Eye medication comes in an ointment or drop form. Drops are usually easier to apply (and all companies produce both dosage forms) so ask your doctor to GIVE DROPS WHENEVER POSSIBLE.

The first step in the application is to wash your hands thoroughly to prevent any new or further infections. Then follow these next steps.

1. Stand in front of the mirror with your head straight (or if you have some assistance, face the person).
2. Make a pocket by gently pinching the skin under the lower eyelid between your thumb and index finger. Pull the lid forward and down gently as shown.

APPLYING EYE
MEDICATION

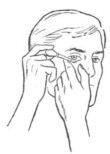

MAKE A "POCKET"
FOR THE DROPS

3. Place the drops in the little pocket. Don't worry about getting too many drops in the eye, the excess will roll down the cheek.
4. As soon as the drops are in, release the lower lid and, with the eyes lightly shut, look up, down and sideways. Don't rub your eye.

5. Keep the eyes shut and lie down for 5 minutes.
6. Wash the hands.

For SMALL CHILDREN follow this application advice:
1.   With the child lying flat on his back, ask him to look up at the ceiling and then close his eyes tightly. (You may need to "mummify" younger children with sheet around arms for restraint.)
2.   Place a drop or two in the corner of each eye while he is squeezing them shut. The new blunt eye droppers make it easy and safe to apply drops. You should also have your ring or little finger (of the hand used to give the drops) touching the face as a safeguard against sudden movement.
3.   When you are finished with the drops, tell him to open his eyes.

There will be no yelling, crying or fear with this method. A cooperative older child can in fact be taught how to apply his own medication.

Nose Drops Nose decongestants are available in nose drops or sprays. The nose drops are generally easier to apply and somewhat less expensive.

1. Lie down and tip your head back over a pillow or towel.
2. Apply nose drops in right nostril and then tilt your head over to the right. Hold it there for one minute while repeatedly saying the letter K (kay-kay-kay-kay).
3. Apply nose drops to your left nostril and then tilt your head to the left and keep it there for one minute. Repeat K-K-K-K-K-K etc.
4. Return your head to the center and repeat the letter K again for 30 seconds. This causes alternating pressure in the sinuses and helps open up the sinus and ear passages that open into the nose.
5. Gargle with hot water. This helps clean out excess nose drops and mucus.

For SMALL CHILDREN AND BABIES, the application is generally the same, but with this variation:

1. The child is held in the lap, head centered and fixed against the abdomen of the mother (or the adult administering the treatment). The child's body is cradled between the mother's legs, while the feet point away from her.

2. The mother holds the child's head on the left in her left hand and applies the drops to the left nostril using her right hand.

3. To instill drops in the right nostril, the procedure is reversed.

NOTE: NEVER use nose drops more than three times per day or for more than three consecutive days. Excessive use of nose drops may cause loss of sense of smell and other adverse changes in the nasal mucosa.

BANDAGES/DRESSINGS

Application Dressing After cleansing the wound and the bleeding is controlled, the wound should be dressed with a 2 x 2 in. or 4 x 4 in. sterile gauze dressing or an ouchless dressing such as Telfa sterile pad. The dressing should be affixed with adhesive tape, roller gauze and tape or Kling.

Butterfly Closure After carefully cleansing the wound and controlling bleeding as instructed, superficial lacerations may be closed with a Band-Aid Butterfly Closure or you can cut your own from ½ in. adhesive tape as shown.

MAKE A BUTTERFLY BANDAGE

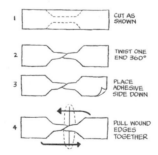

1 CUT AS SHOWN

2 TWIST ONE END 360°

3 PLACE ADHESIVE SIDE DOWN

4 PULL WOUND EDGES TOGETHER

A gauze bandage, Band-Aid or Curan is then placed over the wound and the Butterfly Closure. If the wound is large and pressure is needed, an external roller gauze or elastic gauze bandage like Kling is helpful.

Removal Dressing The dressing may be removed and changed as often as needed if there is much drainage or blood. If possible, however, keep it on 24 hours before the first change.

G84

Removal of the dressing should be lengthwise, as shown in the diagram, so as not to reopen the wound.

BANDAGE REMOVAL

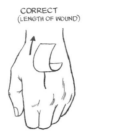

CORRECT
(LENGTH OF WOUND)

INCORRECT
(ACROSS WOUND)

Triangle Sling A convenient arm sling can be prepared with a triangular piece of cloth (55 in. across the base and 36 to 40 in. along the sides) or a large, 30-in. square dish towel folded into a triangle. Apply the sling as shown.

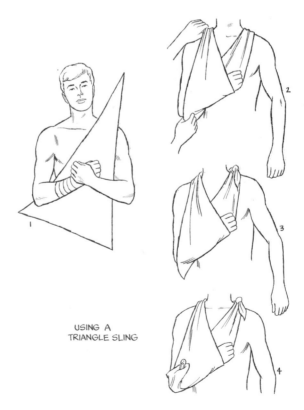

USING A
TRIANGLE SLING

BLEEDING CONTROL

Skin/Scalp Direct pressure to wound is easy, quick and effective in nearly all lacerations.

1. Place a sterile gauze pad or clean handkerchief on the wound.

2. Put your whole hand firmly over the wound and press down hard as shown.

DIRECT PRESSURE FOR BLEEDING

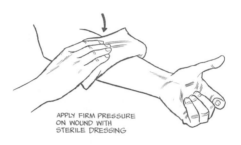

APPLY FIRM PRESSURE
ON WOUND WITH
STERILE DRESSING

3. Keep the pressure on for 3 or 4 minutes.
4. Check to see if bleeding has stopped.
5. Reapply pressure if needed.

Nose The same principle of pressure to control skin bleeding applies to nosebleeds. Prompt control can be obtained by:

1. Taking your thumb and forefinger and grasping your nose as shown in the diagram.

NOSE BLEED CONTROL

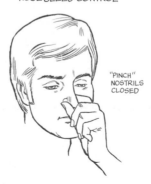

"PINCH"
NOSTRILS
CLOSED

2. Squeeze hard enough to cause pressure but not pain.
3. Continue pressure for 5 minutes without letting go.
4. If still bleeding, resume pressure again for 5 minutes.

COLD APPLICATIONS AND BATHS

Ankle, Wrist, Skin and Sinuses A true "miracle drug" is the ice cube, crushed ice or cold compresses properly applied. These cause the arteries around an injured site, whether bruise or cut, to constrict, slowing both the external bleeding and the internal bleeding that causes swelling.

In general, dry cold is better than wet compresses to control bleeding. A plastic bag filled with crushed ice applied directly to the site is best.

A common type of swelling seen is that which when a child falls off his bike or tricycle and gets a cut lip or cheek. Putting ice to the area may be a tough assignment, but if you have the child apply a popsicle it becomes easy. It is cold and serves the same purpose. By the time the child has consumed a frozen treat or two, most of the danger of swelling has passed. And, don't worry about the swallowing of blood in the process, it won't hurt the child one bit.

Cold compresses for bruises, sinusitis, insect stings and various other injuries can be obtained by placing one or two dozen ice cubes in a pan, mixing it with cold tap water and placing a towel in the pan. Wring the towel out before applying it to the injury. Repeat as often as directed.

For injuries of feet, ankles, wrists, arms and hands direct immersion is preferable. A styrofoam picnic cooler filled as needed with ice and water makes a good container. It is larger than most dishpans and does not allow the cold to dissipate as quickly.

Cool Baths For Fever If there is need for a rapid cooling of the body, as in the case of persistent high fever or fever convulsion, the patient should be quickly immersed in a bathtub half-filled with tepid water. After a few minutes in the water the temperature of the water can then be lowered by the addition of ice cubes. If there is shivering, the bath is too cold. A cool shower is also suitable for prompt dissipation of heat.

An alternate method, if there is some difficulty in transporting the patient to the bathroom, is the application of cold towels to the body. After a plastic sheet or oilcloth is placed under the patient, compresses soaked in a dishpan of liquid containing 2 quarts of water, 1 pint of rubbing alcohol and 1 quart of ice cubes is an effective cooling method.

Keep the sick room as cool as possible if the patient has a fever.

EAR WAX REMOVAL

What makes wax, anyway? Wax is a normal protective secretion, like mucus from the nose or tears from the eyes. It is there to catch bugs, dust, germs and general debris such as skin that has peeled off the external ear canal.

Once the foreign body is caught in the wax, it is gradually worked outward by hair-like cilia (like those in the mucous surface of the lungs). Normally, the particles of wax end up in the external ear and are washed or fall away.

Unfortunately, through ignorance of Mother Nature's "house cleaners," people will jam Q-tips, hair pins, fingers, pencils, etc. into the canal, forcing the wax back in and packing it into a solid mass (and mess!). The wax may then, over many months (or years), change from its normal brown color and soft consistency to a black hard coal-like particle that requires all the skills of the doctor's office for removal. Perhaps it will even take two or three visits for the job!

The thing to remember here is DO NOT USE Q-TIPS, cotton tips or other "pokers" in the external canal! They only give Mother Nature a set-back.

The removal of ear wax is easy if you follow these instructions. After verifying that wax is present (see Testing Index, p. G122–G123) the following plan works in over 75 percent of the cases.

o Apply Debrox each night for 3 or 4 days.

o Put in five drops at bedtime and then apply a hot water bottle or heating pad set at medium high to affected ear for 15 minutes.

o Turn ear over on handkerchief or paper tissue and gently remove excess solution.

o Examine ear with otoscope after 3 or 4 treatments and repeat if necessary for two more nights.

NOTE: If this attempt is not successful and hard wax persists, please see your doctor.

EXERCISES

Back

The following series of relaxing, stretching, yoga-type exercises are indicated for nearly all back problems. It is essential, however, that the exercises be done on a daily basis for long-term benefit. Do them as follows.

1. Find a time in the day, preferably at night, when there are no other distractions such as phones, visitors or family interruptions.
2. Set up a procedure that is almost a ritual. Do it the SAME WAY every night.
3. Wear comfortable, loose-fitting pajamas or leotards while exercising. (Do each exercise 5 times, but for beginners 2 or 3 times are enough.)
4. Spread a large beach towel on a carpeted area (or on a comforter or heavy blanket on a hard floor). Use the same room every time.
5. Keep the lights in the room subdued and turn off radio and television.
6. Do the exercises in a specific sequence: "corpse" position, leg stretches, spinal twist, "cobra" position, and shoulder stand as shown in the following diagrams.

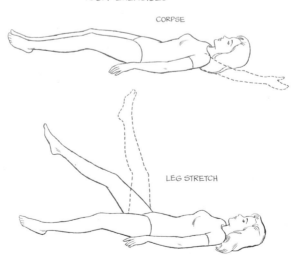

YOGA EXERCISES

CORPSE

LEG STRETCH

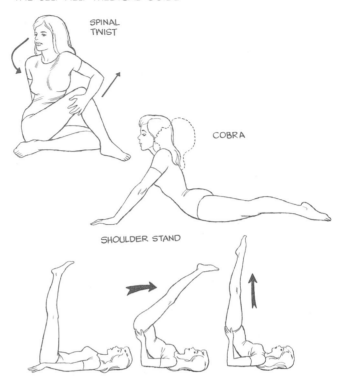

7. The specific instructions are as follows.

Corpse 1. Lie flat on your back with your arms at your sides.
2. As you slowly stretch your arms out from your sides to above head, stretch entire body and take in a slow, deep breath, pulling in your belly. Think only of breathing slowly.
3. Slowly move your arms back to your sides as you exhale, pushing your belly out. Feel your entire body relax.

Leg 1. Lie flat on back.
Stretch 2. Elevate left leg as high as you can with knee straight.
3. Slowly lower to 15° and hold in place for 10 seconds.
4. Replace leg on floor and rest.
5. Repeat with right leg.

Spinal 1. Sit with left leg extended and right knee flexed.
Twist 2. Twist torso and outstretched right arm as much as possible.
3. Repeat in other direction with right leg extended and twist torso.

G90

Cobra 1. Lie on stomach.
2. Support yourself on outstretched arms with elbows "locked" into place.
3. Arch back and neck as far back as possible. Hold this position — looking at ceiling — then relax, bringing head forward.

Shoulder 1. Lie flat on back.
Stand 2. Elevate both legs over head (as if "bicycling").
3. Support hips with hands.
4. One at a time, touch right and left foot to floor above head (if possible).
5. Touch both feet to floor simultaneously above head.
6. Slowly return to supine position.

When doing the exercises remember that each should be accompanied by slow, deep breathing — deeply inhale with the beginning of the exercise, hold the breath and slowly exhale at completion. Work out your own pattern. Take a course at your local "Y" if it is offered.

The entire sequence should take about 30 minutes. You can soon add your variations on the exercises as you increase your flexibility and skills with these basic five. When you have completed the shoulder stand and returned to sitting position, sit on the floor for a few minutes before standing upright. You will feel refreshed and relaxed.

Warning Persons with chronic diseases of heart and vascular system must avoid shoulder stands.

Breathing

The exercises described here will help patients with chronic obstructive lung disease (C.O.L.D.). In general they:
1. Teach you, through breathing through pursed lips (like whistling) to slow your exhalation.
2. Teach you to contract the abdomen only while exhaling.
3. Strengthen your abdominal muscles.

Do each exercise 4 or 5 times morning and night at the beginning and then increase the amount done.

Exhaling While standing or sitting erect, inhale deeply and slowly
Through through the nose taking 4 seconds. Exhale slowly for 8
Pursed Lips seconds through pursed lips, while pushing inward on your abdomen as shown. Do this two times each minute. Relax in-between.

G91

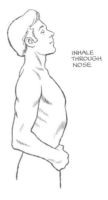

BREATHING
EXERCISE

INHALE
THROUGH
NOSE

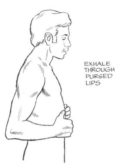

EXHALE
THROUGH
PURSED
LIPS

Abdominal While lying flat on the floor on your back put
Breathing right hand on abdomen and left hand on chest. While slowly
inhaling, push out your abdomen (like a pregnant woman)
and let your right hand visibly rise. Then exhale through
pursed lips and slowly press your abdomen in toward your
backbone. Repeat exercises while slowly raising and lowering
legs, one at a time, to strengthen the abdominal muscles.

ABDOMINAL BREATHING

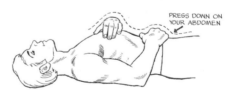

PRESS DOWN ON
YOUR ABDOMEN

Elbow

Do each of the following exercises 5 times each day.

1. Hold arm out to side with palm and thumb up, touch
hand to shoulder and return.

2.   Add weight to hand (books that increase in size are good weights). Repeat (1) above.

3.   "Walk up wall" with fingers while holding the shoulder down or fixed with the other hand.

4.   Turn a door knob while someone is holding it on the opposite side.

5.   Do broom twisting as shown. With injured elbow and arm twist the broom clockwise, then counterclockwise with resistance offered by unaffected hand.

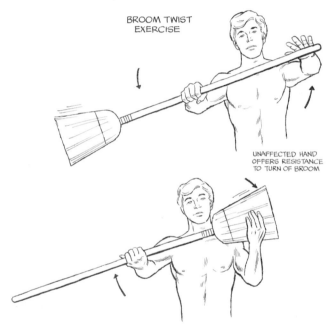

BROOM TWIST
EXERCISE

UNAFFECTED HAND
OFFERS RESISTANCE
TO TURN OF BROOM

Shoulder

Do the "T" exercise to strengthen an injured shoulder. With the hand of the injured arm holding a comfortable weight of 2 or 3 pounds (a rock or a common brick will do), stand erect and stretch both arms out to sides for the starting "T" position.

1.   Swing injured arm forward as shown, and then return to side.

2.   Repeat swing forward and back 10 times

3.   Increase weight (a household iron is about right) and take starting position. If weight is comfortable, do exercise 10

times. If any weight causes pain or uncomfortableness, stop.
Use a lighter weight.

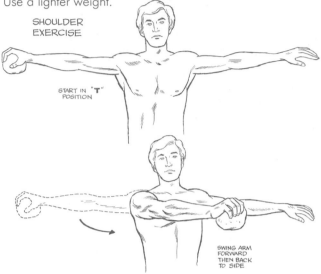

SHOULDER
EXERCISE

START IN "**T**"
POSITION

SWING ARM
FORWARD
THEN BACK
TO SIDE

HEAT APPLICATIONS

Back and Joints   Moist warm heat is of significant help in reducing acute chronic pain in back, arms or legs. Do it in this way twice daily for best results:

1. Take a large towel, wet it thoroughly in warm water, wring it out well, fold it in thirds lengthwise. Wrap it around the joint or lay it across the back.
2. Cover the towel completely with two layers of plastic wrap (or waxed paper).
3. Place a heating pad over the plastic cover (make sure there is no contact with the wet towel). Turn the dial to medium setting. Leave for one hour.
4. Use plug-in radio (NOT a portable) near the heating pad. The radio will give a warning crackle of static if heating pad is getting wet.

Ear   A convenient way to apply heat to the ear of children or adults is as follows.

1. Take several paper towels and soak in hot water. Wring dry.
2. Stuff towels into a small drinking glass that has been warmed with hot water from the faucet.
3. With head held so painful ear is upward, place BOTTOM of glass against ear for 10 minutes. Keep glass upright to avoid

spilling water from the hot, wet paper towels.

4. Repeat for another 10 minutes after rewarming glass and towels.

5. Equally good sources of heat are a heating pad turned to the medium high setting or a hot water bottle.

Eye Wet compresses are easily prepared following these rules.

1. Warm water compresses should be warm, NOT HOT. Test the water on the inner aspect of the forearm. (If the water used is too hot, the soft tissue around the eye will become swollen.)

2. Apply with face cloth or handkerchief for 5 to 10 minutes every three hours if there is a scratchy feeling in the eye and discharge.

3. COLD compresses may feel better if the eye itches or is quite swollen.

4. Apply eye drops AFTER the soaks are completed.

Sinuses Hot, wet compresses will usually give relief to the pain of sinusitis but alternating the hot soaks with ice cold soaks is at times more effective.

1. Soak towel in hot water, wring dry and lay over forehead or cheeks until heat dissipates, usually about 30 seconds.

2. Soak another towel in pan filled with cold tap water and ice cubes. Place on forehead or cheeks until chill is dissipated.

3. Do alternating hot and cold soaks for 10 minutes.

4. Repeat four times daily with last treatment at bedtime.

Throat A time-proven gargle is made by putting 1 tsp. of salt in 8 oz. of hot water. Gargle with this for 5 minutes every 2 hours as pain indicates. Others may prefer gargling with a hot solution of Cepacol or another similar product sold at the drugstore.

Vagina or Rectum The hot sitz bath is an old time treatment that gives much relief of pain in the vagina or rectum. Put enough warm to hot water in the tub to cover the buttocks while sitting in the tub. The temperature should be somewhat warmer than that used for a regular bath.

INSECT STINGS

Tenderizer A home treatment* for bee and wasp stings that, if done

*The mode of therapeutic action in this treatment is uncertain, but it is hypothesized that the venom is protein-like and is dissolved and neutralized by the tenderizer.

immediately, is surprisingly useful is as follows.
1.   Wash off the site with soap and water.
2.   Sprinkle a generous amount of meat tenderizer (a common brand is Adolph's Instant Meat Tenderizer) on a wet handkerchief or 4 x 4 in. gauze bandage.
3.   Apply to sting area for 20 to 30 minutes. Some relief from pain and itching is noted in 5 to 10 minutes.
4.   Check arm. If swelling is still visible, reapply for another 30 minutes.

Tourniquet One of my few indications for the use of a tourniquet is a modified method (see illustration) that restricts surface level lymph drainage. It is helpful in slowing the venom of insect and snake bites.

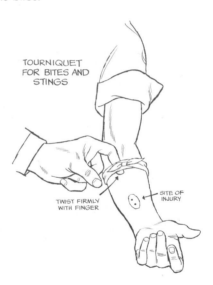

The pressure to the tourniquet is best applied with a gentle twisting by the index finger rather than a stick as in the traditional tourniquet for a severed or partially severed extremity. The purpose of this technique is to slow or stop the superficial lymphatic drainage that spreads the venom.

MASSAGE

Ankle If you have moderate swelling around the outer portion of your ankle but no bleeding, massage is helpful.

G96

TREATMENT INDEX

1. Gently massage above the swelling, then below it with strokes angled up TOWARD the heart.
2. Place the index finger under your middle finger as shown.
3. Stroke the spot of tenderness gently and work it out.

MASSAGING SWOLLEN ANKLE

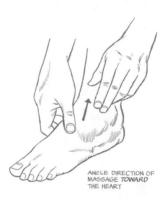

ANGLE DIRECTION OF MASSAGE *TOWARD* THE HEART

4. This same massage method is suitable for swelling on arm, upper leg and elsewhere.

PREPARATIONS

Baking Soda/Ammonia A good home remedy to relieve itching is to make a paste of baking soda and ammonia solution. Mix ½ cup of soda with enough ammonia water (standard household cleaning ammonia) to make a paste. Apply it to the skin.

Gargles The simplest, cheapest gargle is 1 tsp. salt in an 8 oz. glass of water, the temperature of hot tea. Instead of a salt solution, you may prefer a prepared gargle, such as Cepacol.

GI Drink* This inexpensive drink which replaces lost salts from diarrhea, vomiting, etc. can be made as follows:
1. For each quart of boiled water add: 1 level tsp. table salt, 1 heaping tsp. baking soda, 4 rounded tsp. sugar.
2. Stir until clean and add 1 package of sugarless Kool-Aid or similar flavoring product.
3. Make fresh daily and keep in refrigerator.

*This recipe from PATIENT CARE, April 15, 1974, Darien, Connecticut.

Sugar This drink which provides energy while replacing lost
Water fluids is prepared by adding 1 tbs. of sugar or maple or
pancake syrup to 8 oz. of boiled water.

Vinegar 1.   An effective, hygienic douche is made by putting 1 oz. of
Douche vinegar in a quart of warm water.
2.   The douche is applied while you are lying on your back in
the bathtub with douche bag suspended well above the
body.
3.   Insert the tube tip well up into the vagina and release the
clamp.
4.   Allow the solution to flow freely.
5.   Clamp the tube again and let the vagina drain while you
are sitting up in the tub.
6.   Repeat the process until 1 or 2 quarts of solution has been
used.

REMOVAL PROCEDURES

Blood under This procedure, although it appears difficult, is quite
Fingernail easy to do when these directions are followed.

DRILLING THE FINGERNAIL

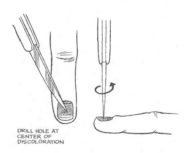

DRILL HOLE AT
CENTER OF
DISCOLORATION

1.   Sharpen the tip of a pocket knife.
2.   Place injured finger or thumb on a table or other firm, flat
surface.
3.   Fix the finger with the help of an assistant so that it will not
move.
4.   Have assistant gently drill hole through the nail at center
of purple discoloration as illustrated.
5.   Absorb blood with tip of handkerchief or gauze as soon
as hole is drilled through the nail.

Fishhook If the barb is imbedded, the fishhook should be removed by a doctor if one is available. If, however, such aid is not available, while on a fishing trip to remote area, the hook can be extracted in the following manner.

1. Have an assistant advance the barb by pushing until it protrudes as shown in the diagram.

REMOVING FISHHOOK

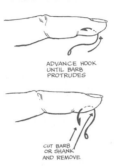

ADVANCE HOOK
UNTIL BARB
PROTRUDES

CUT BARB
OR SHANK
AND REMOVE

2. Using a cutting tool, cut off either the barb or the shank and remove it.
3. Cleanse the wound carefully.
4. Dress the wound.
5. Consult a physician as soon as possible regarding possible infection and booster injection of tetanus toxoid.

Foreign Body in Eye An assistant will be needed to help remove the foreign body. Follow these steps.

1. Observe the eye to locate the foreign body.
2. Pull out the lower lid to see if the object is on the inner surface of lower lid.
3. If it is there, take the corner of a clean handkerchief and touch it to the foreign body to remove it.
4. If the piece of dirt or other substance is not there, it may be lodged beneath the upper lid.

REMOVING A PARTICLE

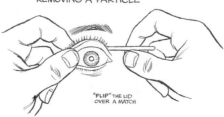

"FLIP" THE LID
OVER A MATCH

5. With the victim looking down, grasp the lash of the upper lid.
6. Pull the upper lid down over the lower lid. The tears and maneuver may dislodge the object.
7. If the particle is still there, "flip" the upper lid with a wooden match or toothpick as illustrated. Pull the lash upward against the matchstick and lift off the particle with the corner of the handkerchief.
8. Wash the eye with water.

RESPIRATORY DISTRESS

Cool Mist or Steam Inhalation Both adults and children can use the umbrella-tent method. (For a baby, the same effect can be obtained by putting a sheet over the crib.)

1. Open a full-sized umbrella and lay it over the pillow at the head of the bed.
2. Drape a sheet over the umbrella and the steamer or cool mist* which should be placed securely on a chair at the side of the bed.
3. Have patient spend 30 to 40 minutes under the tent prior to bedtime and 3 or 4 times during the day.
4. If patient can sleep all night under the tent this is desirable.

Postural Drainage Previous problems with this procedure were related to the difficulty in getting into and keeping the necessary positions, such as lying on a bed with your elbows resting on the floor. Here is an easy series of postures, from a recent PATIENT CARE article, designed to promote drainage.

1. Lie with stomach downward and a pillow placed under body as shown in illustration 1. Hold the position for about 5 minutes.
2. Then turn on right side and lie with hips elevated. See illustration 2.
3. Turn next on left side.
4. Finally, lie on back with pillows under hips as shown in 3. After lying in each position for about 5 minutes, gently cough up sputum.

*Preferred by many physicians. A widely distributed and reputable brand is Kaz Humidifier, 614 West 49th Street, New York, NY 10019.

POSTURAL DRAINAGE POSITIONS

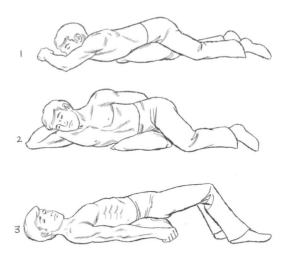

Unconscious Patient and Airway If a patient is unconscious or semiconscious but breathing well, a simple precautionary position change may be all that is necessary to ensure an airway. Roll the patient over on the side as shown. This position will allow mucus or vomitus to drain out without danger of the victim aspirating it.

UNCONCIOUS VICTIM

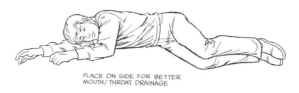

PLACE ON SIDE FOR BETTER
MOUTH/ THROAT DRAINAGE

Cardio-pulmonary Resuscitation

CPR Your own low-cost (about $10.00) CPR emergency kit* should be assembled and kept in your home. It can be

*Developed by Dr. David P. Pilcher of the University of Vermont, Burlington, VT.

G101

stored in a sewing or fishing tackle box or cookie tin. The kit should contain the following.

1. An ear syringe (for children) and for adults a plastic turkey baster. It is used to suck out mucus, vomitus or blood from an accident victim's mouth.

2. Two plastic airways — one for an adult and one for a child (can be purchased at drugstores or hospital supply store).

3. Box of Kling self-adhesive bandage.

4. A large 5 x 6 in. dressing.

5. A pair of scissors.

The A-B-C steps of cardiopulmonary resuscitation are:

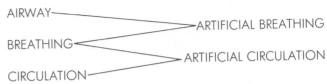

AIRWAY ⟶ ARTIFICIAL BREATHING

BREATHING ⟶ ARTIFICIAL CIRCULATION

CIRCULATION

Airway To find out if the patient is breathing, place him flat on his back and put your ear close to his mouth. If he is breathing you will feel his breath and see the chest rise and fall.

If there is evidence of foreign bodies or dentures in the mouth remove them. Aspirate mucus, vomitus or blood with the syringes and use the large 5 x 6 in. dressing to help clean out the mouth.

When this is completed insert the appropriate size plastic airway. (If available, an airway should be inserted whether the patient is breathing well or not, as a precaution.)

Breathing If the victim has stopped breathing, lift up his neck with one hand and push the forehead down with the other as shown in the diagram. This opens the airway and the person may start to breath. If he doesn't, begin rescue breathing at once. Pinch the victim's nostrils shut with the fingers of one hand and blow air into mouth (see illustration). When his chest moves up, take your mouth away and let his chest go down by itself.

The first rescue breathing should be FOUR QUICK FULL BREATHS without allowing time for full deflation of lungs between breaths.

In rescue breathing for infants and children, the rescuer covers both the mouth and nose of the child with his mouth and uses SMALLER breaths to inflate the lungs ONCE EVERY 3 SECONDS.

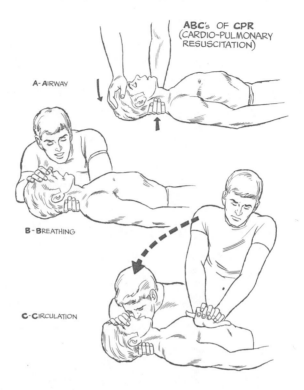

ABC's OF CPR
(CARDIO-PULMONARY RESUSCITATION)

A- AIRWAY

B- BREATHING

C- CIRCULATION

Circulation If unexpected cardiac arrest occurs, the ABC's of basic life support are required in rapid succession.

Cardiac arrest is recognized by pulselessness in the large arteries at the neck near the angle of the jaw and an unconscious patient having a death-like appearance and absent breathing.

Absence or questionable presence of the pulse is indication for external cardiac compression. This consists of rhythmic application of pressure over the lower half of the chest plate (sternum). The heart lies slightly to the left of the middle of the chest and pressure here will compress the heart between your hand and the victim's spine producing artificial circulation.

If there is only one rescuer, he must perform both breathing and circulation using a 15 to 2 ratio (after 15 chest compressions at a rate of 80 per minute, 2 very quick lung inflations). If there are two rescuers, the procedure is somewhat easier. Two lung inflations should be performed, interposed between compressions, for each 5 chest compressions done at a rate of 60 per minute, with no pauses for ventilation.

CPR PROCEDURE

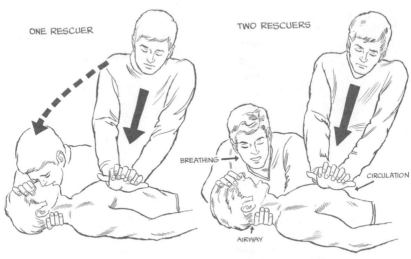

ONE RESCUER

TWO RESCUERS

BREATHING

CIRCULATION

AIRWAY

• 15 CHEST COMPRESSIONS
  (80 PER MINUTE)
• 2 QUICK LUNG INFLATIONS

• 5 CHEST COMPRESSIONS
  (60 PER MINUTE)
• 2 LUNG INFLATIONS FOR
  EACH 5 COMPRESSIONS

The same procedure is followed for infants and children but less force is applied, the compression rate is faster (80 to 100 per minute) and breaths are still applied after each group of 5 compressions.

The rescue procedures should be maintained until the victim has resumed breathing and the heart its beat and pulse or until mechanical resuscitation is available via a rescue squad or other emergency service.

SPLINTING

Ankle An ankle may be splinted by using a towel or pillow as shown.

Toes/Fingers Injured fingers or toes (digits) can be conveniently splinted by taping them to an adjacent uninjured digit using two or three pieces of ½ in. tape.

Wrist An injured wrist can be easily immobilized by using a newspaper or magazine as a splint.

G104

ANKLE SPLINT

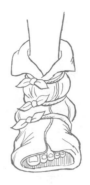

ANKLE OR LEG SPLINT

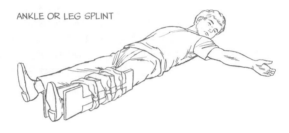

WRIST OR FOREARM SPLINT

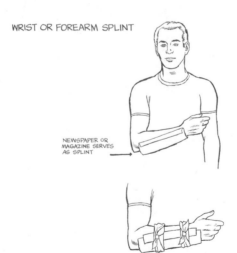

NEWSPAPER OR
MAGAZINE SERVES
AS SPLINT

General Immobilization If there has been a cut or laceration, similar methods should be used to immobilize the area. By using splints, tapes, formed casts, etc. the healing time will be shortened and the chances of infection minimized.

G105

TAPING

Ankle The ankle can be given substantial support by using the basketweave method as follows.

1. Cut 6 strips of 2 in. adhesive tape, each 12 to 15 in. long, and a 7 in. strip.
2. Cover skin with a layer of tincture of benzoin.
3. Place short strip along back of foot starting at heel.
4. Place first long strip HORIZONTALLY along length of foot at level of top of foot.
5. Place the second strip VERTICALLY and to the rear of the foot with the center of the strip passing under the heel.
6. Alternate, placing the next horizontal strip ½ in. further down on the foot and the next vertical strip ½ in. toward the front of the foot to overlap strips as shown.

BASKETWEAVE ANKLE SPLINT

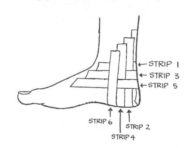

7. Continue tapings to get basketweave effect.
8. Mold the tape to tight fit with warm hands.

Back The back can be given support by strapping with 2 in. tape as follows.

1. Have patient sit on stool with back bare from tail-bone up to midback.
2. Cover back area to be taped with tincture of benzoin.
3. If there is a lot of body hair in the area shave it off.
4. Cut 6 pieces of 2 in. tape in strips 12 in. long.
5. Start with lowest part of back and place tape horizontally.
6. Lay next strip ½ in. higher on the back, etc.
7. Mold tape to back with warm hands.

SYMPTOM/ CONCEPT INDEX

This index has been prepared to give you a clearer understanding of the "body talk" that doctors call symptoms and to improve your insight into some of the basic concepts of health leading to proper treatment and, even better, preventive measures. Briefly, this index will tell you how some parts of your body work and what the body is doing to cause those symptoms.

These symptoms and concepts — a small fraction of those your doctor understands — are selected especially to help you understand and cope with the common illnesses and emergencies already presented in this Self-Help Medical Guide.

ALLERGIC REACTIONS

An allergic reaction occurs when a particle such as ragweed pollen or cat dander (allergens), both common causes of nose allergies, hits the mucous membrane of the nose and eyes of a person allergic to these protein substances.

Then a chain reaction occurs. Allergens entering the body are trapped by antibodies produced by plasma cells of the lymphatic system, while other sensitive cells release histamine. As the histamine is released, this chemical, a powerful vasodilator — that is, it makes the small arteries open up widely — causes the membranes to swell up and become congested.

With the congestion, the little arteries leak fluid into the tissues of the nose and eyes causing the familiar symptoms of reddened eyes, sneezing, runny/stuffy nose, etc.

G107

The symptoms are protective in that they tell you to try and avoid those allergic particles next time. Sneezes also clean out the nasal passages and get rid of the offending allergens.

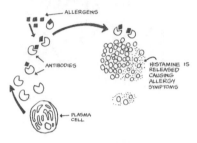

ALLERGIC REACTIONS

Treatment is based on avoiding the allergens, neutralizing the histamine with antihistamine, decreasing the nasal congestion with mild constrictor drugs and building up immunity with hyposensitization injections.

ANKLE AND WRIST INJURY

The basic injury of strain, sprain or fracture depends on the strength of the twisting exerted on the joint. A greater force tears the ligaments and the bone loose causing a fracture. The lesser force tears only PARTS of the ligaments and causes a strain or sprain. It is a matter of degree.

DYNAMICS OF ANKLE FRACTURE

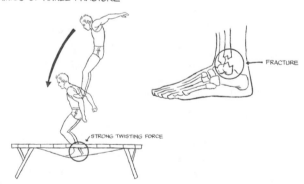

The symptoms are parallel to the degree of tearing that caused the bleeding into the injury site. Swelling, tenderness, pain on movement, discoloration, etc. are the usual symptoms. They are protective in type.

Treatment is based on ice packs, elevation and elastic

wraps to limit swelling of the injured site. This is followed by immobilization with casts, tapes and crutches to allow healing.

ANTIBODY FORMATION

Antibodies are chemicals manufactured by the lymphatic system to counteract such things as viruses and bacteria when they invade the body to cause illness. When antibodies are numerous, a condition called IMMUNITY results — the invading viruses or bacteria are unable to gain a foothold. Antibody formation takes place when you are immunized by your doctor, or when you are recovering from the flu.

Antibodies are formed in the entire lymphoid system. Part of this system is visible at times during infections when such activated lymph nodes become enlarged.

You can help your body, during the formation of antibodies, by getting as much rest as possible so that the manufacturing process is given the number one priority. Your body uses the symptoms of aching, tiredness, fever, dizziness, etc. to encourage rest. You feel so "sick," in fact, that you HAVE to lie down!

Antibody formation takes several days — or longer. That is why limited activity, proper vitamins, food and plenty of liquids are necessary to hasten your recovery from the illness.

BACK/SPINE

Your spine or vertebral column is somewhat like a TV tower. The TV tower requires the support of guy wires to hold it erect and your spine has muscles and ligaments to hold it upright.

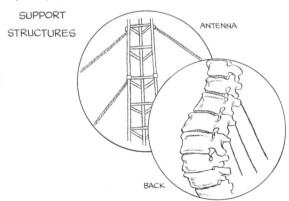

SUPPORT
STRUCTURES

ANTENNA

BACK

If some of the guy wires in your back have pulled loose or become torn, there is an imbalance. This causes symptoms of pain, fatigue and a general aching. The symptoms are protective and encourage you to limit your movement.

They may also be preventive if you "listen" to your back while you are doing something strenuous and quit before serious damage is done.

Treatment is based on rest (done by splinting and braces), heat (to hasten the healing process) and analgesic to relieve pain. Preventive measures are aimed at keeping your muscles regularly stretched and strengthened with daily exercises.

BLOOD PRESSURE

Your heart and arteries are, in the mind of an engineer, the efficient pumping and pipe system shown.

If all parts of your body are to receive oxygen, food and protective blood elements, the pump must maintain a certain pressure level. If the pipes are in spasm because of nervous tension, clogged with fatty deposits of cholesterol or too long because they have to travel through many extra miles of fat tissue, the pump has to work harder.

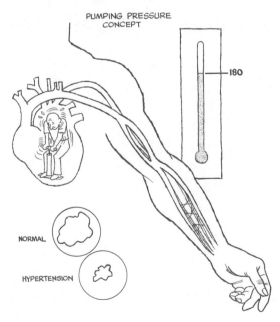

PUMPING PRESSURE
CONCEPT

180

NORMAL

HYPERTENSION

Many of the symptoms associated with high blood pressure can be explained by this extra pumping: fatigue (the pump is tired from working overtime), leg aches (not enough oxygen reaches the leg muscles), skipped or extra beats (the motor misses a few times because it is going too fast), flushed face (extra blood flows into the small vessels near the skin's surface), etc.

Treatment is aimed at relaxing the spasm in the arteries, losing weight, cutting down on fats and cholesterol in diet and slowing the heart.

BLOWING NOSE

The correct way to blow the nose is to close one nostril with the thumb and then GENTLY blow the mucus out of the opposite side. A concept understood by even a small child regarding the effort required to blow GENTLY is this: "Pretend you are blowing out a birthday candle." If the effort more closely resembles BLOWING A BUGLE, it is incorrect!

If you blow the nose too hard, mucus is blown up into the eustachian tubes that lead to the ear. Often flecked with various kinds of bacteria, the mucus lodged there sets the scene for a middle ear infection (otitis media).

Another prevention tip is to stop children from snorting and sniffling when they have a runny nose. This habit also draws mucus up into the eustachian tube. The nose runs to get mucus OUT of the passageways not to be sucked up by useless sniffling and snorting. Give the child his own box of tissues or large clean handkerchief and let him dab or sneeze or gently blow out the mucus.

In over 20 years of medical practice, I have become convinced that 90 percent of middle ear infections, with all the cost and misery associated with them, could be prevented by following the advice given above!

BRUISING AND DISCOLORATION

The black-and-blue mark you get on your cheek when you bang it against the door, the black eye from the unexpected left hook from the three-year-old child you are rough-housing with or the badly discolored ankle after the sprain, are all due to a similar sequence of events.

Initially, the area is injured enough to rupture small blood vessels, both arteries and veins, which bleed into the soft surrounding tissue. When blood doesn't have oxygen, the cells turn quickly from red to blue and the blackish color you see is the result. Depending on the severity of the injury and the speed of first aid given (cold, pressure, elevation, rest), the site will either continue to bleed until the tissue can't hold any more fluids, or the vessels will constrict and bleeding stop.

Obviously, the quicker cold applications (ice or other agents), pressure (elastic wrap or bandage), elevation (blood is mostly water and "runs down hill"), and rest (continuing to use the tissue — muscles, tendons, ligaments — may cause further injury) are brought to action at the site, the less bleeding will result.

Once the bleeding has stopped, healing forces begin and the cleanup progresses colorwise from purple to blue to green to yellow — and finally, in a week, normal.

BURNS

The key thing to note, see illustration, is that the amount of the body injured by the burns causes changes in the whole

RULE OF NINE FOR BURNS

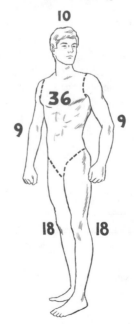

system. Fluid is lost into the tissues causing swelling, pain, heat sensations and damage to the circulation.

The treatment is based on restoring lost fluids, covering the damaged skin with grafts of good skin, blood transfusions to help in the repair work and diet to replace lost protein.

Medical treatment and hospitalization are required if second- or third-degree burns cover a 9 percent surface area in children or a 15 percent surface area in adults.

CHEST AND HEART PAIN

One of the potentially most serious symptoms — and at times most frightening — is that of chest pain. The odds are thrown out of the window when the pain is in YOUR chest. You want to know for SURE.

The chart that follows, modified from a series developed by the Medical Department of Ives Laboratories, Inc. in New York, is a review of some distressing chest pain that is NOT caused by heart attack (acute myocardial infarction).

What are the other conditions that can cause pain similar to heart attack?

Heart Pain (Angina) This pain comes from a lowered blood flow (ischemia) to the heart muscle under exertion. This can happen during physical exertion (like climbing stairs), emotion (anger in a job or family situation), cold weather (walking against the wind on a cold day) and at times when you lie down (particularly after a heavy meal).

Gall Bladder Spasm This pain is caused by irritation from a small gallstone, sludge in the bile or spasm from certain foods. Common dietary causes are butter, rich salad dressings or gravy, spicy foods and at times fresh, raw vegetables or cereals.

Hiatal Hernia The distress of a sliding hiatal hernia occurs when a portion of the stomach slides above the level of the diaphragm, the umbrella-like muscle that divides the chest from the abdomen. The symptoms are, in addition to pain, sensations of burning, bloating and general irritation on centerline under ribs.

Anxiety In today's "Age of Anxiety" it is common to have a variety of vague symptoms in the chest. They are generally precipitated by nervous tension and unresolved conflicts in human relations.

PARAMETERS	HEART PAIN (ANGINA)	GALL BLADDER SPASM	HIATAL HERNIA	ANXIETY
LOCATION OF PAIN	CHEST MIDLINE OFTEN SPREADING ACROSS THE CHEST	UPPER ABDOMEN OFTEN SPREADING CHEST MIDLINE	UPPER ABDOMEN SPREADING ACROSS THE CHEST BUT OFTEN NO SYMPTOMS	OVER LEFT CHEST OR VARIABLE
RADIATION OF PAIN	TO EITHER OR BOTH ARMS NECK OR JAW OR ANY COMBINATION THERE OF	LOWER RIBS TO BACK AND BENEATH RIGHT SHOULDER, SOMETIMES TO LEFT REGION AND SHOULDER	TO EITHER OR BOTH ARMS, NECK OR JAW, OFTEN COMBINATIONS	GENERALLY NONE
DURATION OF PAIN	USUALLY SUBSIDES IN ONE TO FIVE MINUTES	USUALLY STEADY FOR HOURS, SOMETIMES INTERMITTENT (COLIC)	A FEW MINUTES TO ONE HOUR	FROM LESS THEN ONE MINUTE TO SEVERAL HOURS
CHARACTER OF PAIN	PRESSURE OR HEAVY DISCOMFORT	SEVERE, INTENSIFYING RAPIDLY	DULL OR HEAVY DISCOMFORT	SHARP STABBING PAIN OR DULL DISCOMFORT
ASSOCIATED SYMPTOMS	USUALLY NONE BUT OCCASIONALLY INDIGESTION	BLOATING, BELCHING, UPPER ABDOMINAL DISCOMFORT, NAUSEA AND VOMITING, DARK URINE LATER	HICCUP, BELCHING OR HEARTBURN	VAGUE FLOATING WORRIES FLUTTERING SENSATIONS
CAUSATIVE FACTORS	EXERTION, EMOTION, EATING, COLD WEATHER	FRIED FOODS AND VARIOUS VEGETABLES, LARGE MEALS	LYING DOWN, EXERTION AFTER HEAVY MEALS, BENDING OVER	TIREDNESS OR EMOTION BUT OFTEN NONE
RELIEF FACTORS	STOP EFFORT, MEDICATION	WATCH DIET, DRINK FLUIDS	ANTACIDS, DRINKING LIQUIDS, SITTING OR STANDING UPRIGHT	LYING DOWN, SEDATIVES

COUGHING

A cough is an attempt by the body to expel fluids, mucus, dust, and allergens from the lung or throat.

A concept that is helpful is that of thinking of a portion of mucus as a volleyball that is being passed up the bronchioles. Then, the cough is like the spiker who drives the ball over the net.

The symptom of coughing is protective and helps clean out the respiratory tract. Because it is protective it is not wise to take so much cough medicine (antitussive or anti-cough) that it disappears. The cough is there to help.

The so-called "dry cough" comes from dryness and irritation of the lining of the upper respiratory tract rather than mucus being expelled. Nothing comes up with the cough.

Treatment of both dry and loose coughs is aimed at helping liquefy the mucus (vaporizer and lots of liquids by mouth), bed rest (it takes less work to cough lying down than standing or sitting up), postural drainage (help water run downhill by use of pillows to elevate the lower chest and body).

DISC PAIN
Sciatica

The pain associated with disc pain is caused by a pinching of the roots of the sciatic nerve that leads into the leg. It is a mechanical affair that is aggravated by recurring injury to the pad between the vertebrae (intervertebral disc).

This diagram shows what causes the injury and how the pinching takes place.

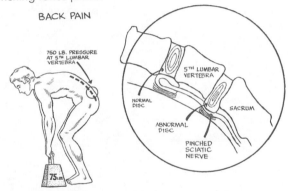

LIFTING 75 LB. = 750 LB. HYDROLIC PRESSURE

Treatment is based on returning the vertebrae and disc to a neutral nonirritating position and then letting the inflammation from the injured nerve subside. Pain medication, heat and massage are aimed at muscle relaxation in the lower back.

Prevention is a key factor in this disorder. Symptoms can play an important role by warning you of bad positions in car seats, bad lifting habits, poor posture, poor physical fitness and limited vertebral joint movements.

FEVER

A fever is an elevation of temperature above your normal level. The average oral temperature is 98.6° F., but your own normal could be slightly above or below that. Your temperature may also vary during the day — registering higher after 5 P.M., and lower in the early morning before you get out of bed.

It is important for you to know your normal oral temperature. Your rectal temperature will register about 1° higher than the oral temperature.

The symptom of fever is not necessarily bad. At times of infection, fever is an important part of the healing process. Just as one sterilizes a baby's bottle by heating it to kill germs, your body turns up the heat (fever) which helps kill the germs and form antibodies faster.

Thus, when you have an infection, don't worry excessively about any fever up to 100° if you are not too uncomfortable. For babies and children under three, fever is a greater concern because their temperature regulator is still not developed completely. Give them aspirin or Tylenol sooner and dress them in lightweight sleepwear in a moderate to cool bedroom.

ITCHING

Itching occurs when infections from skin bacteria, viruses and fungi cause a scaling of the top layers of the skin. This scaling tickles or irritates the nerves in the surface of the skin.

The symptom tells you that the skin surface is not sealed. It is flaking and dry.

Treatment is aimed at sealing the surface with protective creams or ointments and by the applications of soothing preparations that restore moisture to the skin.

It is important to know that most skin medications must be rubbed down through the upper scaling skin in order to be absorbed into the deeper skin layers.

PAIN

Pain is a symptom that is hard to overlook. Its type and location depend on the cause. The causes may be obvious and directly located on the problem — an example is a boil on the neck. Pain may also be indirect or referred from an internal organ. Several common examples of referred pain are shown in the accompanying diagrams.

Pain in the abdomen is especially important to understand because it may herald serious disease that could require hospitalization and perhaps surgery. Common examples of abdominal pain patterns are visualized in the graph below.

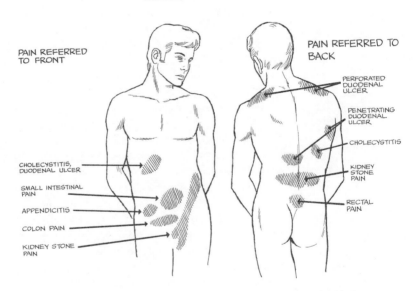

PAIN PATTERNS

TYPE	VISUALIZATION
CRAMPS	
CONSTANT ACHE	
INTER-MITTENT COLIC	
CONSTANT COLIC	

PAIN REFERRED TO FRONT

PAIN REFERRED TO BACK

PERFORATED DUODENAL ULCER

PENETRATING DUODENAL ULCER

CHOLECYSTITIS

KIDNEY STONE PAIN

RECTAL PAIN

CHOLECYSTITIS, DUODENAL ULCER

SMALL INTESTINAL PAIN

APPENDICITIS

COLON PAIN

KIDNEY STONE PAIN

The symptom called pain is usually protective and alerts you to disease. In some cases it may also signal the expelling of unwanted substances such as kidney or gallstones.

Treatment is based on unravelling the cause of the pain through diagnosis and then applying indicated therapy.

TESTING INDEX

The purpose of providing this index is to help you become a better observer of events in common illnesses. Several common testing tools and physical examination methods are necessary for you to more accurately observe these events.

Traditionally, these tools and methods have been in the exclusive domain of your doctor and his office staff. Things have changed over the years and are changing even more today. Although it was relatively rare to find a family with an oral thermometer 25 years ago, most own one today. If five years ago, I'd been told that blood pressure cuffs and stethoscopes would be promoted in my Sunday paper for home use, I'd have scoffed — yet look at the recent ads in PARADE magazine and other such popular publications.

My experiences with several Courses for the Activated Patient have shown me that important and accurate observations can be made by nonprofessionals. So here is the information you need to do-it-yourself. The people who take my classes learn to do these tests after lecture and demonstration sessions — of course, the best way to learn them. However, the methods are safe and presented here in such a way that with a little instruction from your doctor or nurse, AND MUCH PRACTICE, you should be able to do many of these tests at home — on members of your own family.

Keep in mind that the observations I teach you are simple and straightforward. When you are told to examine the ear canal, you are told to look for the presence or absence of ear wax. Nothing complex about that. When you are told to look at the drum, you are asked to observe whether it is red or pearly white. Again, an easy observation. That's as far as we go. You are not expected to make medical observations that require a doctor's training. Maybe you aren't as relaxed with these procedures as you'd like to be, but remember, it's a start. It's also so much more than most people have to work with when they call their doctor.

G118

ABDOMINAL DISTRESS

The only observations that will be emphasized in this section will be those involved with identifying the portions of the abdomen. You will note in the following diagrams that the wall of the abdomen is conveniently divided into several areas, all related to the belly button (navel or umbilicus).

After noting the pain pattern, have the patient lie on a firm surface, naked from the chest to the hair line of the pubis, as comfortably as possible with arms by his sides. Then gently apply pressure to the abdomen. Observe the area of greatest tenderness. Do the exam, if possible, when the pain has subsided. Repeat the examination 2 or 3 times and write down your observation. It might read like this: "Pain and tenderness lower abdomen — right side."

ABDOMINAL LANDMARKS

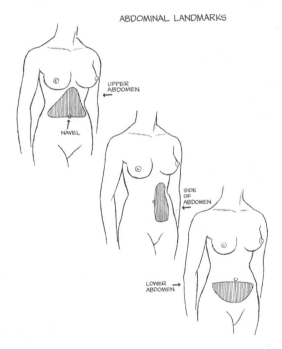

BLOOD PRESSURE
Use of Sphygmomanometer

To take blood pressure you need a stethoscope, blood pressure cuff, a good instruction booklet and some training by your doctor or nurse.

A stethoscope costs $5.00 and up. You can buy them at surgical and hospital supply stores and stores such as Sears and Wards. "Disposable" stethoscopes made for coronary care units cost $3.00 and at times can be obtained free after use. It is best to buy the flat-surfaced diaphragm model rather than the bell-shaped type.

The blood pressure cuff (sphygmomanometer) costs $25.00 and up. It is usually available at the same stores that offer stethoscopes. There are two basic types, the mercury column and the aneroid model. The aneroid is several dollars cheaper than the mercury column.

BLOOD PRESSURE TOOLS

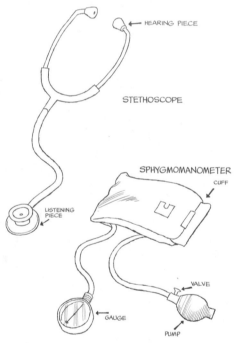

Instruction books that come with these instruments vary. Excellent ones, however, are available. Write for:

HOW YOUR BLOOD PRESSURE IS MEASURED, W. A. Baum Co., Inc., Copaigue, NY 11726.

RECOMMENDATIONS FOR HUMAN BLOOD PRESSURE DETERMINATION, American Heart Association, 44 East 23rd Street, New York, NY 10010.

Concept   Before I go into the how-to-do-it specifics, here are some concepts that will help you. The entire process of testing has to do with the dynamics of the flow of liquids. Think of the flow of blood in the artery of your arm as the flow of water in your garden hose. There is no noise while the flow of water is smooth, but if you step on the hose or kink it you hear sounds of turbulence. When you release the hose to its normal diameter again, the sounds disappear and the water runs smoothly. You could even use a sort of blood pressure cuff to test the pressure in your garden hose. Similarly, when you take a blood pressure of the artery in your arm, you first hear no sounds with your stethoscope. Then, as you increase the pressure by pumping up the balloon in the cuff and narrow the diameter of the "hose" you hear sounds of turbulence. When they disappear completely, the artery is closed by the pressure and we call this point the systolic pressure.

When you loosen the cuff, there is a turbulence as the fluid starts flowing again. At the point that you hear no more noise, the artery is completely open. We call this lower level the diastolic pressure.

Checking   The person whose blood pressure you are checking (NOTE:
Pressure   It is difficult to check your own!) should be seated on a chair next to a table on which the left arm of the person is outstretched. The arm and forearm should be bare.

Loosen the valve (turn counterclockwise) and deflate the cuff completely before you wrap it around the upper arm. The lower edge of the cuff should be 1 in. above the crease where the arm bends. Fasten the cuff snugly.

Put the stethoscope in your ears and place the diaphragm 1 in. below the arm crease on the midline. Do not touch the cuff with the stethoscope.

Place the gauge of the cuff in a position where you can easily read the dial. Close the valve (turn clockwise) and pump the pressure up to a level of about 180. IMMEDIATELY LOOSEN the valve a bit so that the needle starts moving down slowly. NOTE: If you keep the cuff pumped up at 180 or more it is quite painful for the patient.

Watch the dial as you listen with the stethoscope. You will soon hear the pulse sounds. The pressure number on the dial when the sound is first heard is called the SYSTOLIC pressure. A normal example would be 125.

G121

Then, as the needle continues to drop, the sound will again disappear. The pressure number when this occurs is the DIASTOLIC pressure. A normal example would be 70. Then, open the valve completely and let the pressure fall to 0. Remove the cuff.

In the above example, the blood pressure would be recorded as 125/70. A normal reading. An abnormal example indicating the possibility of high blood pressure might be 160/90.

Recheck the blood pressure several times at different times of the day and take an average of at least three readings. This can then be called the person's blood pressure reading.

If it continues to be normal (under 150/90) that is good. If it is elevated, have it rechecked by a doctor or nurse.

BREATHING RATE

This observation is an easy one. It can provide useful help, especially in children during fever or respiratory illnesses.

The only tool needed for this is a watch or clock with a sweep second hand. Place your outstretched hand on the front of the chest. Touch the collarbone with your ring finger and put your thumb two or three ribs lower. Count the number of breaths while the person is sitting in a quiet manner.

The normal, healthy adult and child will have a breathing rate of 18 to 20 breaths per minute. Young children and babies will have a faster rate, perhaps 22 to 24 breaths per minute.

When lung illness or fever are present, the respiratory rate will be faster. It moves up in pace with the fever.

EARS
Use of Otoscope

To examine the ear you need an otoscope or an ear speculum and penlight.

An otoscope will usually cost $25 and up at surgical supply stores. There are some available for less at about $13. (This economy model penlight otoscope, catalog #2314, can be ordered by your doctor through his surgical supply salesman from Medisco, Inc.)

An ear speculum or otoscope cup can be purchased at

surgical supply stores for less than $1. This, when used with a high intensity penlight that costs $2 or less, will give you a fair examining tool.

In doing the ear exam, grasp the middle of the ear as shown and pull the ear back and out. This straightens the canal and makes it easier to see.

Insert the otoscope speculum into the external canal and look for brown or black wax. If wax is present use Debrox to soften and remove it. (See Treatment Index, p. G88.)

TO EXAMINE EAR

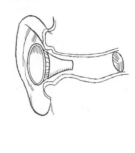

SPECULUM IN EAR CANAL

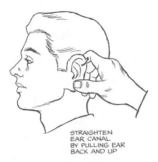

STRAIGHTEN
EAR CANAL
BY PULLING EAR
BACK AND UP

If there is no wax to hide it you will see a shiny, PEARLY WHITE ear drum — if it is normal. If the drum is inflamed, it may be partly or completely RED. This usually indicates an acute infection (otitis media). A BLUISH color on the drum may mean fluid in the middle ear associated with serous otitis media. NOTE: Some people have extremely curved ear canals and the drum is difficult to see. If it cannot be seen easily and without pain, stop the examination.

EYES
Use of Penlight

To examine the eyes for pupil size, the only tool needed is a penlight. Practice eye examination by having a volunteer sit across from you face-to-face. Flash the light on the pupil and it will get smaller. This is a normal protective reflex. The pupil will return to normal size when the light is removed. If a patient is unconscious or has a severe head injury, the pupils may be widely dilated. Quick inspection (see illustration) shows it to you even without the penlight.

G123

PUPIL SIZE

NORMAL   DILATED

   While you are examining your volunteer or patient, look
also at the "whites of the eye." They should appear clear and
white. There may normally be one or two fine red streaks (tiny
arteries on the surface of the conjunctiva) but if the
appearance is "bloodshot" it is called conjunctivitis
(inflammation of the conjunctiva).
(A good disposable, narrow-focus, hi-power beam penlight
is available for about $1 from Hennikers, 1485 Bayshore
Blvd., San Francisco, CA 94124.)

HEART RATE
Use of Stethoscope

If the heart rate (pulse) is so rapid that it can't be counted at
the wrist — as may be the case with a young child with fever
or an adult in shock — use the stethoscope to count the heart
rate over the heart at the chest. Listen in the area just under
the left nipple and above line of the lower edge of the ribs.
   But, before you start listening to heart rates, put the
stethoscope ear pieces in your ears and try them for comfort.
If there is distress, try switching the pieces to the opposite ear.
Then practice listening to things in your house, room or
apartment.
   First, try listening to running water in a pipe, then the pipe
from the furnace. The next step is to get an adult male
volunteer, since a woman's breast can interfere with
inexperienced heart monitoring, or a child and check the
heart rate. Take off the shirt and place the listening piece near
the nipple, about 3 in. from the midline of the chest. If the
volunteer is a male with a hairy chest, you'll hear a scratchy
sound as the hair moves against the plastic listening piece. If
possible, use a patch of skin without hair.
   You will hear the "lub-dub," "lub-dub" sound of the
heartbeat. Listen first for a full minute and count the beats.
Later on, listen for 15 seconds and multiply by four for the
proper rate.

The rate varies with age, temperature (if there is fever), exertion and so on. The usual rate for well adults is 68 to 72 beats per minute. The rate for babies and children is higher. Usually, the younger the child the higher the rate. A young baby may have a rate of over 100 beats per minute and still be normal.

KIDNEY TENDERNESS

To determine if the patient's lower back may be tender in an acute urinary tract infection (pyelonephritis), lightly "punch" the areas indicated in the diagram.

KIDNEY TEST AREA

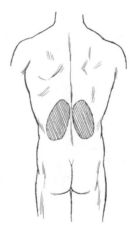

This area over the kidneys may be extra sensitive or tender if the infection has moved up from the urinary bladder into the kidneys.

NOSE
Use of Penlight

With the aid of a high intensity penlight, the nasal mucosa can be examined to give clues about whether a persistent stuffy nose is an allergic reaction. A PALE SWOLLEN water-logged (sometimes even bluish) mucous surface makes allergy a probable cause. The normal color is pink and shiny — look at the mucous lining of the mouth as a comparison. If, on the other hand, the mucosa is bright red and shiny, the stuffy nose is most likely caused by bacterial infection. There may also be streaks of blood in the mucus.

TEMPERATURE
Use of Thermometer

Thermometer A good thermometer costs about $2.00. You can buy one at any drugstore or surgical supply store. (I am always surprised in my courses to find out how few people have a workable thermometer at home. Usually the number is less than half.) There are two types of thermometer, the oral for mouth temperatures and the rectal type for use in children under six years of age. Most young children cannot keep an oral thermometer under their tongues, and some have even accidentally bitten off the glass tip!

There are many good thermometers available in your drugstore. The one we use in our courses is put out by Becton-Dickinson of Rutherford, NJ. It is marked "B-D" and comes with a convenient plastic case. There are now some good quality electronic thermometers coming on the market but most are still too expensive for household use.

Taking Temperature The proper procedure for taking the oral temperature is as follows.

1. With soap and water, wash off the bulb and lower part of the thermometer that will go into the patient's mouth. Then do not touch this area.

THE THERMOMETER

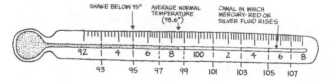

2. Grasp the thermometer at the high-number end and shake until the fluid in the canal falls below the 95° mark. (See the illustration.)
3. Place the bulb under the patient's tongue. Tell patient to close mouth and breathe through nose. Leave thermometer in position for 3 minutes.
4. Remove thermometer and hold up in good light to read where the mercury has stopped.

G126

5.   Read the LONG line immediately left of where the mercury stopped. (See illustration.) This gives you the full degree.
6.   Count the SHORT lines between the long line you have just read and the point where the mercury stopped. Each short line stands for two-tenths of a degree. Adding the long and short line readings gives you the temperature in degrees Fahrenheit.

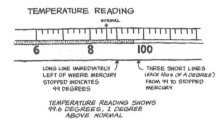

TEMPERATURE READING

NORMAL

6   8   100

LONG LINE IMMEDIATELY ⌡   ⌐ THREE SHORT LINES
LEFT OF WHERE MERCURY   (EACH 2/10 s OF A DEGREE)
STOPPED INDICATES   FROM 99 TO STOPPED
99 DEGREES   MERCURY

TEMPERATURE READING SHOWS
99.6 DEGREES, 1 DEGREE
ABOVE NORMAL

THROAT AND NECK
Use of Penlight

The throat can be examined with the aid of a penlight and a teaspoon. The teaspoon handle may be used as a tongue blade and is preferred by most because it eliminates the dry woody feel that causes some people to gag.

If you have a fussy child, as is common when a three-year-old is sick, who simply can't or doesn't want to open his mouth, ask him to play the Puppy Dog Game. Ask him if he remembers how a puppy pants in the summer time when it's hot. Then have him pretend that he's a puppy dog panting. As he opens his mouth and pants you can take a quick look. The panting elevates the palate enough to see the upper throat.

LANDMARKS OF MOUTH AND THROAT

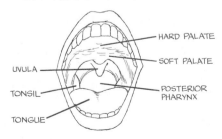

HARD PALATE

SOFT PALATE

UVULA

POSTERIOR
PHARYNX

TONSIL

TONGUE

With the mouth open as shown, the throat and tonsils can be examined. If there is a possible strep throat (bacterial pharyngitis, tonsillitis), the throat will be red with patches of yellow or white exudate. It may have a "cobblestoned" appearance.

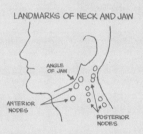

LANDMARKS OF NECK AND JAW

The lymph nodes at the angle of the jaw may be enlarged and tender.

101-PLUS SELF-HELP FREEBIES

There is a great amount of well-written, nicely illustrated health education material available from health associations, pharmaceutical companies, the Department of Health, Education and Welfare, medical associations, county health departments and so on. Much of it is free or available for a nominal fee (25¢ to $1.00).

I have been collecting such material for several years and had a good supply but appreciated the extra shove recently supplied by the American Academy of Family Physicians and the Metropolitan Life Insurance Company. These organizations each put out a fine publication: "Compendium of Patient Education Materials" (AAFP Reprint B-3500) and "Patient Education" (Metropolitan Life). I am indebted to them in part for the materials and organization of this section.

Alcohol/Alcoholism

"About Alcohol" 5½ × 8 in. A 16-page scriptographic booklet. Explains the effects of alcohol, stages of intoxication, alcoholism, dangers of permanent damage and reasons why 32% of the U.S. adult population are nondrinkers. 25¢ each to 99 copies, 19¢ each for 100 to 500. Order from Francis J. Rodovich, Vice President, Channing L. Bete Co., Inc., 45 Federal St., Greenfield, Mass. 01301.

"The Beginning of Wisdom About Alcohol" 8½ × 11 in. A 4-page reprint from *Fortune* (May 1968). Describes corporate programs for salvaging executives and workers. National Council on Alcoholism, Inc., 2 Park Ave., New York, N.Y. 10016.

"The Illness Called Alcoholism" 4 × 8½ in. A 16-page booklet. Explores alcoholism as a disease, attitudes toward alcohol, causes of alcoholism and treatment of the disease. 25¢ each to 99 copies, 15¢ each for 100 to 499. Order #OP-192 from Order Handling Dept., American Medical Association, 535 N. Dearborn St., Chicago, Ill. 60610.

Allergies

"Allergy: Facts and Fiction" 5¼ × 7 in. A 100-page monograph. Intended to be a handy, quick reference guide to allergies. Prepared to be distributed to patients by doctors. Budlong Press Co., 5428 N. Virginia Ave., Chicago, Ill. 60625. $2.00.

Robins "How-To" Series Desensitize a car for the allergy patients. Help create a mold-free home for the allergy patient. Reduce the allergic load for the allergy-prone infant. Tame the outdoors for the allergy patient. A. H. Robins Co., Richmond, Va. 23220.

"Sneezing, Wheezing and Scratching" 8½ × 11 in. Doris J. Rapp, M.D. A simple picture book for children about allergies. Tips to avoid and prevent common allergies. 25ε. Office of Public Health Education & Information, Erie County Department of Health, 953 County Office Bldg., 95 Franklin St., Buffalo, N.Y. 14202.

"You and Your Skin and Your Allergies" 4 × 6 in. Presents a basic understanding of the causes and treatments of skin allergies. Schering Corp., Bloomfield, N.J. 07003.

Arthritis

"About Arthritis" 5½ × 8 in. A 16-page scriptographic booklet. Explains rheumatoid arthritis, osteoarthritis, gout and other types of America's most crippling disease. 25ε each to 99 copies, 19ε each for 100 to 499. Order from Francis J. Rodovich, V.P., Channing L. Bete Co., Inc., 45 Federal St., Greenfield, Mass. 01301.

"Arthritis — The Basic Facts" 5½ × 8½ in. This booklet emphasizes the various kinds of arthritis.[1]

"Home-Care Programs in Arthritis" 8½ × 6½ in. A valuable guide for patients regarding exercises and physical therapy.[1]

"Osteoarthritis (A Handbook for Patients)" 5½ × 8½ in. This describes the common arthritis found in persons over 60.[1]

"Rheumatoid Arthritis (A Handbook for Patients)" 5½ × 8½ in. This describes the symptoms and causes of rheumatoid arthritis.[1]

"Self-Help Manual for Arthritis Patients" 6 × 9 in. This 124-page monograph describes self-help aids, devices and procedures for everyday care and activity. $1.25.[1]

Birth Defects and Hereditary Diseases

"Be Good to Your Baby Before it is Born" 8½ × 11 in. Virginia Apgar, M.D. gives a new look about what to do and expect during pregnancy. The National Foundation — March of Dimes, P.O. Box 2000, White Plains, N.Y. 10602.

"Nutrition & Birth Defects Prevention" 4 × 9 in. An 8-page pamphlet. Stresses the importance of eating right when you're "eating for two." Illustrated chart explains the foods you need, how much each day and why. Free. Order from Health Information and School Relations, The National Foundation — March of Dimes, 1275 Mamaroneck Ave., White Plains, N.Y. 10602.

"Unprescribed Drugs & Birth Defects Prevention" 4·× 9 in. A 6-page pamphlet. Questions and answers about unprescribed drugs (including cigarettes and alcohol) and how they can affect a pregnancy. Free. Order

[1]Single copies, except as marked, are free and may be obtained from The Arthritis Foundation, 221 Park Ave. South, New York, N.Y. 10003.

from Health Information and School Relations, The National Foundation — March of Dimes, 1275 Mamaroneck Ave., White Plains, N.Y. 10602.

Cancer

"About Cancer" 5½ × 8 in. A 16-page scriptographic booklet. Explains some "facts and fiction" about cancer, how cancer develops, how it can be prevented and stresses learning of the seven warning signals. 25¢ each to 99 copies, 19¢ each for 100 to 499. Order from Francis J. Rodovich, V. P., Channing L. Bete Co., Inc., 45 Federal St., Greenfield, Mass. 01301.

"Breast Cancer" 3 × 6 in. 8-page pamphlet. A reprint from *Redbook* explaining who may get breast cancer, self-examination, possible treatments and the importance of a complete examination by a physician. $7 per 100, $17 for 250. Order #R-14 from ACOG Publications, American College of Obstetrics and Gynecology, One E. Wacker Drive, Chicago, Ill. 60601.

"Some Facts Concerning Cancer" 3½ × 6 in. A bright pink leaflet. Facts and statistics of vital interest to every woman about breast and uterine cancer. $1 per 100, order in multiples of 100. Order from Information Resource Dept., American Academy of Family Physicians, 1740 W. 92nd St., Kansas City, Mo. 64114.

Consumerism

"Medicaid-Medicare, Which is Which?" 3½ × 5 in. This 28-page booklet gives general guidelines for coverage under these two federal insurance plans. 25¢. MSA-901-70. Superintendent of Documents, U.S. Government Printing Office, Washington, D.C. 20402.

"Brands, Generics, Prices and Quality" 3½ × 9 in. This brochure brings you information about Rx medicines you need to know. Free.[2]

"The Medicines Your Doctor Prescribes (A Guide for Consumers)" 3½ × 9 in. This 6-page brochure, written by Sue Boe, assistant vice president, Consumers Affairs of P.M.A., suggests ways to save money at the drugstore.[2]

"Statement on a Patients Bill of Rights" (English and Spanish versions) 3 × 9 in. This brochure presents the "Bill of Rights" for the hospitalized patient. American Hospital Association, 840 N. Lake Shore Drive, Chicago, Ill. 60611.

Diabetes

"About Diabetes" 5½ × 8 in. A 16-page scriptographic booklet. Facts about diabetes — symptoms, tests and treatment. Encourages an annual medical checkup, watching your weight and following good health practices. 25¢ each to 99 copies, 19¢ each for 100 to 499. Order from Francis J. Rodovich, V.P., Channing L. Bete Co., Inc., 45 Federal St., Greenfield, Mass. 01301.

[2]May be obtained from Pharmaceutical Manufacturers Association, 1115 Fifteenth St., N.W., Washington, D.C. 20005.

"A Cookbook for Diabetics"   6 × 9 in. A 175-page spiral bound book. A wide variety of dishes and menus for every occasion — an interesting and attractive diet suitable not only for diabetics but for their families and guests. Includes explanation of the six exchange lists, and gives exchange information for each recipe. $1 each, lesser cost in quantity. Order from Jessie H. Raborg, American Diabetes Assoc., 18 E. 48th St., New York, N.Y. 10017.

"Signs of Diabetes"   4 × 10 in. A 3-page guide that gives the signs of diabetes and symptoms of too little sugar or too much sugar. Geigy Pharmaceuticals, Division of CIBA-GEIGY Corp., Ardsley, N.Y. 10502.

Drugs

"About Drugs & Drug Abuse"   (For parents) 5½ × 8 in. A 16-page scriptographic booklet. Aids parents in recognizing symptoms of drug abuse, suggests ways to help children avoid drug abuse and steps to take if parents discover their children are taking drugs. 25¢ each to 99 copies, 19¢ each for 100 to 499. Order from Francis J. Rodovich, V.P., Channing L. Bete Co., Inc., 45 Federal St., Greenfield, Mass. 01301.

"Drugs and You"   5½ × 8 in. A 16-page scriptographic booklet. Explains stimulants, depressants and hallucinogens, ethical use and drug abuse, myths about drugs and federal legal controls. 25¢ each to 99 copies, 19¢ each for 100 to 499. Order from Francis J. Rodovich, V. P., Channing L. Bete Co., Inc., 45 Federal St., Greenfield, Mass. 01301.

Epilepsy

"Answers to Questions About Epilepsy"   3½ × 8½ in. A 16-page booklet. Question and answer format provides detailed information on all aspects of epilepsy. $5 per 100.[3]

"Because You Are My Friend"   4 × 8½ in. A 16-page booklet. Well-illustrated, large-print booklet for primary-grade readers. A first-person narrative explanation of epilepsy. Well done. $6 per 100.[3]

"Can Epilepsy Be Prevented?"   3½ × 8½ in. A 20-page booklet. One of the objectives of the pamphlet is to raise questions and encourage more study on the extent to which many convulsive disorders can be prevented, including epilepsy. $10 per 100.[3]

[3]All booklets may be obtained from Epilepsy Foundation of America Regional Offices nearest you.
    Regions I & II (Connecticut, Maine, Massachusetts, New Hampshire, Rhode Island, Vermont, New Jersey, New York, Puerto Rico)
        101 Tremont Street, Suite 613-614
        Boston, Massachusetts 02108

    Regions III & IV (Delaware, District of Columbia, Maryland, Pennsylvania, Virginia, West Virginia, Alabama, Florida, Georgia, Kentucky, Mississippi, North Carolina, South Carolina, Tennessee)
        1581 Phoenix Boulevard, Suite #10
        Atlanta, Georgia 30349

Eye Care

"Amblyopia — Lazy Eye"   3½ × 6½ in. An 8-page folder. Explains the most frequent cause of poor vision in the young child, with a list of ABCs which suggest the need for an eye examination. Includes instructions on how to test your child's eyes with tear-off stamps for a picture test. $5 per 100.[4]

"Dyslexia — Your Child's Reading Disability"   4 × 9 in. An 8-page folder. Explains dyslexia, what causes it, how it can be recognized, why early diagnosis is important and the best approach in dealing with dyslexia. $5 per 100.[4]

"Eye Cues for Eye Care"   3½ × 6 in. A 6-page folder. Explains the importance of good vision to a child's education, and gives cues which will help identify signs of eye trouble in children. $1.25 per 100, $10 per 1,000.[4]

"Living with Glaucoma"   3½ × 6½ in. A 6-page folder. Outlines seven simple lifetime rules to help patients preserve remaining vision in the glaucomatous eye. 5¢ each, $2 per 100.[4]

"Medical Information on Myopia"   4 × 8½ in. An 8-page folder. Designed to acquaint the reader with the problem of simple myopia. $2.25 per 100.[4]

"Seeing Well as You Grow Older"   4 × 9 in. An 8-page folder. Illustrated, narrative explanation of common vision problems associated with age. Stresses the importance of periodic eye examinations by an ophthalmologist. $2.25 per 100.[4]

"Cataract" — What it is and how it is treated.[5]
"First Aid for Eye Emergencies"[5]
"Home Eye Test for Preschoolers"[5]
"Signs of Eye Trouble in Children"[5]

Family Planning

"A Guide to the Methods of Postponing or Preventing Pregnancy"   5½ × 5½ in. A 34-page book. Points out there is no method of contraception that is

---

Regions V & VII (Illinois, Indiana, Michigan, Minnesota, Ohio, Wisconsin, Iowa, Kansas, Missouri, Nebraska)
343 South Dearborn Street, Suite 1717
Chicago, Illinois 60604

Regions VI & VIII (Arkansas, Louisiana, New Mexico, Oklahoma, Texas, Colorado, Montana, North Dakota, South Dakota, Utah, Wyoming)
1625 Main Street, Suite 305
Houston, Texas 77002

Regions IX & X (Arizona, California, Hawaii, Nevada, Alaska, Idaho, Oregon, Washington)
5665 N. Las Virgenes Road
Calabasas, California, 91302

[4]All items can be obtained from American Association of Ophthalmology, 1100 17th St. N.W., Washington, D.C. 20036.

[5]All items can be obtained from National Society for the Prevention of Blindness, Inc., 79 Madison Ave., New York, N.Y. 10016.

ideal for every woman. Explains various methods, listing advantages and disadvantages. Carries Ortho identification but no product endorsements. Free.[6]

"Intrauterine Contraception" 3½ × 5 in. A 6-page folder. Written as a letter from the doctor explaining what to expect during the "breaking-in" period for an IUD. Contains commercial product mention. Free.[6]

"Questions and Answers about the Pill" (brochure)[7]
"New Hope for Childless Couples" (brochure)[7]
"Voluntary Sterilization for Men and Women" (brochure)[7]

First Aid

"About First Aid" 5½ × 8 in. A 16-page scriptographic booklet. Tests prior knowledge of first aid ability, presents steps to be taken in various situations, stresses when to call the doctor, and encourages signing up for a Red Cross first aid course. 25¢ each to 99 copies, 19¢ each for 100 to 499. Order from Francis J. Rodovich, V. P., Channing L. Bete Co., Inc., 45 Federal St., Greenfield, Mass. 01301.

"First Aid Chart" 11 × 17 in. A two-color chart. Illustrated chart explaining steps to take in common first aid situations. 50¢ each. Order from Ms. Vivian Olson, Dept. "P", American Academy of Pediatrics, P.O. Box 1034, Evanston, Ill. 60204.

"First Aid Manual" 4 × 6 in. A 48-page booklet. General recommendations of the AMA for first aid, designed to supplement instruction in first aid techniques. 30¢ each to 99 copies, 14¢ each for 100 to 499. Order #OP-15 from Order Handling Dept., American Medical Association, 535 N. Dearborn St., Chicago, Ill. 60610.

"Guide to First Aid" 5 × 7½ in. A 23-page booklet prepared by Lois Mattox Miller and Susan W. Thompson for the *Reader's Digest*. 25¢ each. Order from Reprint Editor, *Reader's Digest*, Pleasantville, N.Y. 10570.

Foot Health

"Foot Health and Aging" 4 × 9 in. A 4-page folder. Discusses preventive foot care to avoid ailments which make it difficult and often impossible for older people to live useful, satisfying lives. Single copies free, larger quantities free on certain individual requests. $5 per 100.[8]

"Memo to Parents" 4 × 9 in. brochure. Describes childhood foot problems.[8]

"Step Up to Foot Health" 4 × 9 in. A 4-page folder. Discusses the basic rules of foot care, detailing some common foot problems. Single copies free, larger quantities free on certain individual requests. $5 per 100.[8]

[6]Both items may be ordered from Ortho Pharmaceutical Corp., Rt. 202, Rariton, N.J. 08869.

[7]Items may be ordered from Planned Parenthood Federation of America, Inc., 810 Seventh Ave., New York, N.Y. 10019.

[8]Order from Department of Public Affairs, American Podiatry Association, 20 Chevy Chase Circle N.W., Washington, D.C. 22015.

"So You Have a Foot Problem?" (Bunions) 3½ × 8 in. A 4-page folder. Explains what bunions are, how they develop, and the importance of medical attention. $4 per 100 copies. Order from Henry R. Cowell, M.D., Secretary, American Orthopaedic Foot Society, VA Center, 1601 Kirkwood Highway, Wilmington, Del. 19805.

Handicapped Persons

"Self-Help Clothing for Handicapped Children" 6 × 9 in. 84 pages. Neva R. Waggoner, Eleanor Boettke, Claire Bare. Guidelines for selection or simple alteration of all articles of child's wardrobe. 50¢[9]

"When You Meet a Handicapped Person" 5½ × 8½ in. 15 hints for rewarding relationships. Free.[9]

"The Crippled Child's Bill of Rights" Free[9]

"Airline Transportation for the Handicapped and Disabled" Stanley G. Hogsett. $1.25[9]

"Feeding the Cerebral Palsied Child" Free[9]
"A Guide for Stroke Rehabilitation" Free[9]

Hearing (See Speech & Hearing)

Heart/High Blood Pressure/Stroke

"The Heart and Blood Vessels" 5½ × 8½ in. A 20-page booklet. Well-illustrated explanation of the heart and circulatory system, including a discussion of cardiovascular diseases. Single copies free.[10]

"How the Doctor Examines Your Heart" 3½ × 6 in. A 32-page booklet. Cartoon-illustrated explanation of the procedures involved in a heart examination. Single copies free.[10]

"Reduce Your Risk of Heart Attack" 3½ × 9 in. A 16-page booklet. Explains the major risks of heart attack and what to do about them. Has helpful facts about the heart and circulation, and about atherosclerosis. Single copies free.[10]

"The Way to a Man's Heart" 4 × 9 in. Folder and poster. A fat-controlled, low-cholesterol meal plan to reduce the risk of heart attack, complete with poster of the 5 basic food groups. Single copies free.[10]

"Your Blood Pressure" 3½ × 5½ in. folder.[10]

"How You Can Help Your Doctor Treat Your High Blood Pressure" 8 × 5½ in. A 12-page booklet by Marvin Moser, M.D.[10]

[9]May be ordered from National Easter Seal Society, 2023 W. Ogden Ave., Chicago, Ill. 60612.

[10]Order from American Heart Association, 44 East 23rd St., New York, N.Y. 10014.

"Your Blood Pressure"   4 × 8½ in. An 8-page folder. Graphically illustrated discussion of hypertension, the most common chronic disease in the United States. 15¢ each to 99 copies, 7¢ each for 100 to 499. Order #OP-44 from Order Handling Dept., American Medical Association, 535 W. Dearborn St., Chicago, Ill. 60610.

"Watch Your Blood Pressure"   Theodore Irwin. 35¢. Pamphlet 483, Public Affairs Pamphlets, 381 Park Ave. S., New York, N.Y. 10016.

"Understanding Stroke"   3½ × 8½ in. A 6-page folder. Helpful for families of stroke patients, this folder presents facts about stroke, medical terms to understand and steps to aid in the rehabilitation. $35 per 1,000. Order from Library, National Easter Seal Society, 2023 W. Ogden Ave., Chicago, Ill. 60612.

Lungs (also see Smoking)

"Asthma — The Facts"   3½ × 8½ in. A 6-page folder. Concise discussion of who gets asthma, how it attacks, what causes it, and how it can be treated and attacks prevented. Free.[11]

"Chronic Bronchitis — The Facts"   3½ × 8½ in. A 6-page folder. Explains what it is, how serious it is, who gets it and how it attacks. Lists six rules for any person subject to bronchial infections. Free.[11]

"Emphysema"   3½ × 8½ in. A 6-page folder. Six pointers to remember highlight this discussion of this serious disabler. Free.[11]

"Shortness of Breath"   3½ × 8½ in. A 6-page folder. How can you tell shortness of breath from just rapid breathing? This folder explains how to tell the difference, and that shortness of breath may be a signal of other things. Free.[11]

"Tuberculosis"   3½ × 8½ in. An 8-page pamphlet. "Half of what you heard about TB a few years ago isn't true today. In fact, much of what you hear about it today isn't true." The facts are presented in this pamphlet. Free.[11]

Mental Health

"About Mental Health"   5½ × 8 in. A 16-page scriptographic booklet. States that mental health, like physical health, can be improved by good habits, environment and relationships. 25¢ each to 99 copies, 19¢ each for 100 to 499. Order from Francis J. Rodovich, V. P., Channing L. Bete Co., Inc., 45 Federal St., Greenfield, Mass. 01301.

"Learning About Depressive Illnesses"   5 × 7 in. A 16-page booklet. Narrative discussion of what happens when depression becomes something more than just normal feelings of blues or letdown. Explains what causes depression and how it can be treated. From the NIMH. 20¢ each. Order Stock No. 1724-0235 from Superintendent of Documents, U.S. Government Printing Office, Washington, D.C. 20402.

[11]May order from American Lung Association, 1740 Broadway, New York, N.Y. 10019.

"How You Can Handle Pressure" 4 × 8½ in. A 4-page folder. Suggests three approaches for coping with pressure, as well as ten tension reducing tips. 25¢ each. Order Stock No.1724-00355 from Superintendent of Documents, U.S. Printing Office, Washington, D.C. 20402.

"It's Good to Know About Mental Health" 4 × 8½ in. A 12-page pamphlet. Explains that mental health has to do with the way a person adjusts to life, what symptoms to watch for and how to help yourself to mental health. Excellent overview from the NIMH. 25¢ each. Order Stock No. 1724-00337 from Superintendent of Documents, U.S. Government Printing Office, Washington, D.C. 20402.

"How to Deal With Your Tensions" 4 × 8½ in. A 6-page pamphlet. Free[12]

"A Child Alone in Need of Help" 4 × 8½ in. A 9-page pamphlet. Free[12]

Multiple Sclerosis

"Mental Health and MS" 5¼ × 8½ in. Pamphlet by Molly Harower, Ph.D. Describes the special problems that confront a patient in transition from prior state to multiple sclerosis. Free[13]

"Prescription for Living with MS" 8½ × 11 in. Reprint from *The American Journal of Nursing* (May 1973) by Donna Lynn Jontz, a nurse who is afflicted with multiple sclerosis. Free[13]

"You and Multiple Sclerosis" 3½ × 9 in. A pamphlet for patients. Free[13]

Muscular Dystrophy

"Careers for the Homebound" 4 × 9 in. A 16-page booklet prepared by the President's Committee on Employment of the Handicapped. Free. B'nai B'rith Career & Counseling Services, 1640 Rhode Island Ave. N.W., Washington, D.C. 20036.

"New Hope for Dystrophics" 5 × 7 in. A 28-page pamphlet by Elizabeth Ogg. Describes cause and treatment for the muscle disorders. 25¢. Pamphlet #271S. Public Affairs Pamphlets, 381 Park Ave. S., New York, N.Y. 10016.

"Patient and Community Services Program" A description of the various dystrophys and the Muscular Dystrophy Associations of America. Free. Write MDA, 810 Seventh Ave., New York, N.Y. 10019.

Nutrition (See Physical Fitness & Nutrition)

Oral Health

"Casper Presents Space-Age Dentistry" 5 × 6½ in. A 16-page comic book. The dentist at Cape Kennedy Medical Center explains to Casper, the

[12]Order from National Association for Mental Health, 1800 N. Kent St., Arlington, Va. 22209.

[13]Items may be ordered from National Multiple Sclerosis Society, 257 Park Ave. S., New York, N.Y. 10010.

friendly ghost, how he can keep his teeth in as good shape as the astronauts'. $1.75 for 25 copies. #G47[14]

"Cleaning Your Teeth & Gums" 6 × 6 in. A 12-page pamphlet. Full-color illustrations throughout in this explanation of using floss, basic brushing, toothpastes, mouthwashes, etc. $2.30 for 25 copies. #G38[14]

"You Can Prevent Tooth Decay" 5 × 6 in. A 12-page pamphlet. Line drawings help illustrate how tooth decay occurs, and what you can do in order to prevent it. $1.70 for 25 copies. #P6[14]

Parenthood

"Parents' Responsibility" 6 × 9 in. A 34-page booklet. For parents of young children of preschool and early school age. Discusses the importance of sex education from infancy on, stressing that love is basic. 40¢ each to 99 copies, 24¢ each from 100 to 499. Order #OP-12 from Order Handling Dept., American Medical Association, 535 N. Dearborn St., Chicago, Ill. 60610.

"Child Development in the Home" 5 × 7¼ in. This 20-page booklet describes parents' role in child's learning patterns, self-esteem, responsibility, problem solving and so on. 25¢. #(OHD)74-42, Superintendent of Documents, U.S. Government Printing Office, Washington, D.C. 20402.

"Memo to Parents About Immunization" Instructions and recommendations for immunizations and vaccinations. Schedules given. Free. Metropolitan Life Insurance Co., 51 Madison Ave., New York, N.Y. 10010.

"Children Learn What They Live" 11 × 14 in. Copy of guidelines for framing. Dept. RDA, P.O. Box 688, Ross Laboratories, Columbus, Ohio 43216.

Personal/Family Health Records

"Child Health Record" 6 × 9 in. A 20-page booklet. Provides a continuous and lasting health record of the child from birth through school age, and helps the doctor by giving him a summary of the past medical history of the child. $1 each on single orders, 35¢ each on orders of 10 or more. Order from Ms. Vivian Olson, Dept. "P", American Academy of Pediatrics, P.O. Box 1034, Evanston, Ill. 60204.

"The Personal Health Record" 4 × 8 in. A 6-page health record. Metropolitan Life Insurance Co., 1 Madison Ave., New York, N.Y. 10010. Free.

"Family Medical Record" 8½ × 11 in. Reprinted from *Woman's Day* magazine. Free. The National Foundation — March of Dimes, Box 2000, White Plains, N.Y. 10602.

Physical Fitness & Nutrition

"A-B-C's of Good Nutrition" 5½ × 8 in. This 16-page scriptographic booklet outlines the importance of good nutrition, recommended daily nutrients

[14]Order from American Dental Association, 211 E. Chicago Ave., Chicago, Ill. 60611.

(from the National Academy of Sciences), the four basic food groups for a balanced diet and guidelines for individualized food needs and habits. 25¢ each to 99 copies, 19¢ each for 100 to 499. Order from Francis J. Rodovich, V. P., Channing L. Bete Co., Inc., 45 Federal St., Greenfield, Mass. 01301.

"The ABC's of Perfect Posture" 4 × 8½ in. A 22-page booklet. Cleverly illustrated with the help of a wooden model, this booklet explains patterns of posture and ways to protect your good posture. 25¢ each to 99 copies, 18¢ each for 100 to 499. Order #OP-320 from Order Handling Dept., American Medical Association, 535 N. Dearborn St., Chicago, Ill. 60610.

"Dietary Control of Cholesterol" 7 × 10 in. A 48-page booklet. Provides sample menus for meals low in saturated fat at three different calorie levels, along with many exchange lists which make for a wide variety of meals that meet the requirements of the diet. Carries commercial identification. Free, limit 100. Order from Fleischmann's Margarine, P.O. Box 1407, Elm City, N.C. 27822.

"Exercise Doesn't Have to Be So Bad" 3½ × 6 in. Bright yellow leaflet. Promotes brisk walking as one of the best all-round exercises, suggesting it be incorporated into your everyday life-style. Sample copy free, $1 per 100, order in multiples of 100. Order from Information Resource Dept., American Academy of Family Physicians, 1740 W. 92nd St., Kansas City, Mo. 64114.

"Food & Fitness" 5½ × 7½ in. A 96-page booklet. The basic building blocks of good health, illustrated in full color — how to eat the right foods, what you get out of the food you eat, how you can get and keep yourself in better physical condition. Single copy free, $15.50 per 100 + shipping. Order from Ms. S. C. Restea-Jewell, Communications Division, Blue Cross Association, 840 N. Lake Shore Drive, Chicago, Ill. 60611.

"The Healthy Way to Weigh Less" 4 × 8½ in. A 6-page folder. How to plan an effective weight-reduction program, including the inescapable exercise of turning your back on your food. 20¢ each to 99 copies, 12¢ each for 100 to 499. Order #OP-322 from Order Handling Dept., American Medical Association, 535 N. Dearborn St., Chicago, Ill. 60610.

"Low-Sodium Diets Can Be Delicious" 6 × 9 in. A 40-page booklet. Prepared to make the "taste transition" to a low-sodium diet easier through the planning and preparation of tasty, nutritious and interesting meals. Carries commercial identification. Free, limit 100. Order from Fleischmann's Margarine, P.O. Box 1407, Elm City, N.C. 27822.

"Mr. Peanut's Guide to Nutrition" 6 × 9 in. A 36-page booklet. "Everyone knows that Mr. Peanut is a nut, but maybe they don't know he's an expert on nutrition, too." This guide for young people will help them choose the foods their bodies need each day. Carries commercial identification. Free, limit 100. Order from Fleischmann's Margarine, P.O. Box 1407, Elm City, N.Y. 27822.

"Nutrition — Food at Work for You" 6 × 9 in. A 30-page booklet. A few facts about food and health to form a basis for selecting the foods we eat. Prepared by the U.S. Dept. of Agriculture. 20¢ each. Order #GS-1 from

Superintendent of Documents, Government Printing Office, Washington, D.C. 20402.

"What Physicians Say About Physical Education" 4 × 8½ in. An 8-page pamphlet. Extracts of supporting statements for physical education made to the President's Council on Physical Fitness and Sports. Free by individual request. Order from Public Information Dept., President's Council on Physical Fitness and Sports, 400 Sixth St., S.W., Washington, D.C. 20201.

"Your Age & Your Diet" 4 × 8½ in. A 12-page pamphlet. Every age group has nutritional needs of its own. Presents guides for food habits which will satisfy nutrient needs from infancy through adulthood. 25¢ each to 99 copies, 16¢ each for 100 to 499. Order #OP-31 from Order Handling Dept., American Medical Association, 535 N. Dearborn St., Chicago, Ill. 60610.

Pollution

"Air Pollution — The Facts About Your Lungs" 3½ × 8½ in. An 8-page pamphlet. Explains how we know air pollution is harmful to our health, why we have it, and how we can help stop it. Free. Order from your state or local Lung Association (find address in your telephone directory).

"Don't You Dare Breathe That Air" 7 × 10 in. A 16-page booklet. For students in the primary grades, explains air pollution and has space and suggestions for the students to draw pictures about pollution and health. Free. Order from your state or local Lung Association (find address in your telephone directory).

Pregnancy

"Do's and Don'ts for the Most Important 9 Months in Life" (English and Spanish) 3½ × 6 in. A 4-page folder. Lists things you should know, things you should do, and some things to avoid. Please specify Spanish or English. Free, limit 50 copies. Order from Mrs. Sara W. Kelley, Director of Public Relations, United Cerebral Palsy Association, Inc., 66 E. 34th St., New York, N.Y. 10016.

"So You're Going to Have a Baby" 5½ × 8 in. A 16-page scriptographic booklet. Explains the stages of pregnancy — from conception through birth. 25¢ each to 99 copies, 19¢ each for 100 to 499. Order from Francis J. Rodovich, V. P., Channing L. Bete Co., Inc., 45 Federal St., Greenfield, Mass. 01301.

"What to Do Before Your Baby Comes" 4 × 8½ in. An 8-page folder. Written especially for a black audience, this folder explains the steps to take in order to get the proper prenatal care. 25¢ each to 99 copies, 15¢ each for 100 to 499. Order #OP-193 from Order Handling Dept., American Medical Association, 535 N. Dearborn St., Chicago, Ill. 60610.

"Comfort During Pregnancy" 4 × 8½ in. A 6-page folder. Well-illustrated explanation of how to keep comfortable during pregnancy, including best positions for rest periods. 25¢ each.[15]

"For the Expectant Father" 4 × 8½ in. A 6-page folder. Discusses how learning about the events of a pregnancy and the part a father can play will help reduce some of his apprehension and draw the couple even closer together. 25¢ each.[15]

Safety

"Are You Fit to Drive?"   4 × 8½ in. A 6-page folder. Contains information about conditions that can affect your driving, including emotional upsets, sleepiness and alcohol. 20¢ each to 99 copies, 12¢ each for 100 to 499. Order #OP-302 from Order Handling Dept., American Medical Association, 535 N. Dearborn St., Chicago, Ill. 60610.

"Child Safety Suggestions, Set #1"   5½ × 8½ in. Leaflets, 8 in the set. Prepared by the Accident Prevention Committee of the AAP, these eight leaflets give specific pointers on protecting your child from birth through age twelve. 75¢ per set, $30 for 100 sets. Individual pages may be ordered for $3 for 100. Order from Ms. Vivian Olson, Dept. "P", American Academy of Pediatrics, P.O. Box 1034, Evanston, Ill. 60204.

"Home Accidents Aren't Accidental"   4 × 8½ in. An 8-page folder. Home accidents are the end product of a sequence of events which can be predicted and should be prevented, controlled or minimized. This folder tells how. 25¢ each to 99 copies, 16¢ each for 100 to 499. Order #OP-359 from Order Handling Dept., American Medical Association, 535 N. Dearborn St., Chicago, Ill. 60610.

"Home Safety Round-Up"   3½ × 8½ in. A 6-page folder. A check list to help you spot potential hazards that may exist in all areas of your home. $10 per 1,000. Order from Library, National Easter Seal Society for Crippled Children & Adults, 2023 W. Ogden Ave., Chicago, Ill. 60612.

"Poison and Overdose First Aid Chart"   8½ × 11 in. Quick reference chart for back of medicine cabinet door. Mead Johnson Laboratories, Evansville, Ind. 47721.

"Responsibility Means Safety for Your Child"   5½ × 8½ in. A 24-page booklet. Cleverly illustrated narrative explains steps in teaching responsibility to the infant, preschool and school-age child. 50¢ each. Order from Ms. Vivian Olson, Dept. "P", American Academy of Pediatrics, P. O. Box 1034, Evanston, Ill. 60204.

"Safety Belts Save Lives"   4 × 8½ in. A 6-page folder. The facts about safety belts as extremely effective in protecting you and your family from injury and death from automobile crashes. 25¢ each to 99 copies, 15¢ each for 100 to 499. Order #OP-214 from Order Handling Dept., American Medical Association, 535 N. Dearborn St., Chicago, Ill. 60610.

"Safety Check List for Parents"   3½ × 6 in. A 6-page folder. Prepared with the belief that through protection, discipline and education, parents can keep their children safe from accidents. $10 per 1,000. Order from Library, National Easter Seal Society for Crippled Children and Adults, 2023 W. Ogden Ave., Chicago, Ill. 60612.

[15]Order from Publications Dept., Maternity Center Association, 48 E. 92nd St., New York, N.Y. 10028.

Smoking

"Facts: Smoking and Health"   4 × 9 in. A 14-page booklet. Presents the main facts to remember about the relationship between cigarette smoking and health, including graphs on death rates and heart attacks. Free[16]

Poster: "All You Smokers Who Plan to Quit"   16 × 22 in. Brightly colored images of hoarded cigarettes help illustrate the message that 20 years from now, after 146,000 more cigarettes, it's not going to be easier to quit. Free[16]

"Smoker's Aid to Non-Smoking: A Scorecard"   4 × 8½ in. A 12-page pamphlet. Very clever calendar to help the smoker develop a new habit — not smoking. Has a daily tabulation of how much money you've saved, with encouraging tidbits such as "I feel better already," and "I am not a dummy." Free[16]

"Women & Smoking"   4 × 8½ in. A 6-page folder. Suggests a number of good reasons why women should quit smoking, and offers encouragement through a coupon for more literature. Free[16]

"Me Quit Smoking? How?"   4 × 5½ in. A 24-page booklet. Cartoon illustrations emphasize useful suggestions on how you can join the more than 20 million Americans who have quit smoking. Free[17]

"Hey, Look — a Smoking Puzzle!"   7 × 8½ in. folder. Smoking crossword puzzle complete with a tear-off solution. Such clues as . . . "Smokers often suffer from annoying, chronic_____." Free[17]

"37 Ways to Stop Wasting Your Breath"   A clever self-motivated way to stop smoking. Developed in Europe by Max Planck Institute, Boehringer Ingelheim Ltd., Elmsford, N.Y. 10523.

Speech & Hearing

"About Speech & Hearing Problems"   5½ × 8 in. A 16-page scriptographic booklet. Presents an overview of possible speech, language and hearing problems and their treatment to help guard against communications handicaps. 25¢ each to 99 copies, 19¢ each for 100 to 499. Order from Francis J. Rodovich, V.P., Channing L. Bete Co., Inc., 45 Federal St., Greenfield, Mass. 01301.

"Doctor, Is My Baby Deaf?"   3½ × 8½ in. leaflet. Explains signs which may indicate a hearing loss in babies aged 3 to 24 months, and what to do if these signs appear. Free[18]

"Hearing Alert!" (Packet)   4 × 8½ in. Pack of materials. Varied information concerning early detection and treatment of hearing loss in children. Introduced by Robert Young as ABC's Marcus Welby, M.D., Single copy free.[18]

[16]Order from Health Information Branch, National Clearinghouse for Smoking and Health, 5401 Westbard Ave., Bethesda, Md. 20016.

[17]Order from American Lung Association, 1740 Broadway, New York, N.Y. 10019.

[18]Order from Hearing Alert!, Alexander Graham Bell Association for the Deaf, 3417 Volta Place N.W., Washington, D.C. 20007.

"What to do When Hearing Fades" 4 × 8½ in. A 6-page folder. Stresses consulting your family doctor if you suspect a hearing loss. Explains types of losses and methods of treatment. 20¢ each to 99 copies, 10¢ each for 100 to 499. Order #OP-28 from Order Handling Dept., American Medical Association, 535 N. Dearborn St., Chicago, Ill. 60610.

"First Aid for Aphasics" Joseph S. Keenan, Ph.D. A simplified guide to speech therapy for a person who is aphasic. 35¢[19]

"Speech Therapy for the Cerebral Palsied" Harold Westlake, Ph.D. and David Rutherford, Ph.D. A practical approach to oral language problems of C.P. children. 50¢[19]

Venereal Disease

"About Syphilis and Gonorrhea" 5½ × 8 in. A 16-page scriptographic booklet. Facts about the two most common types of venereal disease. Stresses seeing a doctor or going to a clinic if you feel there is any possibility you are infected. 25¢ each to 99 copies, 19¢ each for 100 to 499. Order from Francis J. Rodovich, V.P., Channing L. Bete Co., Inc., 45 Federal St., Greenfield, Mass. 01301.

"Venereal Disease" 6 × 9 in. A 26-page booklet. Comprehensive, well-illustrated discussion of the diseases, how they spread, detection and treatment. 40¢ each to 99 copies, 26¢ each for 100 to 499. Order #OP-383 from Order Handling Dept., American Medical Association, 535 N. Dearborn St., Chicago, Ill. 60610.

"Venereal Diseases & Birth Defects" 8½ × 11 in. A 2-page flyer. Concise overview of VD and how strongly it can affect the "innocent victims," new born infants. Free in reasonable quantities. Order from Health Information & School Relations, The National Foundation — March of Dimes, 1275 Mamaroneck Ave., White Plains, N.Y. 10602.

"What You Should Know About VD" 5 × 7 in. A 12-page reprint. Factual information on venereal disease reprinted from the Reader's Digest. Carries position statement endorsed by 17 health related associations (including the AAFP) and 3M Company identification. Free while supply lasts. Order from Information Resource Dept., American Academy of Family Physicians, 1740 W. 92nd St., Kansas City, Mo. 64114.

[19]Order from National Easter Seal Society, 2023 W. Ogden Ave., Chicago, Ill. 60612.

A NOTE TO PHYSICIANS[1]

When I was in medical school and consolidating my plans to go into family practice (I should say general practice because when I graduated in the early 1950s we had not yet evolved into the concept we have now) I asked one of my favorite professors at Case Western Reserve which kind of "bedside manner" was best for me.

I had carefully observed during my clinical years the various doctor–patient management styles used by physicians on the staff of the Cleveland hospitals affiliated with Reserve. There were: "The Authoritarian" (popular with surgeons and based on the Germanic model of the Herr Professor), "The Smoothie" (often practiced by gynecologists who wore boutonnieres in their lapels and were impeccably groomed in the latest Brooks Brothers suits), "The Pal." "Father Confessor," "Good Fellow" and so on. Which one should I pattern myself after, I wanted to know. "None," he replied. "Be yourself and patients that like you will come to you. . . . But, if you do want some advice — be a good teacher. Most patients will appreciate it and call you a good doctor!"

That advice, given to me 25 years ago eventually led me into developing a series of patient education programs called Course for the Activated Patient and into writing this book. And I believe that, properly used, my concept can serve you, the physician, as a new clinical resource.

Improved Primary Care Training
Helps Patient Education Methods

Most observers of today's medical scene agree that despite gallant efforts in training programs for family practice and other types of primary care physicians, shortages and annual attrition are such that it will take a decade just to catch up.

During the last few years, state legislators, initially in midwestern states, said to the medical school deans, "Train more family doctors or else!" The deans and faculty there and elsewhere rolled up their sleeves and started turning out in larger numbers better trained family doctors than ever before. As they did, they learned some things that had a direct bearing on patient education.

First, what were the actual training needs in such areas as family practice? Although physicians had for many years been trained as family doctors, some researchers such as Maurice Wood (1) of the Medical College of Virginia and Jack Froom (2) of Rochester University said if we are to set up proper training programs for tomorrow we must analyze today's practice trends and records. They then set up careful studies to provide the data needed.

[1]Adapted from presentation, Delaware Academy of Family Practice, Wilmington, Delaware, March 15, 1975.

The information they obtained accurately portrayed the frequency of illnesses and injuries in family practice settings. These studies called practice analysis made it possible to identify the most common problems. Training programs could then be established to ensure that new doctors and their paramedical staffs were ready to handle the things they would encounter in real-life clinical situations.

This may seem like an unnecessary step, but the realities of medical education for primary care had long been that most students leave medical school and teaching hospitals having spent 80% of their time on medical skills that they will find useful in only 20% of the time when they go into practice. This situation is being corrected by most programs in family practice with such knowledge gained from practice analysis.

The second thing the faculties learned (that can also be applied to patient education) came from the training of paramedics who were to work in the field of primary care. In order to train physician assistants and nurse practitioners, it was necessary to establish clinical protocols. This required detailed study of the logic involved in clinical decision-making by physicians and their staff. The triage protocols that asked questions such as: "Should this condition be considered as an emergency or can it safely be seen by a physician tomorrow?" and "Is this the normal course of a self-limiting URI?" were included in the training manuals. Pioneering work by Komaroff et al.(3) at Beth Israel Hospital in Boston and Vickery (4) at Ft. Belvoir Army Hospital in Virginia led to the development of clinical algorithms.

It was a logical next step to convert such training procedures for paramedic professionals to training procedures for patients (see *The Self-Help Medical Guide* within this book).

Medical Economics of Patient Education

In 1974, two significant things happened that will have a major impact on speeding the development of patient education as a new clinical resource for physicians.

The first was the decision of the American Group Practice Association to collaborate with Core Communications in Health in the development of a series of audio visual packages for patient education under the able direction of Rosiland Hawley of Core Communications and Past President W. Grayburn Davis, M.D. of AGPA. Prototype patient education units were established at St. Louis Park Medical Center in Minneapolis; Lovelace-Bataan Clinic, Albuquerque; Palo Alto Clinic; Denver Clinic; Trover Clinic; Madisonville, Ky. and Medical City, Dallas. These will be used to set the stage for more units at other group practice sites around the United States and encourage the development of Departments of Patient Education in clinics affiliated with AGPA. These departments are designed to be profit centers like laboratories, x-ray and physical therapy departments with specific fees charged to patients for services rendered.

The second thing was the decision of Montana Blue Cross to allow patient education as a billable inpatient service. I predict that other Blues will soon follow suit and selected types of education will be reimbursable in other states by the end of 1975.

The director of family practice training at Riverside Hospital in Newport News, Va., Ed Alexander (5), told me that in America there are two things that make change possible: "Dollars and Coercion." It can also be said that when Third Parties pay for a service, the service soon becomes available in hospitals. Thus, with AGPA opening doors in the outpatient and the Blues in the inpatient sector, patient education will soon become more common.

Anne Somers (6), of New Jersey-Rutgers Medical School, has said about patient education: "Consumer health education is an idea whose time has come! . . . The recent revival of interest is no accident. It is a highly appropriate response to recent developments in both the supply and demand for health care.

"There can be little doubt that a few million dollars spent to teach the consumer-patient to develop a life-style conducive to good health and, when ill or disabled, to understand and cope more effectively with his own health problems, could turn out to be more cost-effective than billions spent on the development of exotic new medical technology and expensive inpatient programs."

For the past three decades the vast majority of our health dollars have been spent on treatment and diagnosis with perhaps 4% on prevention according to the President's Committee on Health Education (7). Despite the fact that many of us were taught in school that all medical care should be based on the triad: DPT (Diagnosis, Prevention, Treatment), the emphasis has been on D and T. Poor "P" (prevention through education) has been given little attention.

What does this mean for most physicians? It means that if they are not currently using patient education as a regular clinical tool, they are missing out on a key part of medical care. What's more, a part of care that more and more patients are expecting — and, in fact, demanding.

In a recent radio interview after his resignation as head football coach at Notre Dame, Ara Parshigian said, "Times are different today. When I started coaching 25 years ago, I simply told the players to do that play, or run that way. No questions asked. Now they want to know 'Why?' and I have to tell them. But, I think it pays off in many ways. Better compliance. Better teamwork and so on. It pays off."

There's a message in there for family doctors. Patient education will also pay off. What are some examples I have found in my own practice?

Phone calls

By giving more explicit verbal directions supplemented by printed instructions for more complex situations or brochures and pamphlets where applicable, labeling prescriptions more completely (including listing the drug name), instructing patients with questions to talk them over with my nursing staff and conducting formal classes for new patients, I was able to have significantly fewer phone calls than my other colleagues had.

Malpractice suits

If you use education as a regular clinical tool and tell your patients what you're doing, why and follow it up with a chance to have them ask questions (and you give honest, direct answers) the chances for legal action and ever increasing premium fees are substantially lessened.

Doctor–patient relationships

Properly used, patient education enhances the traditional good doctor–patient relationship that has been badly eroded in recent years. The goal I have used in education programs is what I call the "Health Partnership." By teaching patients what they can expect from medical care in the *real* world (rather than the idealized world of TV's Marcus Welby), and emphasizing that it is after all the patient's body and that good health measures are *their* responsibility in addition to the doctor's responsibility, I have found vastly improved relationships resulting.

Professional satisfaction

If patient education is used as a regular resource for medical care, it results in a better quality of services. This, in turn, gives a boost to the feeling of professional satisfaction that is important to all doctors. One of the big problems that faces family practice is loss of satisfaction in handling the everyday "garden variety" illnesses and injuries that are seen. Some of my friends in family practice say, "No challenge remains." To that I counter by saying, "Every visit to your office has a great potential for prevention." This involves the highest intellectual challenge possible: motivation methods, patient behavior modification, compliance technics for orders, improved communication skills and so on. If the family doctor can focus on preventive methods rather than intervention — and becomes an expert educator — he will have the same satisfaction that an ophthalmologist has in his challenging eye surgery or the orthopedic surgeon has in his good job on the athlete's knee!

COURSE FOR THE ACTIVATED PATIENT

With this background established, I would like to share with you some of the experiences I have had since my first "Course for the Activated Patient" was established in 1970. I was then affiliated with a small group practice, the Reston-Herndon Medical Center in Herndon, a semi-rural town west of Washington, D.C. in Northern Virginia.

The groundwork for the course had been set by John Renner, M.D., before he left to join the Department of Family Practice at the University of Wisconsin in Madison. I developed a series of 16 two-hour sessions for the 40 housewives, grandmothers and a sprinkling of husbands and other interested men who enrolled in the course. All wanted to know more about good health practices, how to handle common emergencies, illnesses and injuries, the economics of medical care, prescription and O.T.C. drugs, childhood growth and development and a variety of self-help and preventive skills. These early experiences have been described in the literature (8).

Since then I have given courses at the Reston-Georgetown Medical Center, Reston, Va.; the Northeast-Georgetown Medical Center, Washington, D.C. and Fellowship Square House in Reston, Va. The curriculum has been continually improved and revised.

We named our patient education classes after a concept originally described by Vanderbilt University's Vernon E. Wilson (9). The "activated patient" is one whose clinical skills and understanding of his health are such that he becomes an active participant in his own health care in contrast to the passive role traditionally assigned him.

Our courses have had four goals:

(1) To teach patients how to use health care resources more effectively.
(2) To give them a better understanding of self-help and preventive medicine and emphasize the importance of *individual* responsibility.
(3) To train them to do certain easy procedures and make better observations of clinical events in common illnesses and injuries.
(4) To help them save money when purchasing drugs, buying insurance and obtaining medical care.

The courses have been hailed as successful and similar efforts, patterned after the Georgetown series, have now been established in Wyoming, Idaho, Utah, Maine, Virginia, North Carolina, Minnesota, New York and several other states.

Our experiences at Georgetown are being born out at the other sites and evaluations show the following results:

(1) Increased confidence and ability of patients to handle the common illnesses, injuries and emergencies and a parallel lessening of the usual anxieties associated with them.
(2) Some changes in behavior of patients regarding improved eating habits, more regular exercise and efforts to prevent illness.
(3) Savings in drug costs and some types of medical expenses.

A series of seminars and workshops sponsored by the new Center for Continuing Health Education at Georgetown University (Box 7268, Arlington, Va. 22207) have been established to show other health professionals the methods and materials we have developed. The doctors, nurses and health educators who attended the workshops and others are now establishing similar patient-oriented educational programs.

THE FUTURE: WILL YOU BE READY?

In the Sixties, Bob Dylan wrote the words and music for a song that spoke of changes he predicted were "blowin' in the wind."

The changes I see blowin' will be a greatly enhanced interest in patient education. Such skills are being taught to some residents in family practice. I am recommending to directors of training programs that when the F.P. resident leaves tomorrow's training program, he should have in his Black Bag a variety of educational tools, experiences and skills. Just as the urologist can use his sounds and the ophthalmologist his scopes better than other doctors, the family practice specialist should have educational tools that he uses better than others. This will make him a specialist in the skills of patient education and enhance his role as a specialist in preventive medicine.

Another change I see will be the common use of clinical algorithm books that many patients will use when instructed by their doctors. These books will establish the observations and guidelines patients will use before they call the doctor or come in for a visit. Such books will increase the number of appropriate medical visits and decrease the inappropriate and trivial visits that plague many family practice clinics and offices. As the doctor and his staff teach the patients how to use these books, there will be an increased interest in conducting classes similar to the Course for the Activated Patient. Doctors will rediscover, with pleasure, that the French word "*docteur*" means teacher.

A further change will happen as patient education becomes a commonly used resource for family practice (and for the other medical specialties) there will be a gradual shift in the perception of health.

By far the greatest emphasis over the last 30 years has been *intervention* at the professional level. Little time or financial support has been devoted to the individual sector.

In describing things in today's world, Walter Strode (10) of Honolulu with input from 20 other members of the Hawaii Health Net said, "Changes leading to improvement in health can be seen as occurring basically at two levels: *health care system reform* and *conceptual shift*. The problems inherent in the system are so enormous that practically all of us become entangled at the former level, caught up in the demands and counter-demands of different groups of society, with the result that new realities which indicate the need for conceptual change are not understood. For example, even though a national health insurance or service in the United States seems absolutely necessary in order to deal with distribution and cost problems, the adoption of an effective plan of this kind will lock this country into a 'medical care' (health care system) approach to health during the foreseeable future. This may well delay the conceptual changes that are necessary for us if we are to move toward better health. *We must therefore develop the ability to create immediate and effective changes in the system that will facilitate the basic shifts we need and not interfere with them.*" (Italicized by me for emphasis).

Meanwhile, there is an increasing variety of good patient education materials becoming available. Recently the American Academy of Family Practice put out a "Compendium of Patient Education Materials" (AAFP Reprint #B-3500). Metropolitan Life Insurance Company has a similar compendium "*Patient Education* (The Concept, Selected Reading References, Organizational Resources for Patient Education and In-Service and Continuing Education." This book has a section in the glossary that lists educational materials available to the medical profession and the general public at no charge. Some publishing companies, notably the Robert J. Brady Co. (a subsidiary of Prentice-Hall Co., Bowie, Md. 20715) is producing a substantial number of good patient education materials and you may write to them for a catalog.

Further specific information may also be obtained by writing William Carlyon of the American Medical Association's Department of Health Education or Elizabeth Lee, R.N., Department of Patient Education, American Hospital Association, both at Chicago headquarters.

Patient education is a clinical resource that if properly used will save the doctor time from many time-wasting phone calls, prevent possible malpractice suits, enhance doctor-patient relationships and give greater professional satisfaction.

Good patient education must involve more than "Do's and Don'ts" and pamphlets. It will require classes similar to the Course for the Activated Patient and other patient-oriented educational efforts. It will eventually require a change in some traditional medical care methods.

As we move into the Bicentennial Year for the United States, it is worthwhile for us to reflect on the words of Thomas Jefferson. Although he meant it in a political sense, it is appropriate in the perception of the health partnership that can come from patient education. "The secret strength of America will be its informed citizenry."

References

1. Wood, M.: The Way Ahead in Family Practice Records. *J. Clin. Computing,* **2,** 20–28 (1973).

2. Froom, J., Rozzi, C., Metcalf, D.H.: Computer Analysis of Morbidity Reports in Primary Care. *J. Clin. Computing,* **2,** 42–51 (1973).

3. Komaroff, A.L. et al: Protocols for Physician Assistants: Management of Diabetes and Hypertension. *N. Engl. J. Med.,* **133,** 294–299 (1974).

4. Vickery, D.M.: Computer Support of Paramedical Personnel: The Question of Quality Control. MEDINFO **74,** pp. 281–287.

5. Editorial: *Computer Med.* p. 3 (1974).

6. Somer, A.: Educating the consumer, it can mean better health, lower costs. *Amer. Med News,* p.10 (1974).

7. The President's Committee on Health Education, *Report,* Department of Health, Education and Welfare, p. 11 (1973).

8. Sehnert, K.W.: The Patient as a Paramedical. *The Virginia Medical Monthly,* pp. 409–413 (1972).

9. Wilson, V.E.: Smith Memorial Lecture at Rockford (Ill.) Memorial Hospital, December 4, 1970.

10. Strode, W.: Problem/Possibility Focuser, Health: Version Two. *Futures Conditional* (1974).

SUGGESTED READING

Consumerism

1. Health Research Group, *A Consumer's Directory of Prince George's County Doctors*, Public Citizen, Inc., Washington, 1974. 116 p. $2.50. (Health Research Group, 2000 P. St., N.W., Washington, D.C. 20036.)

This directory is a pioneering effort by one of Ralph Nader's Public Citizen groups. It was produced with the help of the National Center for Urban Ethnic Affairs and describes how the directory was compiled and what the information means to an interested consumer. It tells about the doctors who practice in Prince George's County, Maryland. The directory lists type of practice, fees, laboratory facilities, prescribing and immunization practices, education and hospital appointments in addition to office location, phone numbers and other helpful information.

2. Pulver, James A., *The Role of the Consumer in Assuring Quality Health Care*, Albuquerque, N.M.: University of New Mexico Printing Plant, 1973. 134 p. $1.25. (New Mexico Regional Medical Program, 2701 Frontier, N.E., Albuquerque, N. M. 87131.)

This monograph produced by a "working invitational task force" in May 1973 presents the findings of eight work groups on the role of the consumer in improving access to health care, the process of health care, compliance with health care instructions, continuity of health care and outcome of health care. It also describes the consumer's role in overcoming barriers in good health care regarding communications, cultural patterns and cost. In addition to these thought provoking reports, the text includes a keynote address as well as general remarks and comments about consumerism and health care.

Encyclopedias, Home Health Medical References

1. Better Homes and Gardens, *Family Medical Guide*, Des Moines: Better Homes and Gardens Books, 1973. 1088 p. $18.

Designated as a book to "supplement the counsel of one's own personal physician," *Guide* is a useful reference about practical matters of home care, prevention of disease, maintenance of health and recognition of illness. It is well illustrated and has 28 chapters that provide details of physiology and pathology of the body's systems, first aid, specific common diseases, medical genetics, laboratory and x-ray. It also has an illustrated encyclopedia of medical terms.

2. AFE Press, *International Family Health Encyclopedia*, American Family Enterprises, 1971. 3108 p. (21 volumes). $3.98 each.

This comprehensive set of books provides a complete set of medical and health references. It is beautifully illustrated and well written. The encyclopedia gives physiologic and anatomic details, builds understanding of complex body systems, provides historical background for many medical discoveries and insight into social and health problems.

3. Merck & Co., Inc., *The Merck Manual* (of Diagnosis and Therapy) 11th Ed., Merck, Sharpe and Dohme Research Laboratories, West Point, Pa. 1850 p. $10.

This handbook of medical knowledge has been constantly revised since 1899. Originally limited to medical professionals, it is now widely used by laity as a handy resource. Its 366 main chapters and 818 subchapters embrace over 1,000 subjects. Space is devoted to etiology, incidence, physiology, pathology, prophylaxis, prognosis and treatment. Coverage is mainly medical. Many tables and illustrations.

4. *The Concise Home Medical Guide*, Grosset & Dunlap: New York, 1972. 630 p. $9.95.

A useful, and well-illustrated handbook explaining and describing in easy-to-understand language virtually every medical problem that the average person is likely to encounter. In addition to symptoms and treatments of illness and accidents, there are sections on nutrition, personal hygiene, physical fitness, first aid, and recovery and therapy.

Exercises, Physical Fitness

1. Cooper, Kenneth and Brown, Keven, *Aerobics*, New York: M. Evans and Co., 1968. 253 p. $5.95.

This book describes how endurance and fitness increase oxygen consumption, strengthen the heart and improve lung activity. It describes a system of point values for running, swimming, cycling, walking, stationary running, handball, basketball and squash. It provides a graded program for physical fitness and conditioning. Goals and rules are provided to set up programs.

2. Michele, Arthur, *Orthotherapy*, New York: M. Evans and Co., Inc., 1971. 219 p. $4.95.

Written for the general public, the book describes common orthopedic disorders and everyday aches and pains of the musculoskeletal system. Good illustrations show how home programs of exercises can help overcome the ailments. Muscle imbalance, poor seating habits, bad posture, bad mattresses and various causes of common problems are discussed with appropriate plans for corrective exercise.

First Aid

1. American National Red Cross, *Standard First Aid and Personal Safety*, Garden City, N.J.: Doubleday & Co., Inc., 1973. 268 p. $1.95.

This textbook for the general public is the product of many revisions since the first edition appeared in 1910. It provides knowledge and skills needed to meet emergency first aid situations. It incorporates personal safety and accident prevention ideas to acquaint readers with the cause of accidents and to eliminate and minimize the future injuries. Wounds, injuries, shock, emergency respiration, poisoning, drug abuse and rescue methods are only a few of the many topics covered in this well-illustrated book.

Medications, Drugs

1. DiCyan, Erwin, Without Prescription, New York: Simon and Schuster, 1972. 152 p. $2.95.
   This book describes drugs and their effects. It is easy to read. Describes chemical ingredients, generic name and trade name drugs. Allows lay readers to extrapolate newly acquired knowledge about the various medications.

2. Winter, Ruth, "Drugs: The Dangerous Combinations," Woman's Day Magazine. (Dec. 1971), New York.
   A well-prepared article on combinations of common prescriptions to be avoided and concise explanation as to why trouble will result. Commonly used drugs are described.

3. Stern, Edward L., Prescription Drugs and Their Side Effects, New York: Grosset & Dunlap, Inc., 1975. 96 p. $3.95.
   A complete and up-to-date guide to the 150 most frequently prescribed drugs, as tabulated by the New York State Board of Pharmacy, includes precautions, side effects and adverse reactions that may occur.

Nutrition

1. Berkeley Women's Health Collective, Feeding Ourselves, New England Free Press: Boston, 1972. 24 p. $.35. (Berkeley Women's Health Collective, 2214 Grove St., Berkeley, Calif. 94704.)
   This short, yet comprehensive work gives information on digestion, the basic nutrients, special diets, weight reduction, food for pregnant and nursing women, babies, how to conserve time and money, food preparation tips and an annotated list of references. The pamphlet begins with a discussion of the American food industry including the Food and Drug Administration and ends with suggestions for consumer and political activities on food issues. This political content along with its emphasis on natural or organic foods may repel some readers but its approach to nutrition is generally nondogmatic and sane.

2. United States Dept. of Agriculture and Health, Education and Welfare, Food Is More Than Just Something to Eat, 1972. 30 p. Free. (Dept. HEW, Public Health Service, Food and Drug Administration, 5600 Fishers Lane, Rockville, Md. 20852.)

This brochure is clearly written, attractively illustrated and provides basic information on major nutrients and their sources. Nutritional requirements for pregnant women, infants and children, adolescents and senior citizens are presented. There is an explanation of nutritional labeling, processed foods, a daily food guide and discussion of various social, geographical and cultural influences that affect American diets.

3. Life Science Library, *Food and Nutrition*, New York: Time-Life Books, 1971. 200 p. $5.95.

An interesting book written in a concise, clear manner, it provides a useful guide to food problems — medical, scientific, political and humanitarian. Generously illustrated with excellent photos, it provides chapters on digestive processes, vitamins, starvation, dangers of excess food, fads and frauds, food production and manufacturing processes.

Self-Help Medical Skills

1. Griffith, H. Winter, *Instructions for Patients*, 2nd Ed., Philadelphia: W. B. Saunders & Company, 1975. 670 p. $35.

This book is a set of loose-leaf sheets that provide instructions for patients on a variety of common medical problems. The problems are listed in alphabetical order. The materials are prepared for physicians to use in giving better instructions to patients under their care. Information is provided regarding patient activity, diet, medications and general advice. Key signs and symptoms are listed that tell the patient when to get in touch with a physician.

2. Samuels, Mike and Bennett, Hal, *The Well Body Book*, New York: Random House, 1973. 350 p. $5.95.

A book written for laymen gives good instructions on a variety of self-care skills. It tells how a person can become aware of bodily sensations and how to organize these symptoms in a systemic way. Content includes how to take a medical history, health implications of good living habits, common minor illnesses, their recognition and treatment. Good advice is given regarding home treatment and how to use the doctor as a resource. Some reviewers describe the book as a bit "hokey" at times regarding "positive life force" and "visualization exercises" but it is a generally useful book.

3. Kodet, E. R. and Angier, B., *Being Your Own Wilderness Doctor*, New York: Pocket Books, 1972. 173 p. $1.50.

The camper and hiker who has little room left in his backpack will find this a compact source for advice on common injuries and illnesses. Problems such as ingrown toenail, blister, frostbite, heat prostration and poison ivy skin irritation are discussed and treatment suggested. Many practical first aid tips are provided. The contents of light-weight medical kits are identified.

4. Jarvis, D. C., *Folk Medicine: A Vermont Doctor's Guide to Good Health*, New York: Henry Holt and Company, 1958. 165 p. $1.50.

Jarvis explores the effectiveness of folk medicines and self-care skills commonly used in rural New England. It provides insight into folk medicine and gives some generally useful tips.

5. Boston Women's Health Book Collective, *Our Bodies Ourselves*, New York: Simon and Schuster, 1973. 276 p. $2.95.

Described as a book "by and for women" it provides a wide variety of self-help methods with emphasis on gynecologic and obstetrical information. Sections include discussions on nutrition, sexuality, abortion, venereal disease, rape and self-defense, child bearing and menopause. Home delivery methods, women's liberation attitudes and their goals for improved health care are outlined. The book is generously illustrated and makes good use of photographs.

6. Eichenlaub, John E., *A Minnesota Doctor's Home Remedies for Common and Uncommon Ailments*, New York: Dell Publishing Co., 1960. 315 p. $.60.

Muscular backache, foot troubles, rheumatism, constipation and menopause are a few of the many ailments discussed. Brief explanations regarding cause and practical treatments for control or cure are given. Home remedies are suggested.

7. Taylor, Robert B., *A Primer of Clinical Symptoms*, Hagerstown, Md.: Harper & Row, 1973. 220 p. $4.95.

Although written for a medical audience, this book can be read by a layman interested in the role that symptoms play in the medical workup. The information the body "tells" a doctor is the "language" of symptoms. What they mean and where they come from provides a fascinating new dimension for persons interested in developing self-help medical skills.

Yoga

1. Iyengar, B. K. S., *Light on Yoga*, New York: Schocken Books, 1966. 341 p. $9.95.

A book for professionals, it has been described as "the fullest, most practical and profusely illustrated book on Yoga . . . in English." It includes theoretical material on Yoga, definitions of all important terms as well as some explanations of Yoga's spiritual nature. Pictures of 600 postures included. Glossary of terms provided and Yoga philosophy described in Western terms.

2. Brena, Stephen F., *Yoga & Medicine*, Baltimore: Penguin Books, Inc., 1972. 175 p. $1.25.

This book, written for the general public, discusses physiologic concepts of Yoga in medical terms. Concepts and theories are presented in everyday language. Common problems of health, disease and physical and mental hygiene are presented from the viewpoint of an American physician who has studied Yoga and brings out key elements for practical use.

INDEX

abdominal pain, 153, G33, G58–G62, G119

abortions: as cause of death, 144; self, 172; spontaneous, 120

abrasions, 118, G42; medication for, 21, G80

accident-prone personality, 70

accidents, 135; air and space, 144–145; auto, 70, 143–149, 158; avoiding, G47, G49, G69, 319; falls, 144–145, 151; fire, 143–144, G41; firearm, 143–145; machinery, 143–146; motorcycle, 157–158

addiction. See alcohol; caffeine; drug abuse; nicotine

additives, food, 64

adrenal tumors, G24

ages, medical, 126–136

air cleaners, G27, G82

air conditioners, G23, G27

alcohol consumption, 132, 135, G16, G26, G75–G76; and medicines, 24–25, 31–32, G27, G69; teenage, 160; and yoga, 36

alcoholism, 48, 68, 71, 73, 77, 168, 174, G70–G72; as cause of death, 145–148; information on, 307

allergies, 121, 135, 141, G12–G14, G20, G22, G26–G28, G30, G49, G51; food, G61; information on, 307–308; to medicine, 23, 82, 112, G49, G51; nasal, G26–G28, G38, G78–G79; reactions, G49, G51, G107–G108; records of, 82; respiratory, G16; symptoms, 54; treatment, G81–G82

allergy: injections, 158, G14, G22, G28, G108; medication, 20, 21, 26, G13

amphetamines (appetite suppressants), 46, 48, G71, 310

ampicillin antibiotic, 20, 25, 28, G20

analgesic tablets, 21–22, G78

anemia, 47, 141; as cause of death, 143–145

aneurysms (artery wall disorders), G59; dissecting, G17

angina (heart pain), G64, G65, G113

angiograms, 118

ankles, G87; broken, G48–G49, G104, G108–G109; sprained, G55–G56, G108–G109

antacids, 52, G64; and prescription medicine, 29, 30

antibiotics, 20, 22, 28–29, 45, G13, G19, G20, G23; capsules, 25; doctor's opinion of, 92; ointments, 29, G29; liquid, 18, 25, 28; sensitivity to, 118–120; side effects, 24–25, 65, G36

antibody formation, G109

anticoagulants, 30, G78

antidotes, poison, G70, G77

antihistamines, G13, G27, G108; side effects, 23, 31, G27

antinauseant medicine, 21, G77

antipruritic (anti-itching) lotions, 21, G78

anxiety (neurosis), 68; coping with, 69, 72–73, 77; physical symptoms of, 47, 52, G64, G113

appearance, disinterest in, 76, 164

appendicitis, G33–G34, G61; acute, G59

appetite loss: as side effect, G68; as symptom, 48–49, 76, 164, G41, G71

arm pain, G64–G66, G94

arrythmia (irregular heartbeat), G67–G68

arterial disease, 58, 59, 124, G17, G59; as cause of death, 149, 150, 151

arteriosclerosis (arterial hardening), 59, 62; as cause of death, 145–150

arthritis, 141, G11–G12, G39, G54, G66, G68; information on, 308

aspiration, 118, G76, G102

aspirin, 20, 32, G12, G16, G19, G29, G31, G32, G40–G42, G51, G54, G58, G78, G116; allergies to, 23; overdoses, 123, G68

asthma, 131, 134–135, G12–G14, G49, G51; information on, 314; medication, 21

athlete's foot, 168

atrophy, 118

auto safety, 70, 132, 143–149, 158, 175

babies' health problems, 153–157, 166. See also children

backaches, 53, G56–G58, G94; as symp-

FAMILY HEALTH RECORD

EMERGENCY NUMBERS

Fire _____   Pharmacist _____
Family Doctor office _____   Police _____
          After hours _____   Ambulance _____
Gynecologist office _____   Emergency Hospital _____
          After hours _____   Poison Control Center _____
Pediatrician office _____   Other_____
          After hours _____   _____
Dentist office _____   _____
          After hours _____   _____

BIRTH INFORMATION

Family Member	Birth-date	Birth Wt.	Birth Len.	Mother's Health during Preg.	Delivery (normal– abnormal)	Condition at Birth	Type of Feed.	Blood Type
Mother								
Father								
Children 1.								
2.								
3.								
4.								
5.								

FAMILY HISTORY

Blood-related Family members	DISEASE										If deceased, age at death	Cause Of Death
	Cancer	Diabetes	Heart	Hypertension	Mental or Emotional Problem	Stroke	Allergies	Alcoholism or Drug Use	Ulcers	Other		
Grandparents												
Uncles & Aunts												
Parents												
Children												

DENTAL RECORD

Family Member	Date	Age	What Happened

DISEASE AND IMMUNIZATION RECORD

Names	Father		Mother		Children					
	Had or	Date Imm.	Had or	Date Imm.	Had or	Date Imm.	Had or	Date Imm.	Had or	Date Imm.
DPT — Diptheria — First										
Second										
Third										
Boosters										
Tetanus										
Whooping Cough (pertussis)										
Polio — First										
Second										
Third										
Boosters										
Rubella										
Measles										
Mumps										
Diseases for which there is no immunization										
Chickenpox										
Hepatitis										
Strep Throat										
Scarlet Fever										
Rheumatic Fever										
Tuberculosis (note tests for)										
Other:										

347

DRUG RECORD

Date	Family Member	Drug Used	Result/Comment	Any Allergy?

LAB TESTS AND PROCEDURES RECORD

RESULTS

	NAME				
	DATE				
Blood Count (CBC)					
Hemoglobin					
Hematocrit					
WBC					
Differential					
RBC					
Sed. rate					

	NAME				
	DATE				
Blood Chemistry					
Glucose					
Triglycerides					
Cholesterol					
Uric Acid					
Other (list)					

	NAME				
	DATE				
Urinalysis					

	NAME				
	DATE				
Electrocardiogram (EKG)					

	NAME				
	DATE				
X-Ray (type)					

	NAME				
	DATE				
Pap Test					

	NAME				
	DATE				
Other					

ACCIDENTS, SURGERY, HOSPITALIZATIONS RECORD
(or other important medical occurrences)

Family Member's Name	Date	Age	What Happened	Severity	Complications

RECORD OF DOCTORS

Keep a record of all doctors you go to. Note when you change doctors. This can help in assuring that medical records can be quickly located and sent for when needed.

Doctor's name and address	Type of doctor	Hours	Office and after hours phone	Date started with doctor, date ended
1. _____				
2. _____				
3. _____				
4. _____				
5. _____				
6. _____				
7. _____				
8. _____				
9. _____				
10. _____				

AGE/WEIGHT CHART FOR INFANTS

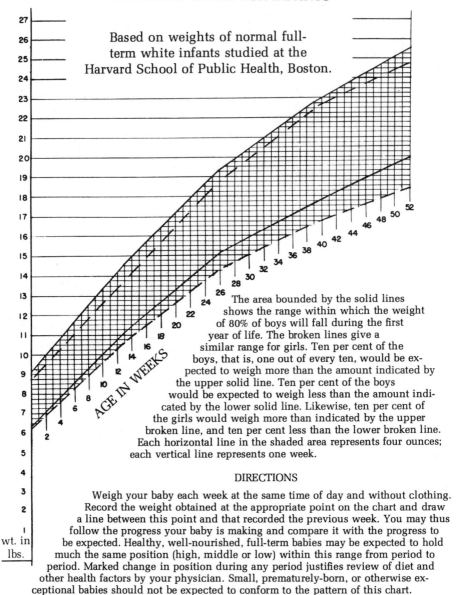

Based on weights of normal full-term white infants studied at the Harvard School of Public Health, Boston.

The area bounded by the solid lines shows the range within which the weight of 80% of boys will fall during the first year of life. The broken lines give a similar range for girls. Ten per cent of the boys, that is, one out of every ten, would be expected to weigh more than the amount indicated by the upper solid line. Ten per cent of the boys would be expected to weigh less than the amount indicated by the lower solid line. Likewise, ten per cent of the girls would weigh more than indicated by the upper broken line, and ten per cent less than the lower broken line. Each horizontal line in the shaded area represents four ounces; each vertical line represents one week.

DIRECTIONS

Weigh your baby each week at the same time of day and without clothing. Record the weight obtained at the appropriate point on the chart and draw a line between this point and that recorded the previous week. You may thus follow the progress your baby is making and compare it with the progress to be expected. Healthy, well-nourished, full-term babies may be expected to hold much the same position (high, middle or low) within this range from period to period. Marked change in position during any period justifies review of diet and other health factors by your physician. Small, prematurely-born, or otherwise exceptional babies should not be expected to conform to the pattern of this chart.